♦ GENES AND GENDER VII ♦

Challenging Racism and Sexism

The Genes and Gender series takes its shape and subject—the critique of genetic determinism—from the diverse work of the activists and scholars who make up the Genes and Gender Collective and contribute to the published proceedings of its conferences. Organized in 1977, the collective advocates responsible scientific and social research and challenges theories holding that genetic processes are primary determinants of human behavior and explain differences.

Also Available from The Feminist Press

On Peace, War, and Gender: A Challenge to Genetic Explanations, Genes and Gender VI, edited by Anne E. Hunter

Series Editors: Betty Rosoff and Ethel Tobach

◆ GENES AND GENDER VII ◆

Challenging Racism and Sexism: Alternatives to Genetic Explanations

Edited by Ethel Tobach
and Betty Rosoff

THE FEMINIST PRESS
at the City University of New York
New York

Published 1994 by The Feminist Press at The City University of
New York, 311 East 94 Street, New York, NY 10128

98 97 96 95 94 5 4 3 2 1

Library of Congress Cataloging-in-Publication Data

Challenging racism and sexism : alternatives to genetic explanations /
    edited by Ethel Tobach and Betty Rosoff.
        p.   cm. — (Genes and gender ; 7)
    Includes bibliographical references.
    ISBN 1-55861-089-8 (alk. paper) : $35.00.—ISBN 1-55861-090-1
    (pbk. : alk. paper) : $14.95
        1. Sexism.   2. Racism.   3. Sex differences.   4. Sociobiology.
    I. Tobach, Ethel, 1921–   . II. Rosoff, Betty III. Series.
BF341.G39   no. 7
[HQ1237]
155.2′34 s—dc20
[305]   94-18179
                                                                         CIP

This publication is made possible, in part, by public funds from the New
York State Council on the Arts. The Feminist Press is also grateful to
Johnnetta B. Cole, Joanne Markell, Caroline Urvater, and Genevieve Vaughan
for their generosity.

Cover and text design by Paula Martinac

Typeset by Creative Graphics, Allentown, Pennsylvania

Printed in the United States on acid-free paper by McNaughton & Gunn, Inc.,
Saline, Michigan

Contents

Preface   vii
Introduction, *Betty Rosoff and Ethel Tobach*   1
Asylum, *Regina E. Williams*   6

◆ **Part I** ◆

**Concepts of Racism and Sexism in Biology, Physiology,
and Psychology**

Race and Sex as Biological Categories, *Ruth Hubbard*   11
Critique of Recent Genetic Research Related to Issues of Racism and
    Sexism, *Ethel Tobach and Betty Rosoff*   22
Can We Draw Conclusions about Human Societal Behavior from
    Population Genetics? *Val Woodward*   35
Race and Gender Fallacies: The Paucity of Biological Determinist
    Explanations of Difference, *Gisela Kaplan and Lesley J.
    Rogers*   66
Racism and Sexism: Comparisons and Conflicts, *Pamela Trotman
    Reid*   93
African-American Women: Derivatives of Racism and Sexism in
    Psychotherapy, *Beverly Greene*   122

✦ Part II ✦

Philosophical and Historical Issues in Racism and Sexism

Race and Gender: The Limits of Analogy, *Linda Burnham*   143
The Genetic Fix: The Social Origins of Genetic Determinism,
    Garland E. Allen   163
Irreducible "Human Nature": Nazi Views on Jews and Women, *Gisela
    Kaplan*   188
When Race and Gender Collide: The Martinsville Seven Case as a
    Case Study of the "Rape-Lynch" Controversy, *Gerald
    Horne*   211

✦ Part III ✦

Contemporary Racism and Sexism in Different
Ethnic Communities

Perspectives of Native American Women on Race and Gender,
    Frederica Y. Daly   231
Educational Policy in Recent History: Reflections on Science,
    Ideology, and Political Action, *Bonnie Ellen Blustein*   256
Growing Up Black in Puerto Rico, *Carmen Luz Valcarcel*   284
School Performance of Asian-American and Asian Children:
    Myth and Fact, *Choichiro Yatani*   295
Feminist Reflections on the Interplay of Racism and Sexism in Israel,
    Simona Sharoni   309

Millennium Foretold, *Georgine Sanders*   332

Notes on the Contributors   333

Preface

In 1989, at the meeting of the American Association for the Advancement of Science (AAAS), J. Philippe Rushton presented a paper in which he said that genes determine the differences among Asians, Europeans, and Africans in regard to intelligence, socioeconomic status, brain size, genital size, and sexual behavior. At that time the media gave these sociobiological statements much publicity, as though there was a consensus about these issues in the scientific community. Members of his audience at that session knew that the Genes & Gender Collective had been active in exposing such pseudoscientific ideas. They suggested that the Collective respond to his statements.

The Collective decided that, rather than engage in a debate, it would be more constructive to present analyses and explanations that are alternatives to genetic determinism. Accordingly, at the next AAAS meeting in 1990 we organized a symposium and invited Garland Allen, Bonnie Ellen Blustein, Linda Burnham, Frederica Y. Daly, Gerald Horne, Ruth Hubbard, Val Woodward, and Choichiro Yatani to address the topic from the viewpoints of their different disciplines.

As the position expressed by Rushton became more widely publicized and featured in popular and scientific venues, we decided that it was important to have our challenges to Rushton's views available in print as the seventh book in the Genes and Gender Series. We then invited others to participate in the volume: Beverly Greene, Gisela

Kaplan, Pamela Trotman Reid, Lesley J. Rogers, Simona Sharoni, and Carmen Luz Valcarcel.

The events of the past two years have unfortunately shown that in scientific and academic circles sociobiology is now the dominant theory in all disciplines, and the beliefs presented by Rushton are still in evidence. The ideologies of racism and sexism continue to be justified by this pseudoscience throughout the world. Racist and sexist policies and incidents are on the increase. The Genes and Gender Collective, together with other anti-racist and anti-sexist organizations, will continue to fight and expose these dangerous policies.

◆ GENES AND GENDER VII ◆

Challenging Racism and Sexism

◆ BETTY ROSOFF AND ETHEL TOBACH ◆

Introduction

The movements to gain equity by people oppressed on the basis of race and gender have found natural allies in each other to an extent that is more or less effective. The scientific community, however, has not always given these struggles sufficient and significant support. One of the reasons for this is the general acceptance of the concept of genetic determinism by the scientific community. Genetic determinism claims that all human characteristics, including behavior, are determined by the functions of genes. This concept, as expressed in the ideology of sociobiology, has permeated all the life sciences and other disciplines bearing on the human condition. The primary tenets of sociobiology demonstrate the fundamental genetic determinist approach of this ideology. These are that the individual organism is the vehicle for the gene, which not only determines all characteristics of all organisms but which also engineers its succession in future generations by programming the cognitive, emotional, and social processes that guarantee this succession.

Many scientists are not patently genetic determinists, and most scientists do not explicate their views on the issues of genetic determinism per se. Their usual position is that the issue of genetic determinism is a nonissue, because no one would dispute that genes and environmental factors interact. Generally, they formulate experimental questions about the relationships between genetic and behavioral processes which ignore the events that intervene between genes

1

and behavior. These experiments then frequently yield answers that do little to change racist or sexist policies and practices.

In this book we present articles that inform us of the history of genetic determinism, that describe genetic function in a rigorously scientific fashion, and that demonstrate the need to fight racism and sexism, not only for the general population but for the scientific community as well. Reflecting many changes taking place in the struggle for equality, the authors have used different terms to describe people. We the editors have not changed the terminology of the chapter authors or those cited.

The papers are organized in three parts. Part I presents evidence of racism and sexism in research and in the distortions of knowledge derived from biology, physiology, and psychology. Part II considers philosophical and historical issues in racism and sexism. Part III discusses contemporary racism and sexism in various ethnic communities.

PART I

Ruth Hubbard, a biologist, discusses the fallacious formulation of race and gender as biological categories, leading to incorrect inferences about individual and group differences. These differences are usually attributed to race and sexual characteristics rather than to factors of class and history. She shows how these attributions reflect the class, race, and gender of the scientists who postulate them.

The critique by Betty Rosoff, an endocrinologist, and Ethel Tobach, a comparative psychologist, examines some contemporary uses of genetics in biomedical research and in studying human evolution. They emphasize the need for researchers to make clear how they have demonstrated what the gene function is which produces the disease state or the characteristics for evolutionary study. Investigators should clearly define populations and what they see to be the limitations and reliability of their generalizations and inferences.

Val Woodward, a population geneticist, rigorously discusses contemporary advances in genetics. He stresses that the understanding of developmental genetics within a specified environment is necessary to describe characteristics of individuals and groups. Simply relying on molecular genetics may lead to misconceptions about these characteristics. He discusses sociobiological interpretations of genetic processes as an example of such misconceptions.

Lesley Rogers, a comparative physiological psychologist, and Gisela Kaplan, a sociologist, discuss unscientific usages of anatomical and physiological traits to explain gender and race differences. In their historical review they criticize sexist and racist theories based on morphology, hormonal processes, and brain size and lateralization. More recent research about homosexuality reveals similar scientific fallacies.

Pamela Trotman Reid, a developmental psychologist specializing in social and feminist psychology, reviews the similarities and differences between racism and sexism and the history of their effects on black women. She draws attention to the need to explicate the complex relationship between racism and sexism in social psychological research, particularly as it affects the development of educational and social policies.

Beverly Greene, a clinical psychologist, calls upon the psychotherapist to understand the collective social plight of African-American women. While it is not necessary for the therapist to be of the same ethnicity, race, and gender as the patient, the therapist must recognize these contexts, as well as sexual orientation, to appreciate the unique community in which the patient lives and the differences in individual experience.

All these papers, in their own ways, make clear that any one aspect of an individual's history, whether it be genetic or societal, is not sufficient to explain the uniqueness of an individual or the shared characteristics of a community.

PART II

Linda Burnham, a writer, activist, and editor in issues of racial justice and gender equity, points out that theoretical questions about the relationship among race, gender, and class are not sufficiently dealt with in feminist movements. One must look at the history of racist and sexist discrimination in a particular society, as, for example, in the United States, by analyzing each type of discrimination independently and interdependently to determine the individual and mutual effects of each on the person and society. More important is the awareness of the scope and the limits of any given analysis that purports to explain a universal, generalized woman.

Garland Allen, a historian of the science of biology, draws on the history of the eugenics movement, from 1890 to 1930, to show societal processes leading to genetic determinism. He critically analyzes research methods used in support of genetic determinism, such as twin studies, the human genome project, and IQ studies. Eugenics was historically used as the basis for repressive social policies such as nationalism and fascism and is contemporaneously used to justify similar societal policies.

Gisela Kaplan, a sociologist and a historian of the Nazi era, discusses the pre-Nazi historical development of anti-Semitism and its use by Hitler. Anti-Semitism was not originally conceptualized as "racialism," but Hitler used a "racialized" anti-Semitism in order to practice eugenics. The Nazi ideology further applied racist policies by extolling the role of women only because they were necessary for the production and continuation of a pure race.

Gerald Horne, a lawyer, author, and Black Studies scholar, presents a historical-legal analysis of the struggle for justice in fighting a false, racist accusation of rape. The politically complex aspect of this struggle for civil liberties is described. The differential treatment by the police and court institutions of the women and the so-called perpetrators involved is based on the color of their skins and leads to the legal lynching of African-African men. Because women are valued as sex objects, another form of property, the supposed rape of a white woman by a African-American man is a most heinous crime. In a white society loss of property to a African-American man is particularly unacceptable and becomes the basis for legal oppression.

The papers in this part illustrate the role of a pseudoscientific theory, genetic determinism, as exemplified in the eugenics movement and how it is used by those in power. The delineation of the similarities and differences between the histories, expressions, and policies of sexism and racism is a profound contribution to the philosophy of feminism. It also provides an important tool for developing strategies for combating racism and sexism.

PART III

In her historical overview of the Native American experience, Frederica Daly, a clinical psychologist, shows how racism murdered Native American women and robbed them of their traditional land use. This economic deprivation continues today. Native American societies are variously organized, including matrilineal societies, and women are often elected chiefs. At the same time, in present-day society Native American women are worn down by poverty and abuse by men. In the silence of the blindness of white society to their oppression of Native Americans, Indian men identify socially with their oppressors today in their treatment of women.

Bonnie Ellen Blustein, a historian of science and teacher of high school mathematics, focuses on the school as a community in which genetic determinist views of ethnicity profoundly affect the educational process. Latino/a children are labeled as incapable of academic success. Employment and wage structures discriminate against Latinos/as as a group. Furthermore, Latino fathers are less likely to be employed than Latina mothers. In the context of such economic exploitation the imposition, through an insensitive educational policy, of rules of obedient conduct and acceptance of discriminatory practices further exacerbates the effects of racism and sexism on Latino/a students.

Carmen Luz Valcarcel, a doctoral student studying counseling psychology, presents the life of a Black woman in Puerto Rico in a vivid demonstration of the effects of racist and sexist practices. Her narrative points out the particular damage to the development of a child in a culture that, by denying its history of slavery, denies the existence of racism. This denial precludes the psychological well-being of dark-skinned individuals, particularly women.

Choichiro Yatani, an industrial/organizational psychologist, criticizes J. P. Rushton's statement that the brains of Asians are the largest and, therefore, that they are more intelligent and better achievers than Europeans and Africans. Yatani points out that the different cultures of Asian countries present a great diversity of educational practices and achievement. In addition, there are differences between Japanese children and U.S. children, not explicable by genetic determinist concepts. The significance of different familial organization and practices, values, and cultural goals as important factors in scholastic achievement is discussed.

Simona Sharoni, a political scientist and an expert in conflict analysis and resolution, describes the intersection between different types of racist and sexist practices against three groups of Israeli citizens: Oriental Jews, Palestinians, and Israeli women. The significance of this interaction for feminist struggles for equity is examined in the particular context of governmental military policies and social practices.

These contributions describe the specificity and generality of racism and sexism in a variety of cultures, demonstrating the validity of the points made in parts I and II. Not any one factor can explain the individual and group differences. The study of the history of the people affected is necessary to understand the causes of racism and sexism.

♦ REGINA E. WILLIAMS ♦

Asylum

for Ernestine Lewis

mourning suns filter thru her
opaque eyes
an inmate clamors
begs, fights for a place
to lay her trauma
straight-jacketed smiles
focus in hallucinated reality.

they say she is mad
this red-maned, red-hued
black woman of piercing eye and probing
she says "i may look broken
but i'm anchored in an ancient ebony frame."
she thinks history splintered &
mutters about an ancestry of cuts
cocks her head and walks
in her own lush garden

she calms my terror
says redmen are passive
only in movies
blackmen only in whitemen minds

sends me to "lie-berries" to read
between lines double-dutches me thru
dual histories
skip-ropes to Now
says tomorrow it's hide & (above all) seek

a bald-faced pharisee
is the rock
shattering her life
so her eyes take on splinters

her life is a legacy
of blood & wired glass
framed
as my window

they say she is mad
and like a mirror
she is.

◆ I ◆

Concepts of Racism and Sexism in Biology, Physiology, and Psychology

◆ RUTH HUBBARD ◆

Race and Sex as Biological Categories

The laws made of skin and hair fill the statute books in Pretoria. . . .
Skin and hair. It has mattered more than anything else in the world.
—Nadine Gordimer, *A Sport of Nature*

Scientists, whose business it is to investigate things that matter in the world, have put a good deal of effort into examining the biological basis of differences not only in skin and hair but also in other characteristics that are assigned cultural and political significance. And they have sometimes made it appear as though the differences in power, encoded in the statute books (and not only those in Pretoria), were no more than the natural outcomes of biological differences. This became critically important in the eighteenth century, when support for the aims of the revolutions fought for liberty, equality, fraternity and for the Rights of Man needed to be reconciled with the obvious inequalities between nations, the "races," and the sexes.

As late as the sixteenth century some authors described the peoples of Africa as superior in wit and intelligence to the inhabitants of northern climes, arguing that the hot, dry climate "enlivened their temperament,"[1] and two centuries later Rousseau still rhapsodized about the Noble Savage. Yet beginning in the fifteenth century Africans became human chattel, hunted and sold as part of the resources Europeans extracted from that "dark and primitive" continent. The industrialization of Europe and North America depended on the exploitation of the native populations of the Americas and Africa, and

11

so it became imperative to draw distinctions between that small number of men who were created equal and everyone else. By the nineteenth century the Noble Savage was a lying, thieving Indian, and Africans and their enslaved descendants were ugly, slow, stupid, and in every way inferior to Caucasians. Distinctions also needed to be drawn between women and men, since, irrespective of class and race, women were not included among "all men" who had been created equal.

Although there are many similarities in the ways biologists have rationalized the inequalities between the races and sexes (and continue to do so to this day), this discussion will be clearer if we look at the arguments separately.

THE RACES OF MAN

Allan Chase[2] dates scientific racism from the publication of Malthus's *Essay on Population* in 1798 and argues that it focused on class distinctions among Caucasians rather than on distinctions between Caucasians and the peoples of Africa, America, and Asia. On the other hand, Stephen Jay Gould[3] points to Linnaeus (1758) for the first scientific ranking of races. Linnaeus arranged the races into different subspecies and claimed that Africans, whom he called *Homo sapiens afer,* are "ruled by caprice," whereas Europeans *(Homo sapiens europaeus)* are "ruled by customs." He also wrote that African men are indolent and that African women are shameless and lactate profusely.

Both dates occur more than two centuries after the beginning of the European slave trade, which became an important part of the economies of Europe and the Americas. But they are contemporary with the intellectual and civic ferment that led to the American and French revolutions (1776 and 1789, respectively) and to the revolution that overthrew slavocracy in Haiti (1791). As Walter Rodney has pointed out,[4] it is wrong to think "that Europeans enslaved Africans for racist reasons." They did so for economic reasons, since without a supply of free African labor they would not have been able "to open up the New World and to use it as a constant generator of wealth. . . . Then, having become utterly dependent on African labour, Europeans at home and abroad found it necessary to rationalize that exploitation in racist terms."

Nineteenth-century physicians and biologists helped with that effort by constructing criteria, such as skull volume and brain size, by which they tried to prove scientifically that Africans are inferior to Caucasians. Gould's *Mismeasure of Man* describes some of the measurements and documents their often patently racist intent. Gould also illustrates the apparent naïveté with which, for example, the famous French scientist Paul Broca discarded criteria (such as the ratio of lengths of the long bones in the lower and upper arm, because it is greater in apes than humans) when he could not make them rank white men at the top. And he shows how Broca and the U.S. craniometer Samuel George Morton fudged and fiddled with their data in order to make the rankings come out as these men knew they must: white men on top, next Native American men, then African-American men. Women were problematic: though clearly white women ranked below white men, were they to be above or below men of the other races? A colleague of Broca's wrote in 1881, "Men of the black races have a brain scarcely heavier than that of white women."[5]

In 1854 an American physician, Dr. Cartwright, wrote in an article entitled "Diseases and Peculiarities of the Negro" that a defect in the "atmospherization of the blood conjoined with a deficiency of cerebral matter in the cranium ... led to that debasement of mind which has rendered the people of Africa unable to take care of themselves."[6] And racialist biologisms did not end with slavery. Jim Crow theorizing and practices survived until past the passage of the Civil Rights Act of 1957. Writing during World War II, Gunnar Myrdal marveled that the American Red Cross "refused to accept Negro blood donors. After protests it now accepts Negro blood but segregates it to be used exclusively for Negro soldiers. This is true at a time when the United States is at war, and the Red Cross has a semi-official status."[7] The American Red Cross continued to separate the blood of whites and African Americans until December 1950, when the binary classification into "Negro" and "white" was deleted from the donor forms. As Howard Zinn remarks, "It was, ironically, a black physician named Charles Drew who developed the blood bank system."[8]

What can we in the 1990s say about the biology of race differences? Looking at all the evidence, there are none.[9] Demographers, politicians, and social scientists may continue to use "race" to sort people, but, as a biological concept, it has no meaning. The fact is that, genetically, human beings *(Homo sapiens)* are a relatively homogeneous species. If Caucasians were to disappear overnight, the genetic composition of the species would hardly change. About 75 percent of known genes are the same in all humans. The remaining 25 percent exist in more than one form, but all these forms occur in all groups, only sometimes in different proportions.[10] Another way to say it is that, because of the extent of interbreeding that has happened among human populations over time, our genetic diversity is pretty evenly distributed over the entire species. The occasional, relatively recent mutation may still be somewhat localized within a geographic area, but about 90 percent of the variations known to occur among humans as a whole occur also among the individuals of any one national or racial group.[11]

Another important point is that, for any scientific measurement of race difference, we first have to construct what we mean by race. Does the least trace of African origins make someone black, or does the least trace of Caucasian origins make someone white? The U.S. census for 1870 contained a third category, "Mulatto," for "all persons having any perceptible trace of African blood" and warned that "important scientific results depend on the correct determination of this class."[12] The U.S. census for 1890 collected information separately for "quadroons and octoroons"—that is, people who have one grandparent or one great-grandparent who is African, respectively, "while in 1930, any mixture of white and some other race was to be reported according to the race of the parent who was not white." Finally, in 1970 the Statistical Policy Division of the Office of Management and Budget warned that racial "classifications should not be interpreted as being scientific or anthropological in nature."[13] We need only look at the morass of legalisms in apartheid South Africa to abandon any notion that there are clear racial differences.

Yet we read such statistics as that "black men under age 45 are ten times more likely to die from the effects of high blood pressure than white men," that "black women suffer twice as many heart attacks as white women," and that "a variety of common cancers are more frequent among blacks . . . than whites."[14] At the same time some scientists and the media keep stressing the genetic origin of these diseases. So, must we not believe once again that there are inherent, biological differences between blacks and whites, as groups?

A closer look again leads us to answer no. What is misleading is that U.S. health statistics are usually presented in terms of the quasibiological triad of age, race, and sex, without providing data about employment, income, housing, and the other prerequisites for healthful living. Even though there are genetic components to skin color, as there are to eye or hair color, there is no biological reason to assume that any one of these is more closely related to health status than any other. Skin color ("race") is no more likely to be related biologically to the tendency to develop high blood pressure than is eye color.

On the other hand, the median income of African Americans

since 1940 has been less than two-thirds that of whites. Disproportionate numbers of African Americans live in more polluted and rundown neighborhoods, work in more polluted and stressful workplaces, and have fewer escape routes out of these living and work situations than whites have. Therefore, it is not surprising to find large discrepancies in health outcomes between these groups.

Mary Bassett and Nancy Krieger, looking at mortality risks from breast cancer, have found that the black-white differential of 1.35 drops to 1.10 when they look at African-American and white women of comparable social class, as measured by a range of social indicators.[15] And within each "racial" group social class is correlated with mortality risk. Thus, although it is true that African-American women, as a group, are at greater risk of dying from breast cancer than white women are, women of comparable class standing face a similar risk within these groups as well as between them. In other words, because of racial oppression, being black is a predictor of increased health risk, but so is being poor, no matter what one's skin color may be.

SEX DIFFERENCE

That having been said, what about sex? Here, too, it can be argued that, since in our society any muting of differences between women and men is intolerable, this insistence may exaggerate biological differences and, therefore, enhance our impressions of them.[16] (Note the use of the phrase "the opposite sex" instead of "the other sex.") In fact, women and men exhibit enormous overlaps in body shape and form, strength, and most other parameters. The diversity within the two groups is often as large as the differences between them. Yet biological differences exist as regards women's and men's procreative capacities. Our society may exaggerate and overemphasize them, but the fact is that people who procreate need to be of two kinds. Therefore, the question I want to look at is to what extent ideological commitments to the differences our society ascribes to women and men in the social and political spheres influence the ways biologists describe the differences that are involved in procreation.

To do this it is useful to start with a quick look at Darwin's theory of sexual selection, which embedded Victorian preconceptions about the differences between women and men in modern biology. Sex is important to Darwin's theory of evolution by natural selection because the direction evolution takes is assumed to depend crucially on who mates with whom. This is why Darwin needed to invent the concept of sexual selection—the ways sex partners choose each other. Given the time in which he was writing, it is not surprising that he came up with the Victorian paradigm of the active, passionate, sexually undiscriminating male who competes with every other male in his pursuit of every available female, while females, though passive, coy, and sexually unenthusiastic, are choosy and go for "the winner." Darwin theorized that this makes for greater competition among males than females, and, since competition is what drives evolution by natural selection, males are in the vanguard of evolution. Females get pulled along by mating with the most successful males. The essentials of this interpretation have been incorporated into modern sociobiology.[17] Only in the last few years feminist sociobiologists, such as Sarah Blaffer Hrdy, have revised this canon and pointed out that females also can be active, sexually aggressive, and competitive and that males can nurture and be passive. Among animals as well as among people females do not just stand by and wait for the most successful males to come along.[18]

I have criticized the Darwinian paradigm of looking at sex differences elsewhere.[19] The point I want to stress here is that, until quite recently, the active male–passive female dyad has been part of biological dogma and is the metaphor that informs standard descriptions of procreative biology at every level.

For example, the differentiation of the sex organs during embryonic development is said to proceed as follows: the embryo starts out sexually bipotential and ambiguous, but early during embryonic development in future males something happens under the influence of the Y chromosome which makes part of the undifferentiated, primitive gonads turn into fetal testes. These then begin to secrete fetal androgens (called male hormones), which are instrumental in masculinizing one set of embryonic ducts so that they develop into the sperm ducts and external male genitalia (the scrotal sac and penis), whereas another set of ducts atrophies. The story goes on to say that, if at this critical point no Y chromosome is present, then *nothing happens.* In that case somewhat later, and without special hormonal input, another part of the undifferentiated fetal gonad differentiates into ovaries, and, since these do *not* secrete androgens, the other set of fetal ducts differentiates into the fallopian tubes, uterus, vagina, and the external female genitalia (the labia and clitoris).

Notice that in this description male differentiation is active and triggered by the Y chromosome and by so-called male hormones; female differentiation happens because these triggering mechanisms are absent.[20] Of course, this cannot be true. All differentiation is active and requires multiple inputs and decision points. Furthermore, the so-called sex hormones are interconvertible, and both males and females secrete all of them and, for considerable parts of our lives, in not very different proportions. Diana Long Hall has described the history of the discovery of these hormones and the ways gender ideology was incorporated into designating them "male" and "female."[21] Anne Fausto-Sterling has noted that the Greek names that scientists gave them are also ideology laden. The "male" hormone is called androgen, the "generator of males," but there is no gynogen, or generator of females. Instead, the "female" analogue of androgen is called estrogen, from *oestrus,* which means "frenzy" or "gadfly."[22]

The standard description of fertilization again follows the traditional script.[23] Ejaculation launches sperm on its dauntless voyage up the female reproductive tract. In contrast, eggs are "released," or "shed," from the ovary to sit patiently in the fallopian tubes until a sperm "penetrates" and "activates" them. Given that fertilization is an active process in which two cells join together and their nuclei fuse, why is it that we say that a sperm *fertilizes* the egg, whereas eggs are fertilized? In 1948 Ruth Herschberger caricatured this scenario in her delightful book *Adam's Rib,*[24] but that did not change the standard biological descriptions.

Of course, both sessile eggs and sprightly sperm are fabrications. Eggs, sperm, and the entire female reproductive tract must participate if fertilization is to take place, and infertility can result from the malfunctioning of any one of them. Also, a good deal goes on in eggs both before and after fertilization. It is interesting that modern biologists have been so focused on the role of the sperm and on chromosomes and genes that they have paid much more attention to the fact that, during fertilization, eggs and sperm contribute the same number of chromosomes than to the important part the egg's cytoplasm plays in the differentiation and development of the early embryo. The egg contributes much more than its nuclear chromosomes; it contributes all its cell contents—the cytoplasm, with its complement of cytoplasmic DNA and its subcellular structure and metabolic apparatus.

Finally, let us turn to the surely objective realm of DNA molecules. Here we find an article, published in December 1987 in the professional journal *Cell* and immediately publicized in the weekly scientific magazine *Science* and in the daily press, entitled "The Sex-Determining Region of the Human Y Chromosome Encodes a Finger Protein."[25] The authors claimed, and the magazines and newspapers promptly reported, that sex is determined by a single gene, located on the Y chromosome. The X chromosome, the authors wrote, has a similar gene, but it has nothing to do with sex differentiation. Reading the article more closely, we see that the authors identified a region of the Y chromosome which seemed to be correlated with the differentiation of testes. When this region was missing no testes developed; when it was present they did. By this argument the presence or absence of testes determines sex: people who have testes are male; people who don't are female.

More recently, in December 1989, two other groups of scientists claimed that the region on the Y chromosome which the previous group had identified as "determining sex" does not "determine" either maleness or sex because males can develop testes in its absence,[26] but that has simply refocused the search for *the sex* gene elsewhere on the Y chromosome. None of these authors points out that being female implies more than not having testes and that the differentiation of sex organs, whether female or male, requires processes of differentiation in which many genes as well as other metabolites must be involved.

CONCLUSIONS

I have selected these examples to illustrate the ways in which our particular cultural preoccupations with race and sex penetrate the biological sciences. But I do not want this analysis to suggest that it is useless to attempt to describe nature or, indeed, society in scientific ways. In fact, throughout this article I have drawn on scientific work to argue against scientific claims that exhibit racial or gender bias. Science remains one of the better ways we have of trying to understand what goes on in the world. But when we use it to investigate subjects such as race and sex, which are suffused with cultural meanings and embedded in power relationships, we need to be wary of scientific descriptions and interpretations that sustain or enhance the prevailing political realities.

To look critically at these kinds of data and interpretations, we need to bear in mind that in any society that is stratified by gender or race the fact that we are born with "female" or "male" genitals and "black" or "white" skin means that we will live different lives. Yet our biology and how we live are dialectically related and interpenetrate each other. The differences in our genital anatomy or in the color of our skin affect the ways we live, and our ways of life affect our biology.

For these reasons the scientific methodology of research into sex or race differences is intrinsically flawed. Scientists cannot vary genital anatomy or skin color and hold the environment constant, nor can they switch the cultural conditions that differentiate the environments of African Americans and whites or of women and men. Therefore, scientists cannot sort the effects of biology from societal influences. Scientists can catalog similarities and differences between women and men and between African Americans and whites, but they cannot establish their causes.[27]

One last point: I have looked at race and sex as separate categories, but we must not forget that they have also been combined to generate the cultural images of the eroticized, exotic African, male and female, and of the debased, sexualized African American, the black rapist, pimp, and whore. Social scientists and philosophers have only begun to explore the significance and ramifications of this melding of racism and sexism.[28] Scientists, and indeed all of us, need to become aware of the multiple meanings of these images and metaphors and to grasp the extent to which they penetrate our consciousness, collectively and as individuals, if we are to free the ways we think about race, sex, and gender from the subtle as well as the more blatant stereotypes that permeate our culture.

NOTES

1. Londa Schiebinger, *The Mind Has No Sex? Women and the Origins of Modern Science* (Cambridge: Harvard University Press, 1989), 165.

2. Allan Chase, *The Legacy of Malthus: The Social Costs of the New Scientific Racism* (New York: Alfred Knopf, 1977).

3. Stephen Jay Gould, *The Mismeasure of Man* (New York: W. W. Norton, 1981), 35.

4. Walter Rodney, *How Europe Underdeveloped Africa* (Dar-es-Salaam: Tanzania Publishing House, 1972), 99–100.

5. Gould, *Mismeasure of Man,* 103.

6. Cited in Dorothy Burnham, "Black Women as Producers and Reproducers for Profit," in *Woman's Nature: Rationalizations of Inequality,* ed. Marian Lowe and Ruth Hubbard (New York: Pergamon Press, 1983), 35.

7. Gunnar Myrdal, *An American Dilemma: The Negro Problem and Modern Democracy* (New York: Harper and Brothers, 1944), 1367.

8. Howard Zinn, *A People's History of the United States* (New York: Harper and Row, 1980), 406.

9. Leo Kuper, ed., *Race, Science and Society* (Paris: UNESCO Press, 1975).

10. R. C. Lewontin, Steven Rose, and Leon J. Kamin, *Not in Our Genes:*

Biology, Ideology, and Human Nature (New York: Pantheon, 1984), esp. 119–29.

11. Richard Lewontin, *Human Diversity* (New York: Scientific American Books, 1982).

12. Janet L. Norwood and Deborah P. Klein, "Developing Statistics to Meet Society's Needs," *Monthly Labor Review* (October 1989).

13. Norwood and Klein, "Developing Statistics."

14. Nancy Krieger and Mary Bassett, "The Health of Black Folk: Disease, Class, and Ideology in Science," *Monthly Review* 38, no. 3 (July–August 1986): 74.

15. Mary T. Bassett and Nancy Krieger, "Social Class and Black-White Differences in Breast Cancer Survival," *American Journal of Public Health* 76, no. 12 (1986): 1400–1403.

16. Suzanne J. Kessler and Wendy McKenna, *Gender: An Ethnomethodological Approach* (Chicago: University of Chicago Press, 1978).

17. Edward O. Wilson, *Sociobiology: The Modern Synthesis* (Cambridge: Harvard University Press, 1975).

18. Sarah Blaffer Hrdy, "Empathy, Polyandry, and the Myth of the Coy Female," in *Feminist Approaches to Science,* ed. Ruth Bleier (New York: Pergamon Press, 1986).

19. Ruth Hubbard, *The Politics of Women's Biology* (New Brunswick, N.J.: Rutgers University Press, 1990), 87–118.

20. Anne Fausto-Sterling, *Myths of Gender: Biological Theories about Women and Men* (New York: Basic Books, 1985).

21. Diana Long Hall, "Biology, Sex Hormones, and Sexism in the 1920s," in *Women and Philosophy: Toward a Theory of Liberation,* ed. Carol C. Gould and Marx W. Wartofsky (New York: G. P. Putnam's Sons, 1976), 81–96.

22. Anne Fausto-Sterling, "Society Writes Biology / Biology Constructs Gender," *Daedalus* 116 (1987): 61–76.

23. Emily Martin, "The Egg and the Sperm," *Signs* 16 (1991): 485–501.

24. Ruth Herschberger, *Adam's Rib* (New York: Harper and Row, 1948).

25. David C. Page et al., "The Sex-Determining Region of the Human Y Chromosome Encodes a Finger Protein," *Cell* 51 (24 December 1987): 1091–1104.

26. M. S. Palmer et al., "Genetic Evidence that ZFY Is Not the Testis-Determining Factor," *Nature* 342, nos. 21–28 (December 1989): 937–39; Peter Koopman et al., "Zfy Gene Expression Patterns Are Not Compatible with a Primary Role in Mouse Sex Determination," *Nature* 342, nos. 21–28 (December 1989): 940–42.

27. Hubbard, *Politics of Women's Biology,* 128–29, 136–40.

28. Angela Y. Davis, *Women, Race, and Class* (New York: Random House, 1981); Henry Louis Gates, Jr., ed., *Race, Writing, and Difference* (Chicago: University of Chicago Press, 1986); Sander Gilman, *Difference and Pa-*

thology: Stereotypes of Sexuality, Race, and Madness (Ithaca: Cornell University Press, 1985); Donna Haraway, *Primate Visions: Gender, Race, and Nature in the World of Modern Science* (New York: Routledge, 1989); Nancy Stepan, "Race and Gender: The Role of Analogy in Science," *Isis* 77: 261–77.

◆ ETHEL TOBACH AND BETTY ROSOFF ◆

Critique of Recent Genetic Research Related to Issues of Racism and Sexism

A fundamental need in formulating research regarding the expression of genetic functions in human physiology and behavior is clarity in the meaning of the terms used. *Race, ethnicity, population, sex,* and *gender* are rarely defined in research reports and are used without precision, sometimes interchangeably. Even when they are defined by the authors, the criteria used to delineate groups or membership by individuals in the groups are frequently not given. For example, the terms *ethnicity, population,* and *race* are used to specify groups. Ethnicity is based on the cultural history, geography, and language of a people. A population is defined by parameters deemed relevant to the interests of the researchers carrying out the investigation, for example, defined in terms of blood type (Lewontin, 1982); of ethnicity (Aleuts); of geographical location (sub-Saharan people); of species (Mus musculus). Race is usually based on biological characteristics such as melanin in the skin. The groups are then described as having various physiological, hormonal, structural, or behavioral characteristics in common. Frequently, these traits have not been demonstrated to have any genetic relationship to the presumed markers of ethnicity, population, or race.

An examination of these practices reveals that implicit assumptions are being made about genetic processes, assumptions that are not tested in the research carried out. One of these assumptions is that the traits used to form the group are the expressions of a gene or genes probably shared by all the individuals in the group. Another is that evidence for the expression of one gene is assumed to be predictive of other characteristics for which a "gene" or "genes" have not been demonstrated. For example, a shared similarity of degree of melanization is used to project shared similarities of cognitive skills or social behavior.

Such extrapolations are derived from genetic determinism, an ideology that states that all aspects of the individual are seen as primarily determined by genes. This ideology ignores the development of structure and function which is derived from the integration of environmental and genetic processes. The history of this development and its outcome produce a unique organism, each with its own genetic, morphological, and functional characteristics. As categories such as races, ethnicities, and populations are defined by experimenters on the basis of characteristics that are relevant to their study, the groups so constituted become a conglomeration of unique individuals. In most cases individual differences are overlooked or consigned to statistical triviality.

An example of this type of extrapolation is the work of J. P. Rushton (1988). He has continued pursuing his genetic determinist ideology within an evolutionary context, applying it to such societal issues as the AIDS epidemic (1990).

The concept of race (see Woodward, Allen, in this volume) originated in societal usage and was then given a biological meaning in the eighteenth century to designate subpopulations or subtypes of plants and animals. It was this latter tradition that led the early biologists and anthropologists to attempt to classify the human species into different races, primarily based on morphological characteristics. This biological designation derived its negative history from the practices by those in power who benefited from derogating groups based on their races in order to justify their economic and social exploitation. Before the sophisticated instruments of genetic description came into use, the usual means of operationally defining such groups was by the color of the skin and craniofacial configuration. No gene or group of genes thought to be responsible for any of these morphological entities has been shown to be related to behavioral or societal patterns. Rather, such racial classifications have been used to justify oppression based on supposed inferiority of cognitive or social characteristics.

When investigators study the relationship between sex and gender and gene function, the problems of definition differ from those of race and ethnicity. The gender of the individual, a societally defined characteristic, is usually assumed to be the result of the individual's self-identification and is evident in clothing, name, and so forth. It is further assumed that the physiological and morphological characteristics usually associated with the gender presented exist in the individual. Rarely is this determined by morphology and hormonal status. Although most feminist scientists distinguish sex from gender in that sex refers to genetic, hormonal, morphological, and physiological aspects of reproduction, while gender is a societal designation based on the relationship of the individual to society, some do not make that distinction.

Females and males carry different numbers of X and Y chromosomes, but there is no evidence showing that the genes on those chromosomes produce the behavioral differences of women and men. The genetic determinists, not accepting the fact that there is a developmental history in which genes and their functions are integrated in the individual through physiological, social, and societal processes, continue to seek the genetic basis for the differences. Their agenda is to reduce all explanations to the genetic level.

There is an extensive and controversial literature on twin research and other methods used in attempts to define a genetic basis to behavior. This type of research has been critically reviewed, and, while there is an ongoing debate about the validity of the concept of behavioral genetic determinism, there has been no such critical examination of medical genetics.

The value of medical genetic research for finding a gene or genes responsible for diseases or deficiencies cannot be disputed. Medical genetics, a subdiscipline of human medicine, frequently investigates the presence or absence of particular molecular configurations in a racial, population, or ethnic group. Inferences then are drawn about the likelihood that some individual who has been thus societally assigned to a group is thought not only to have a genetic configuration similar to those of the other members of the group but also to have a strong probability of succumbing to a particular disease or having a particular deficiency. Because it is believed that the gene is responsible for the disease, other factors are overlooked as well as other medical conditions that might require attention. There are no data offered about the genealogy or history of the individual (e.g., were they and their parents and grandparents born and reared in that geographical area as members of that ethnic culture?). The issue of the source of individual variations is not considered relevant to the investigation of genetic processes because of the view that genes are "conservative, unchanging, stable."

A sizable industry has developed from the ingenious genetic research techniques now available for mapping human genes. Genetic processes in other organisms are used to elaborate proteins in forms that can be given to people who are deficient in them. The cost of such research programs is primarily born by the U.S. government, and to recoup part of that cost the government has become an entrepreneur offering patented genes for use by industry. The identification of genes that are responsible for various diseases and the therapeutic genetic measures that are becoming available will soon be market items, just as, for example, organs for replacement are now. The effect of the control of the obtained knowledge by the scientific-industrial complex in a society in which the military-industrial complex maintains its power is to deprive those sectors of society which cannot afford to pay for these new cures.

Although the need for caution when these techniques are discussed in terms of human characteristics has been expressed, we cannot be assured that genetic techniques will not be used to "engineer" human beings. The increasing educational triage in the light of economic difficulties results in the lack of decent training for people of color, for the working and lower middle classes, and for women. Contemporary economic difficulties are creating the same need for triage in medical care, and the availability of basic health procedures will again be restricted on the basis of race, gender, and class. The investment of effort, time, and money in the development of new knowledge in genetic research will make little difference for the health of these groups.

Research exemplifying some of the issues of race and gender is discussed in the following annotated bibliography.

REFERENCES

Lewontin, Richard. 1982. Human diversity. New York: Scientific American Books.

Rushton, J. P. 1988. Race differences in behavior: A review and evolutionary analysis. *Personalities and Individual Differences* 9: 1009–24.

———. 1990. Race, evolution and aids: What Rushton really said. Ed. Paul Fromm. Toronto: Citizens for Foreign Aid Reform.

ANNOTATED BIBLIOGRAPHY

The following articles are presented in alphabetical order by the first author's name, except in the case of the discussion of the study of hypertension in African Americans. This list is not exhaustive, but it is representative of the literature.

Ghanem, Nada, Catherine Buresi, Jean-Paul Moisan, Mylene Bensmana, Paul Chuchana, Sylvia Huck, Gerard Lefranc, and Marie-Paule Lefranc. 1989. Deletion, insertion, and restriction site polymorphism of the T-cell receptor gamma variable locus in French, Lebanese, Tunisian, and Black African populations. *Immunogenetics* 30: 350–60.

In this standard analysis of the frequencies of genes in different populations, the authors rely on the usual imprecise definitions. They refer to "Black Africans"; no cultural, geographical, or other criterion is used to define this general group. The authors rely, instead, on ethnic and political designations (e.g., Tunisians, French) to establish populations. Evidence of the history of the individuals (e.g., genealogy) as the basis for their classification would be more enlightening.

Gibbons, Richard J., Andrew O. M. Wilkie, David J. Weatherall, and Douglas R. Higgs. 1991. A newly defined X-linked mental retardation syndrome associated with alpha thalassemia. *Journal of Medical Genetics* 28: 729–33.

A disease with symptoms that overlap with other diseases featuring slow development, feeding and muscle difficulties at birth, and mental retardation "is rare in northern Europeans although it is frequently seen in Mediterranean and Oriental racial groups." It is readily diagnosed by hematological genetic analysis. The authors urge such determinations be made in boys with severe mental retardation and in their women relatives. They say that the test is not sufficiently sensitive to identify all carriers, and there is no discussion of the relevance of this test for genetic counseling. Here again the statistical criterion of frequency count is the basis for defining the relevant populations, which are described in terms of geographical location and race.

McColley, S. A., B. J. Rosenstein, and G. R. Cutting. 1991. Differences in expression of cystic fibrosis in blacks and whites. *American Journal of Diseases of Children* 145: 94–97.

Although the genetic configuration responsible for cystic fibrosis has been identified, it only occurs in approximately 70 percent of white and 37 percent of black cases. This study investigated differences in the expression of cystic fibrosis in white and black patients. They found that there were some significant population differences in such items as number of hospitalizations for pulmonary exacerbations, which were lower for blacks than for whites. Hyponatremic dehydration and peptic ulcer diseases were greater in blacks than in whites. There is no discussion about socioeconomic differences (e.g., available hospital care) or life stress (e.g., presence of peptic ulcer disease). Nonetheless, they conclude that individual differences may be due to genetic heterogeneity of the two populations.

Politzer, William S., and J. Anderson. 1989. Ethnic and genetic differences in bone mass: A review with a hereditary versus environmental perspective. *American Journal of Clinical Nutrition* 50: 1224–59.

These authors introduce their review with a set of definitions.

> The term ethnic group has come to supercede race chiefly because of the unfortunate connotations and harmful effects of the concept of race. . . . The rise of genetics changed the concept of race from a typological to a populational one. People with common ancestors who interbreed among themselves more than with other groups share the same gene pool and, thus, show similar inherited characteristics. . . . Today physical anthropologists view race not as static, qualitative, and absolute with rigid geographical boundaries but rather as dynamic, quantitative, and variable, with clines or gradients in inherited trait, such as skin color or the frequency of a blood group. (1244)

> It is more a social convention than a biological reality that we continue to designate groups by terms of pigmentation. In the real world all is not black and white. Labels are justified when they help us understand biological processes, and, thus, serve human needs. (1245)

> Race implies a population identified by its genes, i.e., genetic differences. Ethnic group implies a population identified by difference but makes no firm commitment as to whether they are due to genetic or environmental causes. . . . Genes do not determine destiny but they set the stage upon which the environment operates. What is inherited is far from obvious. Proof of genetic causation cannot be inferred from the fact that a particular condition runs in families . . . or [from the fact] that a characteristic is far more frequent in monozygotic twins who have 100% of their genes in common than in dizygotic twins who have 50% in common. With this background in mind, we shall explore the question of whether ethnic differences in bone mass . . . are primarily genetic or environmental in origin. (1245).

In their analysis of the "contributions of the four major determinants of BM [bone mass] . . . ethnic-genetic, dietary, physical activity, and hormonal determinants" (1244), however, the authors confuse ethnicity with genetics. Ethnicity is a sociohistorical category distinct from biological categories.

Politzer and Anderson's interest in this topic is occasioned by the fact that postmenopausal osteoporosis is "the major health problem . . . " of Caucasian and Oriental women" (1244). It may be said that they use *Caucasian* and *Oriental* because of the terms' acceptance in the literature, but their definitions would suggest the desirability of using more precise terms and showing respect for the dignity of the people studied by using the names they themselves prefer.

This sensitivity to racism and sexism in science attempts to mitigate the serious problem of typological thinking in approaching the problem of how different people are more or less likely to develop osteoporosis or bone breakage. The differential treatment offered to people of color, to those who are poor, and to women is based on the statistical likelihood of the cost and risk factors of the disease involved (triage). Nowhere in the article is there any evidence of the development of a policy based on individual differences which would challenge the triage approach.

The probability of developing an equitable preventive program derived from the approach that "both genes and environment are important" should be considered in the light of the type of studies cited by Politzer and Anderson. They seem to accept such statements as "Findings show a greater genetic determination for the lumbar spine in premenopausal life but that environmental factors are of increasing importance after menopause in Caucasian women" worth reporting, even though at the same time they state that "the method of calculating correlations and subsequent heritability is open to question" (1256).

The authors conclude, nonetheless, that the genetic factor is ultimately the determining process for the higher incidence of osteoporosis in white and Asian women than in black women. They underplay the significance of diet and exercise, which reflect the culture of the ethnic groups. Their article yields no information about the genes responsible for the osteoporotic bone and certainly does not suggest any research that would elucidate why these characteristics should be defined in populations characterized by skin color or geographic and cultural histories. The view that a particular gene is solely responsible for a particular condition is derived from a misunderstanding of the genetic process: genetic function is involved in every condition. The problem is to understand how these functions are expressed in different experiential conditions (diet, stress, activity, climate, etc.) and in the individual's history at different stages of development.

Ranney, Helen M., Gwen H. Rosenberg, Martin Morrison, and Thomas J. Mueller. 1990. Frequencies of band 3 variants of human red cell membrane in different populations. *British Journal of Haematology* 76: 262–67.

According to administrative hospital records, in this study, ethnicity was appropriately defined by the patients. The participants are described as Hopi, Navajo, African American, Caucasian, Chinese, Filipino, Mexican, Cambodian, Laotian, and Vietnamese. The purpose of the study was to define frequencies of particular membrane proteins in these populations.

Saxena, Samita, and Edward T. Wong. 1990. Heterogeneity of common hematologic parameters among racial, ethnic and gender subgroups. *Archives of Pathology Laboratory Medicine* 114: 715–19.

In their abstract these authors state: "This study was performed to determine whether hematologic indexes might show heterogeneity among different subgroups of the population and, if differences were found, to develop reference ranges for each subgroup. . . . We concluded that the complete blood cell counts and leucocyte differential counts exhibit marked heterogeneity and that reference ranges that reflect the proper racial, ethnic, and sex group should be developed for these parameters" (715). This laudable effort to refine the diagnosis of blood function is unfortunately not paralleled in a refinement of such terms as *White, Black, Latin American,* and *Asian* and by the use of *sex* and *gender* as equivalent terms. The authors present differential and complete blood cell counts for each of the four populations and for the two sexes and state that these are statistically different, yet the values for each of the subgroups (populations) overlap. This overlap presents a problem for developing reference ranges for groups, when the criteria for defining a group are not precise. While there is a need for some normative data to assist in efficient diagnosis, the individual variations that result from different life histories must be taken into account.

Spurdle, Amanda, and Trefor Jenkins. 1991. Y chromosome probe p49a detects complex pvull haplotypes and many new taql haplotypes in Southern African populations. *American Journal of Human Genetics* 50: 107–25.

This study was done to understand "genetic distance between populations" and revealed "a basic split between African and non-African populations." Further, they say that

> the Y chromosome represents the specific paternal contribution to the male genome, and Y-specific RFLP's [restriction fragment length polymorphisms, a tool used in mapping genetic characteristics] would thus be useful for studying the male gene flow. Southern Africa is a particu-

larly interesting area in which to conduct gene flow studies . . . [be-cause] its people represent three of the major races of mankind . . . negroid, caucasoid and Khoisan [Khoisan: a group of African peoples speaking Khoisan language, . . . e.g., Hottentot, and related to others such as Sandawe and Hatsa *(Webster's Unabridged International Dictionary,* 3d ed.)]. . . . Present theories on the ancestry of these populations and on the admixture between them are based on archaeological, linguistic and some genetic data. . . . [T]he resulting frequency data were used to assess the affinities of the populations and to elucidate the nature of the historical interactions between them. (107–8)

In the description of "subjects" the authors refer to language, morphological characteristics (such as "hooked nose" in the Lemba, whom they later discuss in regard to a possible relationship to Jews), ritual practices (kosher killing of cattle), having "typical negroid features" (the Dama), and skin color (the Khoi and the San). The Caucasoid group "includes people of western European and Asiatic Indian origin, as well as Ashkenazim Jews from eastern Europe; *"colored"* refers to mixed ancestry of "negroid people," and trekboers (European farmers), and Dama women. Nowhere in the article is there any discussion about the relevance of any of these characteristics to the genetic configurations they are studying. The use of the terms referring to race, nationality, ethnicity, and culture are given equal weights in defining the populations. Further, the implication is that understanding the genetic characteristics of these people will elucidate their history.

The populations studied consist only of men, and the choices of the Y chromosome and its flow as the basis for elucidating history is not discussed. The authors are clearly aware of the variations within the groups observed because frequencies are the primary bases for similarities and differences that explicate the genetic and historical relationships among these peoples, and none of the frequencies are 100 percent present or absent. This statistical typology is mirrored in the typological thinking about the linguistic criterion for defining the populations, which the authors also recognize as limited in validity ("the present language classification of a group may not reflect its genetic past" [120]). The same problems in group definitions are seen in a later article (see A. Spurdle, M. B. Ramsay, and T. Jenkins. 1992. The Y-associated XY275 low allele is not restricted to indigenous African peoples. *American Journal of Human Genetics* 50: 1301–7). The authors are from the Medical Research Council of Witwatersrand, Johannesburg, South Africa.

Tielsch, James M., Alfred Sommer, Joanne Katz, Richard M. Royall, Harry A. Quigley, and Jonathan Javitt. 1991. Racial variations in the prevalance of primary open-angle glaucoma. *Journal of the American Medical Association* 266: 369–74.

This study was conducted in the eastern and southeastern health districts of Baltimore, Maryland. In it patients were given an opthalmologic screening examination. There is no description of the method used to determine who among them were Black and who were White. The researchers found a significantly higher incidence of this type of glaucoma in the Black population in both women and men; they conclude that "additional efforts are needed to identify and treat this sight-threatening disorder in high-risk communities" (369). In this article, the needs of the community are primary in the discussion, and the usual genetic versus environmental factors are not invoked. As in the case of the incidence of hypertension and kidney disease, these types of studies are useful.

Ward, R. H., Barbara L. Frazier, Kerry Dew-Jager, and Svante Paabo. 1991. Extensive mitochondrial diversity within a single Amerindian tribe. *Proceedings of the National Academy of Sciences* 88: 8720–24.

A study based on maternal inheritance of mitochondrial DNA presents data showing that there is as much genetic diversity in the Amerindians as in the Japanese and sub-Saharan Africans. The term *sub-Saharans* is imprecise and a "remnant of colonial notions of Africa as comprising two separate autonomous worlds" (L. C. Jackson. 1989. HLA diversity within the context of general human heterogeneity: Anthropological perspectives. *Transplantation Proceedings* 21: 3869–71). The authors conclude that "the migratory expansion of early human populations that led to the formation of major ethnic groups most likely did not result in substantial genetic differentiation between groups" (8724).

Wienker, Curtis W. 1990. Birth weight in an African-American population living under moderate ecological stress. *Human Biology* 62: 719–32.

This study was undertaken in consideration of the fact that "one vacuum in the literature addressing environmental stress on humans is the lack of information on responses of African-American populations to ecologic conditions other than those found in the African tropics. . . . Few African-American communities are found at high altitudes, which itself may be indicative of historic and prehistoric failures at acclimatization and adaptation by African and African-derived populations" (720). Wienker cites work by others who report that African slavery failed under the Spanish in Peru, where slaves worked at high altitudes, and that most of the slaves brought to the Western hemisphere came from West African countries, which have a warm climate and low elevations. He also points out that, in general, babies born in elevations above 1,500 meters and higher usually were low in weight at birth. The author, therefore, obtained records of the birth weights of African-American babies born after moderately warm and severely cold winters in McNary, Arizona, at an elevation of 7,300 feet, and compared them with African-American babies born in New York City; Nashville, Tennessee; Oakland, California; Washington, D.C.; and in the United States generally. He found that the weights of the babies born in McNary were not different from those recorded for the entire United States and were heavier than those born in New York City but lighter than those born in Nashville, Oakland, and Washington, D.C. The babies born in Washington, D.C., were the heaviest. There is no discussion of the economic conditions of the populations in those cities, the prenatal care available, or the health of the mothers and fathers, although the author does indicate that he did not obtain any information about smoking or alcohol consumption in the McNary population.

Wienker describes the town of McNary as a company lumbering town, in which virtually all families occupy decaying, company-provided wooden houses with wood stoves or gas or electric heaters; food is purchased at the company store and is supplemented by locally obtained game and fish; the community received free health care at the company-operated hospital until 1970, at which time health care was provided fifteen miles away. No description of that health facility is given. The author states that gross infant mortality was moderately lower in McNary than in the rest of the United States for African Americans and concludes from this that the African-American community maintains comparatively good health because of the easily accessible free health care. There is no discussion about the significance of his findings for the relevance of studying African Americans because they came from a section of Africa that was warm and of low elevation.

Hypertension among African Americans

Wilson, Thomas W., and Clarence E. Grim. 1991. Biohistory of slavery and blood pressure differences in Blacks today: A hypothesis. *Hypertension* 17 (supp. 1): 122–28.

This article presents a hypothesis that a gene for salt sensitivity can explain why American Blacks are more likely to have hypertension than African Blacks by invoking evolutionary theory. The authors propose that a "kidney defect" would cause less excretion of sodium and, therefore, that more sodium would be retained, leading to greater increase of blood volume and higher blood pressure. Further, they suggest that this defect is controlled by a particular gene and that this gene was selected for during the stressful conditions of transporting slaves from Africa to the Americas, where they lived under equally stressful conditions on plantations. They suggest that the major causes of death were salt-depletive diseases such as diarrhea, fevers, and vomiting. Those who had the "defective gene" for greater salt retention would survive to reproduce, while others would die. According to this theory, this gene would not be selected for in Africa, and, thus, this would explain the difference in the incidence of hypertension in American and African Blacks. This hypothesis has been challenged by other scientists in regard to the methods used in determining the relationship between salt sensitivity and hypertension and in regard to the ways in which genetic and evolutionary theories were applied.

The three articles that follow deal with the methods of studying salt sensitivity and hypertension. The first presents a group of studies of this relationship, and the two subsequent articles discuss and criticize the methods.

Luft, Friedrich C., Judy Z. Miller, Clarence E. Grim, Naomi S. Fineberg, Joe C. Christian, Sandra A. Daugherty, and Myron H. Weinberger. 1991. Salt sensitivity and resistance of blood pressure: Age and race as factors in physiological responses. *Hypertension* 17 (supp. 1): 102–8.

Four methods were used to study hypertension and salt sensitivity, as defined by an increase in blood pressure after ingesting high quantities of salt, in different populations, which varied according to age, race, sex, and zygosity (fraternal and identical twins). The same proportion of normotensive white and black women and men were salt sensitive. Hypertensive black men were more salt sensitive when compared with white men. The salt sensitive individuals in both black and white groups were older than those who were not salt sensitive. The zygosity of the twins, that is, whether they were fraternal or identical, was determined by similarities in blood characteristics. The authors then show that there was a correlation between degree of zygosity (being "identical") and salt sensitivity and hypertension. The demonstration of a correlation does not validate a causal relationship between similarity of genes for a blood characteristic (haptoglobin) and genes for salt sensitivity or hypertension.

Flack, John M., Kristine E. Ensrud, Stephen Mascioli, Cynthia A. Launer, Ken Svendsen, Patricia J. Elmer, and Richard H. Grimm, Jr. 1991. Racial and ethnic modifiers of the salt-blood pressure response. *Hypertension* 17 (supp. 1): 115–21.

These investigators make three principal criticisms: (1) skin color is an inaccurate criterion for establishing groups; (2) the method of determining blood pressure changes after ingesting sodium is inadequate; and (3) many other factors should be studied, such as stress, diet, and hormonal characteristics. They cite their study of third-grade children, in which they showed that under stress black children had higher cardiovascular activity than white children.

Grobbee, Diederick E. 1991. Methodology of sodium sensitivity assessment: The example of age and sex. *Hypertension* 17 (supp. 1): 109–14.

Grobbee points out that in studies of these phenomena there are usually insufficient controls, such as diet, physical activity, and social stress and that more studies of women are needed, especially since using oral contraceptives can produce a sodium sensitive effect on blood pressure. "A systematic approach to the assessment of factors and mechanisms responsible for sodium sensitivity in some subjects is needed to determine who might benefit most. Until more data are available there is little basis to discriminate sodium sensitive from sodium resistant hypertensive subjects. Tailoring of individual therapy and monitoring of the response remains a mainstay in the treatment of primary hypertension" (I-113).

Finally, the following article by Jackson gives a historical and theoretical overview of the problem.

Jackson, Fatimah Linda Colier. 1991. An evolutionary perspective on salt, hypertension, and human genetic variability. *Hypertension* 17 (supp. 1): 129–32.

In her review of the history of human salt intake Jackson points out that the modern U.S. diet is much higher in salt intake than was true during the early period of human evolution. She suggests that those individuals who do not develop hypertension on this high-salt diet "are more promising for study because they have a high probability of evidencing important and successful adaptations to the new selective pressure imposed by consistently elevated dietary salt intake" (131). She also discusses Wilson and Grim's hypothesis and suggests that the conditions of the Middle Passage and slavery led to great environmental stress and that this stress caused a number of genetic changes, such as modification of DNA bases, rate of genetic recombination, and presence of mobile genetic elements. "Stresses, including those characterizing middle passage clearly appear capable of producing at the molecular level a new spectrum of combination variation" (131). Finally, she emphasizes that survivors of the Middle Passage were exposed to a new environment and to opportunities for gene flow with Europeans and Amerindians. While Middle Passage effects are significant, it is difficult to believe that this particular forced migration led to selection of a gene for salt retention and that this is the complete answer to the present-day higher incidence of hypertension among American Blacks.

◆   VAL WOODWARD   ◆

Can We Draw Conclusions about Human Societal Behavior from Population Genetics?

The title question was put to me by the editors of the Genes and Gender series. Many geneticists may respond to the question with a tentative yes, but my answer is "Not yet and possibly never." I was asked to write this essay in an attempt to explain my answer.

A great deal has been written about the ideological similarities between communities of science and the larger societies within which these communities find a niche. It has been amply documented that the measures of sexism, racism, and nationalism found within the greater societies are reliable indices of their magnitude within the smaller science communities.[1]

Only one aspect of the many kinds of interaction between science and society is discussed here, namely, the influence exerted by science upon the characteristics of its parent society. Specifically, the science is genetics, and, more specifically, the discussion focuses on the gene—the gene as geneticists know it and as it has been modified to explain individual and societal behavior. To understand how genes are said to influence the greater society it is necessary to understand *the gene as metaphor,* an abstract gene with magical influences upon individual and human societal behavior. While a parent society may provide a niche within which metaphoric genes are comfortable— mainly by protecting them from criticism—the gene as metaphor

Terms that may be unfamiliar to readers are identified in a glossary at the end of this essay.

returns the favor by explaining the characteristics of the societal infra-structure that protects it.

The controlling class's response to metaphoric genes has been en-thusiastic; what better news could it want than that the downtrodden classes are but ordinary and natural adjuncts to the human condition, not the outcomes of societal inequities? As Darwin penned *The Origin of Species* (1859), Herbert Spencer penned and preached "social Dar-winism," the view that Britain's colonial peoples lacked the biological wherewithal (read intelligence) which the British ruling class was able and willing to provide. The U.S. ruling elite (Rockefeller, Carne-gie, Hill, and others) embraced Spencer "into its very bosom."[2]

The gene as metaphor has been called upon to explain nervous tics, criminality, shyness, international relations, war, differences in learning ability, and the emergence of social classes. From this it is not hard to imagine that the gene as metaphor has been invited into the theoretical constructs of economics, psychology, sociology, cul-tural anthropology, and even history. We may smile at the popularity and many uses of the metaphoric gene ("My genes made me do it"), but, as we smile, we should consider the possibility that its merger with comedy may divert our attention from its immense and growing explanatory power.

Kenneth Bock, in a response to sociobiology, said: "The human historical perspective is a fragile and perishable thing. It has been abandoned again and again in the search for immutable forces that lie behind the bewildering complexity of events that make up the lives of peoples. The attempt to locate such forces in genes is only the most recent among repeated circumventions of historical empiricism."[3]

While this essay is not about historical empiricism, it is about us-ing genes to circumvent it. Not the gene as we know it (Mendelian unit of inheritance and molecular unit of transcription) but, rather, the gene as metaphor—genes that have been empowered to transmit their messages beyond the cell and the individual to minds and from minds to human cultures.[4] The essay includes a discussion about some characteristics of the science of genetics which allow genes to be redesigned; genes as we know them are then compared with "genes" that have been modified to circumvent historical empiricism; finally, I will discuss whether real genes belong back in the organism and, if so, how they should be studied in that context.

WHITHER SCIENCE DURING A SCIENTIFIC REVOLUTION?

Scientific institutions are societal institutions. Science is a societal activity. Scientists and nonscientists share societal fears, ambitions, superstitions, and foibles. To remove science and scientists from this context is to invite idealist explanations of both.

"The history of science is dynastic," according to Horace Freeland Judson. Judson compares "the most interesting sciences of our day" with "early-modern European states" undergoing "turbulent overthrow of [their] ruling houses even while the possibilities and the problems, both domestic and foreign, confronting the rulers change only slowly: revolution takes place within a frame of comparatively unyielding continuity."[5]

Two "revolutions" in modern biology fit Judson's model; the first was the "takeover" of biochemistry by molecular biology, a coup that is key to Judson's model. Toward the end of that revolution Francis Crick proclaimed that "molecular biology is anything that interests molecular biologists,"[6] a definition that invites struggle for political leadership but fails to advance our understanding of molecular biology. (But remember, as Lewis Carroll put it in *The Hunting of the Snark*, "What I tell you three times is true.")

This is not to say that molecular biology was run amok by not having a definition; to the contrary, our collective understanding of genes grew rapidly during its reign. But it still is not obvious from its successes that the main questions of biochemistry required "turbulent" displacement by the questions of molecular biology. If biochemistry had been expanded and integrated into the molecular biological perspective rather than overthrown, would molecular biology's contributions have been compromised? Why the interesting questions of biochemistry were "tabled" for two decades requires a political, not a scientific, answer.

The second revolution is called "pop sociobiology" by Philip Kitcher.[7] One of the themes of this essay is that both revolutions, which include the *successes* of molecular biology and the *promises* of pop sociobiology, were initiated by desires to commandeer the gene.

Molecular biologists went after the gene to learn more about its character, and they did not step outside the paradigms of the physical sciences to make their discoveries. Pop sociobiologists went after the gene to modify its character and to extend its powers beyond cells and organisms, even beyond populations, into societal phenomena,[8] a leap that took them beyond the physical sciences to engulf all theretofore existing paradigms of social and societal behavior.

If Judson's model is sound, we can expect that science and discovery will proceed apace while scientists struggle within their fiefdoms for membership in new ruling elites. Science is the calm within the political storm. But Judson's model may not be sound. Indeed, the *scientific ideology that has been developed for understanding nature* could become distorted by battle so as to yield only heat, not light. Understanding could become secondary to the quest for social status. Pop sociobiologists appear to exert far more effort trying to commandeer the gene than they do trying to discover the *processes* of emergence and transformation of individuals, societies, and cultures.

In 1975 E.O. Wilson suggested using the word *sociobiology* as a symbol for a new dynasty promising to take over the study of the *evolutionary histories of all animal social behavior,* including human societal behavior.[9] This appeared then, as it does now, to be a more ambitious takeover than that of molecular biology. According to Arthur Fisher in "A New Synthesis Comes of Age," sociobiology has achieved its goal and with high marks.[10] Is Fisher correct?

A few differences between the two revolutions must be kept in mind if we are to answer this question. Molecular biology had its roots in structural chemistry, biochemical genetics, the "Phage school" of genetics, and in the study of gene regulation. The borders of molecular biology did not extend beyond physics, chemistry, and biology; molecular biology did not select from history's cache of unexamined, self-evident truths a few that would obviate the need for data and for a data-based theory.

The coup of pop sociobiology has a qualitatively different character. It alters the theory of the gene almost beyond recognition by twentieth-century geneticists; it thereby modifies the theory of evolution to accommodate the new powers of the gene, claiming that evolution theory explains the evolution of human cultures (market economy, religion, laws and law enforcement, racism, sexuality and social sex roles, nation-states, war and love of war, and, yes, the origins of fundamental philosophical foundations); in short it purports to explain *human nature.* The laws of evolution are credited with explaining human cultures as they are said to explain industrial melanism in moths.

Here's the catch. It turns out that the richness of cultural histories cannot be reduced sufficiently to match the gene's repertoire of tricks, that is, replication, regulation, and transcription. Therefore, it has become necessary for pop sociobiologists to endow genes with new powers in order for them to explain cultural evolution, and pop sociobiologists have done this prior to developing so much as an algorithm of cultural evolution.

To identify a beachhead on the Pangaean landscape staked out by pop sociobiologists, from which to explore the entire continental mass, is difficult. Only a few have attempted it,[11] but no one has succeeded in constructing a social theory that licenses the use of genes for its support.

CHARACTERISTICS OF GENETICS THAT INVITE A REDESIGN OF ITS GENES

Mathematicians chide physicists, physicists chide chemists, and chemists chide geneticists for being too descriptive, too historical, and not rational. Geneticists chide themselves for their physics envy. But the fact is that genetics is a historical science, not a rational one. Development is a feature of individual histories, evolution is a feature of species histories, and these histories are contingent processes (we cannot predict the next mutation, its fate, its phenotypic consequences, the climate to which it must adapt, etc.). Emergent processes include chance events. Brian Goodwin suggests that it will be a long time before biology becomes rational because "there can be no adequate evolutionary theory without a causal account of [biological] reproduction."[12]

The absence of causal accounts of ontogeny and phylogeny leave genes vulnerable to redesign, and in addition a few accidents of history have contributed. One of these accidents is the concept of dualism (mind and body) made popular by René Descartes.[13] Examples of dualisms that have become ingrained within genetics are somatoplasm and germ plasm, genotype and phenotype, organism and environment.

Descartes was an influential architect of modern science ideology. He described nature (including biological nature) in machine terms. Organisms are machines; limbs, organs, and tissues are machine parts. Human machines differ from other machines, however, in that they are endowed with creative faculties that cannot be reduced to mechanism. These creative faculties, he said, express themselves through language. Creative faculties within body machines make it necessary to ignore mind (known only to the creator) while studying the body. This style of dualism is alive and well today.

Years later August Weismann set out to determine whether acquired characters are inherited,[14] as had been claimed by Lamarck. Weismann discovered that cutting the tails off mice generation after generation did not dissuade later generations of mice from being born with tails. He concluded that acquired characteristics are not inherited. From this he developed the thesis that organisms are composed of immortal germ line cells and mortal somatic cells. Weismann's thesis later encouraged geneticists to study only the germ line cells and to ignore the study of ontogeny, the development of bodies that will die at the end of each generation. The germ line idea was so powerful that the early studies of genetics became partitioned from studies of development. Following suit, studies of population genetics became separated from studies of speciation. In other words, the gene was partially separated from two of the most significant processes in all of biology, development and evolution.

Geneticists have chided biologists who study biology for not getting to the heart of the matter, the chemical basis of life. Reverse charges take the form of chiding geneticists for ignoring the heart of the matter, the developmental processes, life cycles, and the integrative aspects of organisms and their environments. This chiding still goes on, even though geneticists are now moving rapidly into the uncharted domains of development, armed, of course, with the old ideology that development will fall into discrete and measurable steps, as did metabolism in the 1940s, after it has been sufficiently punctuated by gene mutations. The one gene: one enzyme slogan now reads, one gene:one developmental step.

It is easier for those who study germ line cells than it is for those who study life cycles to adopt Cartesian machine models of cells and organisms, especially since the germ cells are alleged to carry genetic blueprints for guiding the development of new machine bodies. But as those who have studied development and speciation have learned, the most interesting aspects of organisms are the ways in which they differ from machines.

After Mendelism came of age Weismann's ideology took on even greater meaning by providing "Mendel's genes" a home in germ line cells. Until the present time the ideological focus of genetics has been upon the gene. The organism has become the genes' way of making more genes, and it serves as a mirror reflecting exotic phenotypes said to testify to the exotic powers of the gene. That is, the processes of development and evolution are reduced somewhat to mechanical cascades triggered by genes.

Bodies as machines and minds as secrets of the gods—what better way could have been found to insure that science would continue to be nourished through its mythical roots? Many have argued that the theory of evolution is but a social construction, and who can deny the similarities between Darwin's explanation of speciation and nineteenth-century social Darwinism, colonialism, and economics? Who can deny the similarities between social Darwinism and pop sociobiology? With this history it should not surprise us to find genes made over to explain these embarrassments.

GENES AS WE KNOW THEM

Two very different methods have been used for "sighting" genes. Indeed, the methods have given rise to different names and different definitions of genes. The first method was discovered by Gregor Mendel. The genes discovered by Mendel's method are called Mendelian genes. Sometimes Mendelian genes are called units of inheritance in that they are "sighted" by inheritance patterns of contrasting phenotypic traits. In humans a phenotypic trait may be eye color and its contrasting forms blue and brown. Or ear lobes, a trait, may exist in two contrasting forms called "attached" and "unattached."

Mendelian genes are never observed directly. Each gene is postulated as the causative agent of a contrasting pair of phenotypic traits. The gene said to cause eye color exists in two forms, one form giving rise to brown and another form to blue color. The two forms of the eye color gene are sighted by observing the inheritance pattern of eye color; the gene is a postulate derived from the inheritance pattern.

The second method for sighting genes is chemical. The history of the discovery that genes are segments of DNA (deoxyribonucleic acid) molecules is a benchmark of twentieth-century science. The molecular gene is a unit of transcription, which is to say that the information contained within the chemical structure of the gene is transcribed, not onto a compact disc but, rather, onto another molecule similar to DNA, that is, RNA (ribonucleic acid). RNA is a transcript of a gene, and a gene is a "template" upon which transcription takes place; that is, a gene is a segment of DNA upon which a messenger RNA molecule (transcript) is synthesized.

RNA transcripts are translated (by enzymes) into amino acid sequences of proteins. DNA base pair sequences, then, specify the sequences of amino acids in proteins, significant in that all biological work is done by proteins. By the time a protein has assumed its working shape, however, it is impossible to trace either the shape of the molecule or what the molecule does backward to the information it received from a gene, as can be done from the sequence of its amino acids.

Even though it is impossible to trace the primary information of genes beyond the amino acid sequences of proteins, we know that genes influence some of the phenotypic variation observed within human populations. These genes can be identified, however, only if they exist in two or more allelic forms, only if the two allelic forms lead to contrasting forms of a phenotypic trait, and only if the inheritance patterns of the contrasting traits obey Mendel's law of inheritance.

Today enough is known about molecular genes to make accurate associations between them and Mendelian genes. We also know the relationships between the contrasting proteins encoded by contrasting alleles and contrasting metabolic, physiological, or morphological phenotypic traits. That is, the two definitions of a gene have melded into one. In the language of genetics, a pair of alleles includes one said to be normal and one said to be mutant; normal alleles encode normal proteins, and mutant alleles encode mutant proteins. Mutant alleles arise as mutations of normal alleles.

While a great deal is known about genes and gene expression, less is known about development. In some cases the "tremors" initiated by a mutation will be felt throughout development—for example, the mutation that leads to phenylketonuria (PKU). Metabolism, physiology, morphology, and behavior are altered as a consequence of inheriting two copies of the mutant allele (such an individual is homozygous). Indeed, the argument has been made that, since mutant genes do in fact alter behavior, genes must encode behavior. This is a specious argument; in this case the normal allele of the mutation that leads to PKU does not encode normal behavior but, rather, the amino acid sequence of normal phenylalanine hydroxylase, the enzyme that catalyzes the transformation of phenylalanine into tyrosine. In the presence of the mutant allele, which misspells the amino acid sequence of the enzyme, thereby leading to its misfunction, phenylalanine accumulates in the blood. From the blood it is distributed throughout the body. In some tissues it inhibits the actions of at least a few enzymes. It appears that one or several enzymes of the central nervous system are inhibited by phenylalanine (hence, mental retardation for untreated PKU children), which is to say that the metabolic consequences of the mutant allele are to inhibit normal brain development, which in turn leads to mutant behavior. The normal allele, however, does not encode normal behavior, only the amino acid sequence of a protein.

Both methods for sighting genes have yielded reliable results. But the Mendelian method is sometimes abused. Recall that much of the phenotypic variation observed within populations is influenced by environmental factors; therefore, the observation of contrasting phenotypes is not prima facie evidence for the existence of contrasting alleles.

GENES THAT HAVE ENRICHED EVOLUTION THEORY

There exist hierarchies of biological complexity—this is not disputed. Macromolecules are structurally and functionally simpler than genes, genes are simpler than chromosomes, organelles are simpler than cells, and so on through organisms, kinships, breeding populations, species, higher taxa, and ecosystems. Interrelationships among hierarchies are disputed, however, as are their historical antecedents.

Evolution theory signifies an attempt to unify our knowledge about phylogenetic histories insofar as histories reveal relationships among hierarchies; population genetics has provided important insights into these attempts, in particular at the hierarchical level of breeding populations within species. This last statement is based upon what geneticists refer to as the distilled essence of Darwin's theory; namely, there is variation within populations, some of the variation is hereditary, and some of the variant types are more reproductively successful than others. Thus, the three principles of Darwin's theory are variation, heredity, and selection.

Population genetics is to a large extent the study of genetic variation, the fraction of the population's phenotypic variance which can be attributed to genetic variance (the phenotypic variation caused by genetic differences among the individuals within the population). Population geneticists have developed methods for distinguishing between variation caused by genetic differences and variation caused by environmental and experiential differences among individuals, and they have amplified Darwin's intuitive feelings about heredity by providing ample evidence that, for populations to change through the generations, the frequencies of the genes that contribute to population variance must change.

Darwin proposed that natural selection is the driving force of evolution. In simple terms natural selection results in differential reproductive success; some parental types leave more offspring than others. Since Darwin it has been observed that natural selection is not the only force that contributes to allele frequency changes within population gene pools through time. In fact, the role of natural selection in evolution is hotly debated. In addition to the forces of natural selection, allele frequencies change as a result of migration (individuals enter and leave populations, sometimes in large numbers); allele frequencies change as a result of chance, as in the packaging of alleles into gametes, as in the chance meeting of gametes at the time of fertilization, and as in the chance occurrence of new mutations.

One of the tasks of the population geneticist is to identify the forces that give rise to allele frequency changes and to estimate the relative importance of each force. These estimates are then integrated into the phylogenetic history of the relevant population. A temptation usually avoided by geneticists, but not by pop sociobiologists, is to guess the circumstances surrounding the adaptation of particular genes during the early history of a population. If one believes that natural selection is the main determinant of gene pool changes, one will be tempted to guess what the selective advantages of the contemporary phenotypes were. (One example used by many pop sociobiologists has to do with the evolutionary histories of coy female and macho male behavior. It has been suggested that women are coy because they produce only a few, and therefore precious, eggs and that they prefer not to waste any of them on the sperm of inferior males. On the other hand males have sperm to spare and are willing [anxious?] to have them fertilize any egg in the neighborhood.)[15]

The contributions made by population genetics to evolution theory have enhanced the explanatory capacity of the theory to explain conservative events that lead to gradual changes within gene pools, but there is controversy about whether population genetics has helped the theory to explain gregarious (punctuated) events and divergence as great as that between the higher taxa.

Of Darwin's three principles variation is the easiest to verify with an untrained eye. Every large population consists of individuals that differ from one another by physiology, morphology, and behavior. It is the sum of these differences that make up a population's phenotypic variation.

Heredity, the second principle, became the focal point of genetics in the 1920s. The expected relationship between heredity and evolution is simple in that, for evolution to occur, some of the phenotypic variation must be heritable. We know that this is so; genes influence phenotypic variation, and genes are transferred from parents to offspring.

The third principle appears self-evident but, in fact, turns out to be even more problematic. We take it as a given that some variant types are more reproductively successful than others and that, as a result, members of modern generations must look like the successful survivors of prior generations. Yet there are not many solid examples that show clearly that natural selection is responsible for a population's genetic composition and phenotypic appearance (it can be demonstrated that targeted gene pools can be engineered by artificial selection regimens [domestic plants and animals], but in natural populations the relationships between genotypes and the environments within which genotypes "struggle for survival" are not well understood).

The role played by natural selection in determining which among competing genotypes will survive is problematic, in part because geneticists do not yet know what it is that natural selection "sees"; the units of selection haven't been identified to everyone's satisfaction. A few biologists have begun to question whether the idea of natural selection is retained merely as an accommodation to Darwin's theory and to Weismann's germplasm-somatoplasm dualism. For example, Goodwin rather minimizes the role of natural selection, saying, "Thus the organism is effectively a transparent shop window with genetic goods displayed directly to the naturally selective shopper, who chooses appropriate articles ('characters') and thus effectively creates the specific packages of goods we call the members of a species."[16] While Goodwin's is an extreme view, he is not the only one to draw attention to the weaknesses of Darwin's main thesis. True, Darwin developed the theory of evolution without knowledge of genes. His understanding of heredity was nil; his major contribution was that natural selection is the driving force behind the elimination and preservation of heritable differences among individuals within species. This idea is being contested today.

The fact that evolution has happened and is happening is not in question; this fact has gotten support from geology, anthropology, paleontology, chemistry, and physics. But the kinds of support provided by these disciplines does not shed light on the role of natural selection during the course of evolution. During the 1920s and early 1930s, however, population genetics, developed by R. A. Fisher, J. B. S. Haldane, and S. Wright,[17] became the most popular explanation of all three of Darwin's principles, including selection. Population genetics gave Darwin's theory a boost and a new name, the neo-Darwinian synthesis.

The contributions made by population genetics to evolution theory gave the Mendelian gene a bigger role in biology, but this bigger role *did not change the character of the gene.* The Mendelian gene's sphere of influence was extended from "inheritance patterns within families" to a place within population gene pools. Genes within gene pools whose frequencies change through time added "muscle" to the abstract "bones" of evolution theory.

Darwin's descriptions of natural selection seemed to caricature its forces as "acts of aggression" upon individuals and species. Darwin divided the whole of nature into niches, each with its own cadre of "aggressors," and within each niche some variants were reproductively successful, and others were not. The reproductively successful variants were called fit, and the unsuccessful ones were called unfit. Early on population geneticists described their task as the study of the genetic bases of fitness; today many of them, having debunked Darwin's metaphor of nature, describe their task as the study of the "interdependence of genotypes and environments."

Thus, while Mendelian and population geneticists define genes the same way, they often describe the gene's role within biological systems differently. For example, the tradition within Mendelian genetics has been to describe "genes *for* this or that trait," a phrase that suggests that traits are "typed" out during development in the mechanical way that letters are typed out during the development of an essay. But population geneticists who seek evidence of the interdependence of genes and their environments are more likely to regard genes as elements within larger systems which influence and are influenced by other elements within those systems. This view is more in tune with the concept of processes during which things (genes, organisms, species) are becoming what they are not and are ceasing to be what they are.

The tradition of viewing genotype-phenotype relationships as simple cause-effect phenomena has been easier for population geneticists than for Mendelian geneticists to debunk, for yet another reason. Population geneticists study a type of variation which cannot be analyzed by Mendelian methodology, namely continuous variation. Many important aspects of phenotype vary continuously within populations, for example, height, weight, rates of growth, reproductive potential, body shape, and running speed. Unlike blood proteins, which can be defined by universally agreed-upon criteria, continuous variation cannot be specified except in terms of *ranges* and *frequency distributions.*

Since many economically important phenotypes of domestic plants and animals vary continuously, geneticists have striven to develop methods for assaying correlations between these kinds of phenotypes and genotypes. With designed programs of artificial selection the frequency distributions and ranges of continuously varying phenotypes can be altered, and the extent to which they can be altered is a measure of the genetic component of phenotypic variation, called heritability. Heritability never accounts for all of the phenotypic variation of any continuously varying phenotype, which is to say that complexes of genetic and nongenetic inputs must combine throughout development to influence such phenotypes.

There is no reason to believe that genes identified as "genetic components of population variance" are different from classical genes, even though the methods of quantitative genetics are of little value to the study of classical genes. What is at issue are the roles played by such genes during the emergence of continuously varying phenotypes.

HOW HAVE GENES BEEN MODIFIED, AND BY WHOM?

The core of the history of molecular biology appears in the form of a "mad pursuit" to discover the structure of the gene.[18] A Mendelian concept of the gene existed prior to molecular biology, and molecular biologists were conscious of the fact that the unknown structural properties of the gene would be called upon to explain its Mendelian properties. The triumph was a good correspondence between the Mendelian and the chemical gene; the explanatory power of the gene theory was expanded many times over.

Pop sociobiologists have treated the gene differently. The theory of the gene has not been enlightened by sociobiology. To the contrary, the suppositions and hypotheses of pop sociobiology have had the effect of transmogrifying the gene. The gene's structural and functional properties were treated as abstractions, as it was being endowed with powers to encode gene > brain > societal behavior circuitry.[19]

To understand the kinds of genes needed by pop sociobiological theory it is informative to examine the tasks genes have been asked to perform. A few quotes will set the stage: In *The Extended Phenotype* Dawkins says: "Having devoted most of this book to playing down the importance of the individual organism, and to building up an alternative image of a turmoil of selfish replicators, battling for their own survival at the expense of their alleles, reaching unimpeded through individual body walls as though those walls were transparent, interacting with the world and with each other without regard to organismal boundaries, we now hesitate. There really is something pretty impressive about individual organisms." The organism, however, "is a physically discrete machine, usually walled off from other such machines." And, he says: "The many-celled body is a machine for the production of single celled propagules. Large bodies, like elephants, are best seen as heavy plant and machinery, a temporary resource drain, invested in so as to improve later propagule production [attributed to another author]." "The importance of the difference between growth and reproduction is that each act of reproduction involves a new developmental cycle. Growth simply involves swelling of the existing body."[20] This book and Dawkins's more recent *Blind Watchmaker* (1986) are rather fun mind games but, unfortunately, mind games billed as substitutes for reality. Indeed, Dawkins's elephants, eels, and egrets—even the earth upon which these "pretty impressive" organisms live—are caricatures. (At one large university library I was somewhat surprised and greatly amused to find Aldous Huxley's *Ape and Essence* cataloged under zoology; it would surprise and amuse me less to find Dawkins's *The Blind Watchmaker* cataloged under modern mythology.)

In a slightly different context James L. Gould and Carol Grant Gould (in *Sexual Selection*) express similar ideas: "Relationships in most of the animal world begin to look as if they have been designed by a hardworking team of bankers, economists, real estate speculators, and advertising executives. Is our own species any different when it comes to courtship and bonding? Does our remarkable capacity for culture and language allow us to override nature, to become a special creature of our own making, or does our limitless capacity for guile and deceit simply make it possible for us to explore the full depths of our innate tendencies unperceived?" "In fact," they add,

> much of our thinking about the role of sexual selection in shaping modern human behavior is paralyzed by the difficulty of separating the effects of nature and nurture. But if the sexual differences in brain organization are really programmed in by nature, what will the evolutionary logic turn out to have been? What aspects of the hunting our male ancestors must have perfected would select for a more dichotomous brain, in which spatial and analytic functions are kept separate? What requirements of the gathering our female forebearers practiced might favor a more integrated mind? These [are] questions, for which many inventive solutions have been proposed.[21]

These views debiologize organisms to present them as Cartesian machines. Either bodies coexist with but are not integrated with minds, or minds become machine parts. Bodies are partitioned into genetic and somatic components, the former being a conduit to immortality, while the latter, after propagating its propagules, dies. Bodies are simply vehicles sculpted by replicators to insure the survival of replicators. The replicators get on well together (primitive altruism), and cultures develop against a tide of natural (devious) tendencies.

With this scheme the social status quo is the natural order. To break with the societal traditions set in motion by genes (e.g., racism, sexism, and nationalism) is to risk defeat by nations/states that take their genes more seriously. Indeed, if we take the Goulds seriously, biological research ought to be turned over to the Hoover Institute and the Heritage Foundation.

This metaphoric approach to genetic determinism is further compounded by equating patterns of organismal and societal behaviors with discrete "traits," analogous to the metabolic, physiological, and morphological traits studied by geneticists. Patterns of behaviors are then broken into apparently measurable bits, after which a gene is invoked to explain each bit as if it were an authentic Mendelian trait. These contrasting bits of behavior, then, become prima facie evidence for genes.

Evolutionary histories of authentic genes are not easy to come by. We simply do not know the cicumstances of the coming into being and survival of contemporary genes (units of inheritance and transcription). But there are a few genes whose histories appear explicable. For example, the Duffy negative allele (which provides resistance to vivax malaria by failing to encode the protein component of an antigen found on normal red blood cells through which the malarial parasite gains entrance into those cells) appears in gene pools of populations that have lived for centuries in tropical (malaria-infested) regions of Africa. We simply do not have the necessary historical evidence to provide analogous explanations of "phenotypes" such as shyness, altriusm, attitudes toward incest, and religious preferences.

UNITS OF SELECTION REVISITED

Going beyond guessing-game relationships between genes and phenotypes, pop sociobiologists have tinkered with the gene in another significant way. Out of Darwin's emphasis upon natural selection as the driving force of evolution a great deal of concern has been given to identifying what it is that the forces of natural selection actually see.

We return to the question "What are the units of selection?" An interesting treatment of this problem is outlined by Leo Buss. Buss argues that the phylogenetic history of contemporary biological hierarchies is a history of transitions from simple to complex units of selection. "From cell to individual is one such transition." Preceding this transition, "there must have been the origin of self-replicating molecules, the association of autonomously replicating molecules into self-replicating complexes," and so on.[22]

In contrast to this view, George C. Williams (in 1966) introduced the idea that the gene is the unit of selection.[23] Since one of Williams's aims was to put down the idea that groups (of individuals) are units of selection, many evolutionists misread him to say that individuals are the units of selection. Ten years later Richard Dawkins popularized Williams's gene selection idea.[24] The antagonist of Dawkins's gene selection thesis is the individual organism.

Dawkins argues that there are no other units of selection, neither cells nor individuals. All higher units, he says, are vectors programmed by genes to transport them into the next gene pool. Dawkins personifies genes by attributing to them a totally selfish character, with the convenient corollary that it is not necessary to ask how their vectors develop.

Dawkins begins his discussion of genes by referring to them as units of inheritance, but he drops this definition to define genes as replicators ("The replicators that exist tend to be the ones that are good at manipulating the world to their own advantage . . . an important aspect of the environment of a replicator is other replicators and their phenotypic manifestations. . . . The world therefore tends to become populated by mutually compatible sets of successful replicators."[25]

While Buss suggests that an early unit of selection might have been a self-replicating molecule, he does not say that this molecule was a gene. It could have been two or more genes. Complexes of self-replicating molecules could have been precursors to chromosomes. At any rate such a complex will include more than one unit of inheritance while itself serving as a unit of selection.

Richard Lewontin suggests that any unit of biological organization, regardless of complexity, is a potential unit of selection if it is propelled through time by the principles of Darwin, that is, if it replicates, if it generates genetic variation, and if the variants are differentially successful at reproducing themselves.[26]

By redefining genes as replicators, it is impossible to explain how lethal, recessive genes remain invisible to natural selection when they exist in the heterozygous state and how neutral mutations enter and leave gene pools other than by chance.

While I agree with Buss that differences between gene and hierarchical selectionists are in part semantic, semantics is not the only issue. Gene selectionism is in direct opposition to the view expressed by Lewontin that any unit of biological organization is a potential unit of selection. If Lewontin is correct, then all units of selection will consist of more than one unit of inheritance. And if this is so, units of inheritance within units of selection must have a synergistic relationship to the whole—such that changes within units of inheritance will tend to be conservative while the units of selection must remain flexible and interact directly with their environments. Changes in the character of units of selection, then, will be tempered by requirements imposed by survival. The metaphoric replicators of Dawkins are assigned both roles, units of inheritance and units of selection.

ON RETURNING GENES TO THE ORGANISM

Simplistic cause-effect progression from gene to protein to a cascade of actions that culminate in altered phenotypes is an insufficient explanation of ontogeny. Even if the tremors of a mutant gene reach all the way from altered mRNA (messenger RNA) to an altered behavior, the tremors still do not tell us *how normal behavior develops.*

As Goodwin puts it:

> If we could read [the] instructions in the DNA we [should] know how organisms are made. But we know enough about these instructions now. . . . There is an enormous gap in our understanding between these and organisms. This gap tends to be papered over by descriptive devices and metaphors such as referring to the instructions in the DNA as a "genetic program" for generating an organism. Covering our ignorance in this way involves smuggling in some kind of undefined organizing principle that puts all the molecules together in the right order to make an organism.[27]

He then shows the "family history" of this modern "organizing principle" all the way back to body and soul.

An attack upon the mythology of dualisms in biology does not require throwing out the baby with the bathwater. No one is suggesting a ban on DNA just because enthusiasts claim to have sighted "blueprints" therein for making adult organisms. Knowledge of base pair sequences within the human genome will not tell us how human zygotes develop into mothers and fathers, secretaries and scientists, plumbers and presidents. Base pair sequences of DNA tell us only about the amino acid sequences of proteins (so far DNA sequence data do not even reveal how proteins fold into their tertiary [working] structures or how they do their biological work after assuming their tertiary structures).

In other words, we still do not understand ontogeny and phylogeny. Perhaps in order to learn more about these processes it will become necessary to integrate genes back into the larger biological systems from which dualism separated them. Goodwin suggests that "it is not specific molecular composition that is the determinant of form, either in inanimate matter or in organisms . . . The same form can arise out of different molecules, while different forms can be made out of the same molecules. . . . [T]he challenge of development is to understand the dynamic principles of organismic tranformation that underlie the processes of evolution."[28]

Population genetics grew up in the chuch of dualisms but switched from water to wine for the sacrament. Germ line cells, genes, and DNA sequences retain primary status over the soma, but for a peculiar twist; neo-Darwinists posited individuals as units of selection. The somas of individuals are examined for rejection or approval by forces external to them; genes tag along. The question of how survivable somas develop, then, becomes necessary to the understanding of evolution.

But this was not the main concern of population genetics and neo-Darwinism; the main concern was to develop a means for measuring variability and gene flux within gene pools. Indeed, population geneticists tend to explain evolutionary change in terms of the ebb and flow of allele frequencies within and between gene pools. This is where the problem rests in much of population genetics today. (More and more genes are available for study, however, as are more and more primary structures of genes and proteins; this information has greatly expanded our knowledge of genetic variation within populations.)

Fluxes of allele frequencies within and between gene pools do not tell us how species arise. Speciation has been modeled (e.g., Darwin suggested that within-species populations [breeding populations] must be separated by geographical isolating events and remain separated until such time that they become reproductively isolated, at which time they will have become two new species), but the models have little or no predictive value; that is, from them, or from knowledge of gene pools of related but geographically isolated populations, it is impossible to predict what it will take for the two populations to become two new species. Even the biology of reproductive isolation is unknown—how many mutations and how much biological difference is necessary for speciation?

From our ignorance of the processes of speciation it should be obvious that population genetics sheds little light upon the evolutionary histories of higher taxa, except through extrapolation from speciation models. What is needed is a more complete understanding of dynamic transformations whose forces of motion include the "friction" generated by emergent internal tendencies of cells and organisms struggling against the limits imposed upon them by the external forces about them and, of course, how the whole changes through time in response to these struggles.

REDUCTIONISM IS NECESSARY, BUT IS IT SUFFICIENT?

As zygotes begin their emergence into adults, they initiate transformations among the external forces about them, and these return the favor by initiating changes within the zygote embryos. Organisms and their environments become elements within larger systems, systems within which all of the elements act and are acted upon and are thereby changed. While dynamic systems may be informed by transcripts, they are not specified by them: transcripts act and are acted upon.

As has been stated, tremors of some mutations may reverberate throughout the development of an organism. The recessive PKU allele and the dominant mutation leading to achondroplasia (short stature resulting from short long bones in the legs) illustrate the point. *But what about tremors initiated by nongenetic stimulants?*

Observations of norms of reaction leave us with the inescapable conclusion that a single genotype may initiate a wide range of phenotypes—if development occurs in a wide range of different environments. For example, cuttings of a single plant of milfoil, *Achillea millefolium,* grown at different altitudes (but in similar soil, watering, etc.) may exhibit very different growth and flowering patterns—same genotype but very different phenotypes. (See Jerry Hirsch et al., for a detailed discussion of norms of reaction.)[29] The full range of phenotypes which can be expressed by a single genotype over wide ranges of environment is that genotype's norm of reaction (fig. 1).

Norms of reaction give lie to the idea that organisms are formed by their genotypes alone. As Mae-Wan Ho puts it: "An organism is not uniquely defined unless its environment is specified. The environment exerts necessary formative influences on development." Then, bringing development into the picture of evolution: "As evolution is in essence a series of organized changes in development, it follows that development contains the potential for evolution."[30]

Studies of environmentally induced phenotypic changes that mimic mutation-induced phenotypes (called phenocopies) have been studied for years in the laboratory of Mae-Wan Ho. The exposure of wild type *Drosophila melanogaster* to ether, for example, will bring about the development of an ensemble of phenocopies that look almost exactly like mutant phenotypes.

While it would be fruitless to try to match every mutation-induced phenotype with an environmentally induced phenocopy, it is even more absurd to continue to believe in Weismann's "barrier" (information flows from germ plasm to somatoplasm but not in the reverse direction), the idea that only germ line cells and their contents participate in evolution, and that the development of adult bodies from zygotes is of no consequence to evolution (fig. 2). The issue of Lamarck versus Weismann is dead; we have learned a great deal during the century which separates that battle from us. But the ideology lingers. As mentioned earlier, geneticists are jumping into the arena of development but with the idea that development, like a metabolic

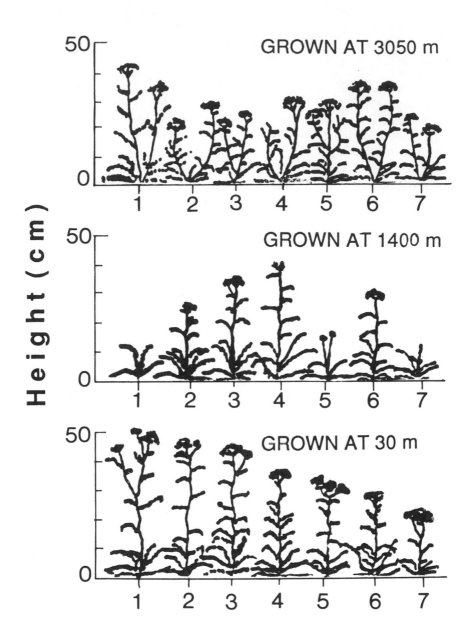

Fig. 1. On Estimating Norms of Reaction. Seven genetically different plants were cloned, and a member of each clone was grown at three different altitudes, as shown. Plant 1 grew tall and flowered at the low elevation, grew short and did not flower at the intermediate elevation, and grew tall and flowered at the high elevation—different phenotypic expressions of one genotype. This figure shows three phenotypes of seven genotypes in three environments.

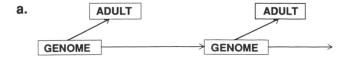

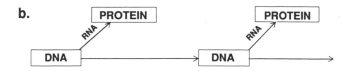

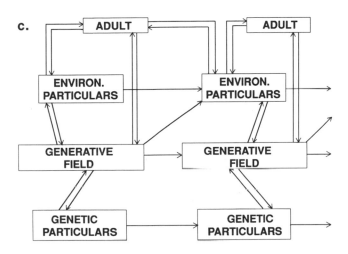

Fig. 2. Different Ways of Viewing Relationships between Genes and Phenotypes. (a) The Weismann barrier idea that information flows from genomes to
bodies but never from bodies to genomes. Continuity between generations is
achieved by information flow from one genome to another. (b) The formaliza-
tion of Weismann's barrier by way of molecular genetics. Information flows
from DNA to RNA to protein and never in the reverse direction. Continuity
between generations is achieved by information flow from DNA to DNA via
DNA replication (DNA synthesis). (c) A schematic illustration of relationships
among genomes, adult bodies, environments, and continuity from one generation to the next. In this scheme environmental and genetic particulars feed
back and forth with generative fields that symbolize the many inputs and
their interactions that provide generation continuity. Both environmental particulars and genetic particulars, however, are transferred from one generation
to the next. You will realize the need for many more arrows linking these
boxes if you extrapolate from the formula, $(pq)!/(p!)(q!)$ = number of interactions, where p = number of genotypes and q = number of environments.

pathway, can be unpacked by highlighting its stages with mutant genes.

It is difficult to follow the information carried by DNA base-pair sequences beyond the point of amino acid sequences of proteins; how much more difficult will it be to follow the path between base-pair sequences and development, behavior, and in particular societal behavior? Will we learn from genes how children learn mathematics in school? or how the use of fire for cooking and of flowers for burial become societal activities? What is the best explanation for a nine-year-old performing a 360-degree slam dunk? We needn't exhume Lamarck for the answers, but at the same time we can't rely on Weismann or Mendel. What we can say is that the information needed for these behaviors is not to be found in DNA base-pair sequences (see fig. 2).

There are those who analogize ideas with genes by ascribing to the sum of ideas the Darwinian principles of variation, heredity, and selection.[31] This argument in fact reduces ideas to the level of molecules through the belief that ideas, like inborn errors of metabolism, are by-products of incorrigibly selfish genes.

Population genetics cannot transfer its expertise with Darwin's principles of variation, heredity, and selection to the evolutionary histories of ideas. This, no doubt, is because (1) the genetic component of idea variation cannot be estimated and is probably zero; (2) the inheritance of ideas is Lamarckian; and (3) the forces of selection acting upon ideas arise mainly from economic necessity and political power. If these conclusions are wrong, there will be pop geneticists in the wings willing and ready to construct demographic maps of mutant ideas and a classification scheme that will tell us whether the mutants are good, neutral, and deleterious.

Extensions of the logic that allows one to identify genes through observations of contrasting phenotypic traits also allows one to analogize human societal histories with the histories of hemoglobin chains, fibrin proteins, radial symmetry, and insect societies. These analogies transcend a data base, which is to say that the paradigm within which explanations of societal histories are formulated does not overlap with the paradigm of population genetics. This fact has long since been clear to most population geneticists. If overlapping, interactive, and integrative boundaries do exist between population genetics and culture they have yet to be discovered (except to assert that the evolution of human societal behavior was postponed until after the evolution of the biological capability of developing culture).

But the lust for an explanation of societal histories is powerful, and what could be a speedier way to find one than to extend gene tremors beyond RNA to individual and societal behavior? This extension may not look like cheating if the explanatory power of population genetics is quietly grafted onto the existing paradigms of historical empiricism, anthropology, sociology, and psychology. It doesn't require the genius of Miss Marple, however, to discover the mischief that reductionism has wrecked upon genes and the theory of evolution.

GLOSSARY

Amino acids

Small building block molecules of proteins. Each is both an acid and a base, the acid being a carboxyl (COOH) and the base being an amino (NH₂) group. All proteins are digested into amino acids, and all proteins have specific sequences of amino acid residues encoded into their primary structures.

Breeding population (BP)

Within-species population so defined because its members are more likely to find breeding partners within the population than from different populations. BPs are not closed to other populations, but they are considered to be the "units of evolution" in that their gene pools can change independently of other gene pools within the species.

Continuous variation

Sometimes called *quantitative variation.* Whereas variation among earlobe types, whether attached or unattached, is discontinuous, variation in height from the shortest to the tallest is continuous.

Enzymes

All enzymes are proteins, and all are biological catalysts. A catalyst is anything that speeds up one or more chemical reactions but is not changed by the reaction. Enzymes are encoded by genes, each by a different gene, and each speeds up a unique biochemical reaction.

Fit	Name used by Darwin to describe individuals, couples, kinships, and larger groups that are reproductively successful.
Gene	A Mendelian gene is defined as a unit of inheritance, which means that it is recognized only if contrasting phenotypic traits show specific patterns of inheritance within family lines. A molecular gene is a segment of DNA which transcribes its information into RNA transcripts, which in turn translate the information into amino acid sequences of proteins.
Gene pools	The sum of genes carried within the genomes of all individuals within a species or breeding population with the potential of being included within the next gene pool.
Gene regulation	Most genes are inactive most of the time, but within specific tissue cells specific genes are active some of the time. Gene regulation describes the events and processes that determine how and when genes are "turned off and on" during cell and organism life cycles.
Germ line cells	Cells that give rise to sex cells (eggs and sperm). Germ line cells carry the chromosomes and genes that will become included within sex cells, and hence the next gene pool. Specifically, primary oocytes and primary spermatocytes.
Heritability	The proportion of the total population variance (phenotypic) that can be attributed to genetic variance (genetic differences among the individuals within the population). While fairly accurate estimates of heritability have been made of variance within farm plant and animal species, it is impossible to make meaningful estimates of heritability of continuous phenotypic variation in our own species.

Heterozygous

Mendelian genes are recognized only if they exist in two or more forms, usually called mutant and normal forms of a gene. If *A* symbolizes the normal form and *a* the mutant form, then individuals with two *A*s, AA, and two *a* forms, aa, are homozygous (same allele), while persons with one of each form, Aa, are heterozygous.

Homozygous

See heterozygous. Individuals who carry identical forms of the same gene (e.g., AA and aa).

Industrial melanism

In England it is said that the light-colored pepper moth adapted to the increasing dark coloration inflicted by coal soot by changing its own color, from light to dark. Since the dark pigment is melanin and since the change took place during the industrial revolution, the name industrial melanism was used to describe the adaptation. The color change is ascribed to a mutant gene that led to the synthesis of more melanin, a classic example of Darwinian evolution—if the story is true.

Kinship

A family. Biologically related individuals, kin. A kinship may be as small as one family or as large as an extended family of many small families.

Metabolism

The sum of chemical reactions taking place within cells and organisms. Usually, metabolism is divided into anabolism, synthetic chemical reactions, and catabolism, degradative (digestion) reactions.

Morphology

The study or science of general body form; the forms and structures of cells, tissues, organs, and organisms.

Mutant

A gene, cell, or organism carrying a gene that is different from the original (normal) gene.

Mutation	The process of a gene changing from one type (normal) to another type (mutant). Sometimes a mutant gene is referred to as a mutation.
Neutral mutation	A mutant gene that does not alter the phenotype of the cell or organism within which it resides such that the "forces of natural selection" can recognize the difference between mutant and normal. The word *neutral* means with respect to natural selection.
Norm of reaction	The range of phenotypic variation exhibited by a population of genetically identical individuals that have lived in a wide range of environments. The range of phenotypes than can be expressed by one genotype.
Ontogeny	The development of an organism from zygote until death.
Organelle	Structures within cell cytoplasms with specific functions, for example, mitochrondria, chloroplasts, and nuclei.
Phage school	Phage (short for *bacteriophage*) is the name given to viruses that infect bacteria; the phage school of geneticists is the name given to a group of geneticists, many of whom were physicists who stressed the need to work with the simplest biological systems (viruses) in order to discover the "fundamental particles of biology" (genes).
Phenotype	The observable properties of an organism, such as size, shape, color, or composition.
Phenylalanine	One of the twenty naturally occurring amino acids, the building blocks of proteins.

Phenylketonuria	A genetic disease characterized by the inability to transform phenylalanine into tyrosine. The mutant gene misprograms the enzyme that catalyzes the reaction; thus, phenylalanine accumulates in the blood and urine and subsequently inhibits the activity of other enzymes, some of which may be essential to mental health.
Phylogeny	The complete developmental history of a population (e.g., species, order, or phylum).
Physiology	The study of the basic processes underlying the functions necessary to maintain the health of a species—specifically, the study of organ functions or of hormonal functions, etc.
Population genetics	The study of genes within populations—in particular, the study of genetic changes within populations, the forces that induce these changes, and the roles of these forces in the evolution of species.
Proteins	Polymers, or long chains, of amino acids. Proteins do biological work, whether catalysis (enzymes) or force and displacement (muscle).
Replication	A chromosome, gene, or molecule of DNA is said to replicate when a new copy of itself is synthesized upon an old copy (i.e., upon the original template).
Social Darwinism	The nineteenth-century view espoused by Herbert Spencer that social organization and societal hierarchies are biological in origin: in particular, British Society is superior to all others in that the British ruling class is superior to all other ruling classes.
Sociobiology	The study of the biological bases of all social behavior in all animal species.
Somatic cells	Soma means "body"; somatic cells are body cells.

Species
Populations of like but not identical organisms which are reproductively isolated from members of all other species.

Structural chemistry
The study of the structures of molecules. The structural chemists who helped usher in molecular genetics studied the structures of large polymers (e.g., DNA, RNA, and protein), mainly by means of X-ray crystallography.

Taxa
Taxonomy began as an attempt to classify all plants, animals, and microorganisms into hierarchies; the hierarchies are taxa (sing. *taxon*). For example, all animals were fitted into the animal kingdom, the highest taxon. These were divided into phyla, the next largest taxa, and so on down to species, of which there are estimated to be more than two million on the earth today.

Transcription
The sum of chemical steps by which information carried by the base pair sequences of DNA (the DNA constituting one gene) are transferred to RNA—specifically, the synthesis of RNA molecules on DNA templates.

Translation
The sum of chemical steps by which the genetic information encoded within mesenger RNA molecules is transferred to protein molecules—specifically, the translation of the language of nucleic acids into the language of proteins.

Tyrosine
One of the twenty naturally occurring amino acids.

Unfit
In Darwinian terms individuals and couples who are unable to reproduce or who are at least somewhat reproductively unsuccessful.

Unit of inheritance

A Mendelian gene. Actually, Mendel never observed a unit of inheritance but inferred it from the inheritance patterns of contrasting phenotypic traits in peas. If the inheritance pattern obeyed the laws of chance, he postulated that one gene initiates the trait and that a different form of the gene initiates each of the forms of the trait.

Units of selection

If natural selection is responsible for reproductive success, or failure, then natural selection must recognize some aspect of an organism, group of organisms, or species. What is it that natural selection "sees"? The gene? Blocks of genes? Cells? Organisms? Families? Species? The actual units of selection have not been identified, and there are some biologists who disclaim the entire notion of natural selection. In science, as in life, there is an inverse correlation between sound knowledge and loud noise.

NOTES

1. R. C. Lewontin, S. P. Rose, and L. J. Kamin, *Not in Our Genes* (New York: Pantheon, 1984).

2. R. Hofstadter, *Social Darwinism in American Thought* (New York: Houghton Mifflin, 1959), 31–50.

3. Kenneth Bock, *Human Nature and History: A Response to Sociobiology* (New York: Columbia University Press, 1980), 2.

4. C. Lumsden and E. O. Wilson, *Genes, Mind, and Culture* (Cambridge: Harvard University Press, 1981).

5. Horace Freeland Judson, *The Eighth Day of Creation: The Makers of the Revolution in Biology* (New York: Simon and Schuster, 1979), 201.

6. Francis Crick, "Molecular Biology in the Year 2000," *Nature* 228 (1970), 2.

7. Philip Kitcher, *Vaulting Ambition: Sociobiology and the Quest for Human Nature* (Cambridge: MIT Press, 1987); Bock, *Human Nature and History;* Barry Schwartz, *The Battle for Human Nature: Science, Morality, and Modern Life* (New York: W. W. Norton, 1986), 14.

8. Richard Dawkins, *The Extended Phenotype* (Oxford: Oxford University Press, 1982).

9. E. O. Wilson, *Sociobiology: The New Synthesis* (Cambridge: Harvard University Press, 1975).

10. Arthur Fisher, "A New Synthesis Comes of Age," *Mosaic* (National Science Foundation) 22, no. 1. (Spring 1991), 2.

11. Kitcher, *Vaulting Ambition;* Bock, *Human Nature and History;* Schwartz, *The Battle for Human Nature.*

12. Brian C. Goodwin, "A Relational or Field Theory of Reproduction and Its Evolutionary Implications," in *Beyond Neo-Darwinism,* ed. Mae-Wan Ho and Peter T. Saunders (London: Academic Press, 1984), 1.

13. René Descartes, *Discourse on Method,* trans. John Veitch (1637; reprint, Chicago: Paquin Printers, 1962).

14. August Weismann (1883), reprinted in *A Source Book in Animal Biology,* ed. T. W. Hall (New York: Hafner, 1964); August Weismann (1885), reprinted in *Readings in Heredity and Development,* ed. J. A. Moore (Oxford: Oxford University Press, 1972).

15. P. Van den Berghe and D. P. Barash, "Inclusive Fitness and Human Family Structure, *American Anthropologist* 79 (1977): 809–23.

16. Brian C. Goodwin, "Organisms and Minds: The Dialectics of the Animal/Human Interface in Biology," in *What Is an Animal?* ed. T. Ingold, 100–109 (London: Allen and Unwin, 1988).

17. R. A. Fisher, *The Genetical Theory of Natural Selection* (Oxford: Clarendon Press, 1930); J. B. S. Haldane, *The Causes of Evolution* (London: Harper and Brothers, 1932); S. Wright, "The Genetical Theory of Natural Selection" (review), *Journal of Heredity* 21 (1930): 329–56.

18. Francis Crick, *What Mad Pursuit* (New York: Basic Books, 1988); J. D. Watson, *The Double Helix* (New York: Atheneum, 1968).

19. Lumsden and Wilson, *Genes, Mind, and Culture.*

20. Dawkins, *Extended Phenotype,* Chapter 14.

21. James L. Gould and Carol Grant Gould, *Sexual Selection* (New York: W. H. Freeman, 1989), 241.

22. Leo W. Buss, *The Evolution of Individuality* (Princeton: Princeton University Press, 1987), 171–72.

23. George C. Williams, *Adaptation and Natural Selection* (Princeton: Princeton University Press, 1966).

24. Richard Dawkins, *The Selfish Gene* (Oxford: Oxford University Press, 1976).

25. Dawkins, *Extended Phenotype,* 264.

26. Richard C. Lewontin, *Annual Review of Ecological Systems* 1 (1970): 1–18.

27. Goodwin, "Organisms and Minds," 1–21.

28. Ibid., 1–21.

29. J. Hirsch, T. R. McGuire, and A. Vetta, "Concepts of Behavior Genetics and Misapplications to Humans," in *The Evolution of Human Social Behavior*, ed. J. S. Lockard (New York: Elsevier, 1980).

30. Mae-Wan Ho, "Environment and Heredity in Development and Evolution," in *Beyond Neo-Darwinism*, ed. Mae-Wan Ho and Peter T. Saunders (London: Academic Press, 1984).

31. Lumsden and Wilson, *Genes, Mind, and Culture.*

♦ GISELA KAPLAN AND LESLEY J. ROGERS ♦

Race and Gender Fallacies: The Paucity of Biological Determinist Explanations of Difference

INTRODUCTION

Over the past two decades we have seen the rise of the New Right. When the National Front supporters rally in the streets of London, the neofascists rampage in Leipzig and Berlin, and The Navigators, a fundamentalist religious sect, call for stoppage of Asian immigration to Australia, they invoke the supremacy of the white male, and they use arguments of genetic determinism to justify their position. To them race is not a social construct but, rather, a natural order ultimately determined by our genes. Equally, to the mounting band of patriarchs who have reacted in backlash to the gains made by the feminist movements in the 1970s and 1980s male privilege is not a social construct but a "natural," innate manifestation of biologically determined difference. The claim is that human behavior is the consequence of biochemical events in cells and that these are in turn determined by the action of the genes within those cells. Biological determinism is used as an arbiter of social issues. According to the biological determinist, all human behavior, and even society itself, is fixed and controlled by the genes.

This essay deals with the role that biological determinism plays, and has played, in influencing general opinion and public wisdom on issues of race and gender. Racism and sexism are two phenomena of persistent prejudice, and here we will discuss how theories of inheritance have helped to perpetuate them. By using science as a supposedly value free, or objective, method for understanding reality, new discoveries and measurements have helped old beliefs to be dressed up in a new garb. Seemingly objective evidence in the field of biology has consistently been used as justification for racism, imperialism, and sexism. Far from being *value free,* much biological research reflects the prejudices and ignorance of its time. To quote Steven Rose, "Biology is inexorably a historical science in a way that chemistry and physics have no need to be" (1988, 161). This is not to say that chemistry and physics have been, and are, without controversy and influence from social forces or religious attitudes (cf. the resistance to reexamining Newtonian physics) but, rather, that the biological sciences are in constant interface with the social attitudes of the time.

Recognition of phenotypes distinguishing broad categories of skin color and eye or nose shape (i.e., purely anatomical and physical features) may appear to be merely descriptive and harmless enough. Equally, the recognition that women are anatomically different from men in certain respects (reproductive organs) apparently does little harm and merely reflects facts. Yet neither research nor social norms have ever left "difference" at that. There are countless examples of the way in which these "harmless" categories and findings in biology were and are being used to explain complex behaviors of the human species. Giant theoretical somersaults have been performed in both the disciplines of biology and sociology in order to pander to prejudices in an apparently scholarly fashion. If the goal was to prove inferiority of "races," the female sex, or the working classes, a whole catalog of beliefs concerning abilities and generalized psychological characteristics was extrapolated from a few physical differences. As is frequently claimed today, complex human behavior is *reduced* to biological explanations at the level of a physical trait or the genes.

In a recent publication entitled *The Sociology of Race* Richardson and Lambert argue that "the sociologist can safely leave biology aside and concentrate on how race is socially constructed" (1986). This, however, is incorrect. Social constructions of reality cannot safely leave behind biology. Indeed, much of that construction is *based* on biological arguments. The processes of genetic determinist support for racist and sexist views are still active in our society today and in the last two decades have even gone through a period of reactivation. It therefore remains an urgent task in each new generation to point out the fallacies and, in view of the social implications, the enormity of these academic transgressions. Biological, or genetic, determinism is politically, socially, and morally dangerous. First, unitary theories are readily popularized and gain widespread publicity. Second, these theories lend legitimation to a range of undesirable prejudicial beliefs that are at odds with modern political thinking of social democracies, civil liberties, and citizenship. Third, they tend to slow down the frontiers of knowledge because the sludge that they create requires "cleanup" and diverts energies.

The dialectic relationship between the development of biological determinist thinking and the socioeconomic and political environment is no more readily demonstrated than in the second half of the nineteenth and early twentieth century. Industrialization, the development of nation-states, their ensuing imperialism and expansionary aims, and the formation of movements such as pan-Slavism and pan-Germanism coincided with the formation of new theories of races and gender. Based on Adam Smith's economic theories of laissez-faire and on Malthus population theory (let the poor die because they represent human surplus), industrialization then entered its most brutal entrepreneurial stage. In racial and gender research much of the new "scientific evidence" for the so-called inferiority of any *Homo sapiens* who was not male and white first appeared in the second half of the nineteenth century. In other words biological determinist arguments entered into these socioeconomic events at this point. They infused the interpretation of reality with new "scientific" ideas in such a way as to remove any accountability or responsibility from those in power.

Among the most respected proponents of racist imperialist ideas were Joseph Arthur, Comte de Gobineau (1816–82), and Houston Stewart Chamberlain (1855–1927). In 1855 Gobineau presented his fatefully poular work *Essai sur l'inegalité des races humaines.* His notorious oeuvre stands out in its simple doctrines and the far-reaching consequences of his views. He used a simple and dangerous weapon: he praised the superiority of the white race, which he claimed was superior to the "black" and "yellow" races, even stating that civilization had progressed only when Aryans had been involved. And he invoked fear. His apocalyptic vision of the decline and death of the white race as a result of being swamped by "inferior races" occupied Gobineau and one of his most prominent pupils, Comte Vacher de Lapouge (1854–1936). Allegedly, even strong "races" and civilizations die when infiltrated by foreign elements. And indeed, as we shall see, scientists proceeded to "prove" the validity of Gobineau's arguments, among them Lapouge, who, unlike his teacher, attempted to prove the inferiority of other races by using skull measurements. Houston Stewart Chamberlain, a British writer, was largely responsible for introducing the Nazi theoretician Alfred Rosenberg to his own views of race. In 1899 Chamberlain published the widely influential book *The Foundations of the Nineteenth Century.* Like Gobineau, he moved to

Germany. Chamberlain married Richard Wagner's daughter and became a German citizen. Chamberlain's theories, just as Gobineau's, were internationally acclaimed.

Gobineau's theories, largely through his friendship with Richard Wagner and the Bayreuth circle, became very influential in Germany. In 1894 one of the members of the Bayreuth circle founded the Gobineau Society. This might seem surprising, since in Germany Gobineau's message of the inferiority and degenerating effect of the so-called yellow and African inferior races never took hold as it did in France or Britain. This had to do with the timing of Germany's acquisition of overseas colonies. Germany took African colonial possessions only in 1884 and a Chinese holding in 1897. Nevertheless, Gobineau's Aryan message and the warning of the degenerative and "diluting" effect of other races were highly usable and could be adapted to the German situation. In one sense it fueled the pan-German movement by "reawakening the Aryan Germanic soul"; in another it became a powerful weapon in the hands of anti-Semites. In the absence of the "yellow and black perils," Germans used the Jew as the one "polluting" race (Mosse 1978, 56).

Craniology flourished in the second half of the nineteenth century, and after Gobineau there were many crude attempts to draw a close association between blacks, women, and apes (see Gould 1981). Arguments that were propagated to justify the domination of men over women and the domination or enslavement of one "racial" group by another often equated women and black people. Thus, sexism and racism were linked aspects of genetic determinist thinking (Richards 1983).

There were two beliefs to which theorists held firmly, one being that the white brain was better developed than the black and the other that the male brain was better developed than the female. Women were said to lack the center for intellect, and blacks too were seen to have inferior intellect. Putting it the other way around, Charles Darwin stated that "some at least of those mental traits in which women may excel are traits characteristic of the lower races" (Darwin 1871, 569). He also referred to the "close connection of the negro or Australian and the gorilla" (Darwin 1871, 201). To make the logical connection that he, perhaps deliberately, leaves to conjecture, women in his opinion must also be closer to gorillas.

Some of the most reputable scientists of the time concerned themselves with finding scientific evidence to support the belief in the inferiority of women and blacks, and they became obsessed with measurement of cranium size and brain weight. The assumption (shown later to be incorrect) underlying this approach was that smaller brain size and weight indicates lower intelligence. Negro and female brains were considered to be not only smaller and lighter in weight but also underdeveloped. Thus, the anthropologist E. W. Huschke wrote in 1854: "The Negro brain possesses a spinal cord of the type found in children and women and, beyond this, approaches the type of brain found in higher apes" (cited in Gould 1981, 103). Similarly, another anthropologist McGrigor wrote in 1869 that "the type of female skull approaches in many respects that of the infant, and still more that of the lower races" (cited in Lewontin et al. 1984). The French craniologist F. Pruner embodied the pulse of that time when he wrote: "The Negro resembles the female in his love for children, his family and his cabin. . . . The black man is to the white man what woman is to man in general, a loving being and a being of pleasure" (1866, 13–33). One notes here the equation of the "negro" *he* with the white *she*. The black woman was apparently considered too worthless to even feature in these debates, and so, for better or worse, she was relegated to oblivion.

The famous neuroanatomist Broca (1824–80), founder of the Anthropological Society of Paris, gathered much data demonstrating that the male brain is on average heavier than that of the female. The motivation for this work is clearly apparent in the following statement of a coworker of Broca, G. LeBon, written in 1879. LeBon was one of the founders of social psychology, crowd behavior in particular, and he influenced the thinking of Mussolini. He opposed higher education for women:

> In the most intelligent races, as among the Parisians, there are a large number of women where brains are closer in size to those of gorillas than to the most developed male brains. This inferiority is so obvious that no one can contest it for a moment; only its degree is worth discussion. All psychologists who have studied the intelligence of women, as well as poets and novelists, recognize today that they represent the most inferior forms of human evolution and that they are closer to children and savages than to an adult, civilized man. They excel in fickleness, inconstancy, absence of thought and logic, and an incapacity to reason. Without doubt there exist some distinguished women, very superior to the average man, but they are as exceptional as the birth of any monstrosity, as, for example, of a gorilla with two heads; consequently we may neglect them entirely. (LeBon 1879, quoted in Gould 1981, 104–5)

To compare the occurrence of an intelligent woman with that of a gorilla with two heads is no less astounding than is the claim that the

Parisians are a race. Apparently, his views went entirely unchecked and uncriticized.

Nevertheless, quite early in the era of brain size measurement scientists had run into a number of problems, which they had either to dismiss or argue around. For example, Broca's theory of brain size and intelligence was momentarily shaken when he found that "Eskimos, Lapps, Malays, Tartars and several other peoples of the Mongolian type" had larger cranial capacity than "the most civilized people of Europe" (1873, 38). To circumvent the problem of, as he saw it, some "lowly" races having large brains he saw fit to claim that the relationship between brain size and intelligence may not hold at the upper end of the scale, because some inferior groups have large brains, but that it did hold at the lower end. That is, small brains belong exclusively to people of low intelligence. By this means he felt that he was able to hold on to "the value of a small brain size as a mark of inferiority" (Broca 1873). As Gould (1981) points out, Broca did not fudge his actual numbers, although some other scientists of the time did so; rather, he reinterpreted them in a way that allowed him to uphold his original, preconceived notions, even if this required the most incredible feats of logic.

It became fashionable to measure the brains of eminent men after their deaths. The brain weight of several of these men were above the European average and were taken as evidence of their superior intellect (e.g., Baron Georges Cuvier and Ivan Turgenev), but those of others were embarrassingly less than the European average (e.g., Walt Whitman and Franz Josef Gall, the founder of phrenology). Undaunted by these figures, Broca continued to claim that those with lower weight had died at an older age, were smaller in build, or that their brains had been poorly preserved. At the time Broca did not know that his own brain weighed only very slightly above the European average. From the hindsight of our present knowledge that up to 80 percent of the brain's volume is extracellular space and that preserving (fixing) methods are particularly variable in the amount of shrinkage which they cause, we are able to see how extremely unreliable was all of this early data on brain weight and volume.

Much was made of this claimed difference in brain weight between women and men until it was realized that no sex difference occurs when brain weight is expressed in relations to body weight. Then attention was shifted to structural differences in the skull or differences in subregions of the brain, such as the frontal lobes or the corpus callosum. The arguments of brain size and cranium shape held sway to support racial, sexual, and indeed class oppression until 1901 when Alice Leigh applied new statistical procedures to the analysis of the data and showed that there was no correlation between cranial capacity and intelligence or brain weight and intelligence. Nevertheless, it was in 1903 that the American anatomist E. A. Spitzka published a figure showing the brain size of a "Bushwoman" as intermediate between that of a gorilla and the mathematician C. F. Gauss and the number of convolutions of the surface of the brain of the Bushwoman as being closer to that of the gorilla (see Gould 1981, fig. 3.3). It is worth noting that the lower "white" classes were also slotted into having inferior, undeveloped brains (see Gould 1981), although this issue does not directly concern us here.

OTHER MORPHOLOGICAL MEASUREMENTS

Many other parts of the human body can be measured, as indeed they have been, in attempts to show the inferiority of blacks, women, and the lower classes. One such example was Broca's measurement of the ratio of the size of the radius bone in the lower arm to the humerus bone in the upper arm, the theory being that a higher ratio means a longer forearm, which, in turn, is more characteristic of the ape. While blacks were found to have a higher ratio than whites, Broca encountered an impasse for his ideology when he found that Eskimos and Australian Aborigines had a lower ratio than whites. He concluded that "it seems difficult for me to continue to say that elongation of the forearm is a character of degradation or inferiority" (1862, 11). In other words, the approach was to hold on to the belief that Europeans rank above races with darker skins and to count as irrelevant the particular nonfitting measurement that was going to be used in support of it. As with his data on brain size, he continued to adhere to a belief and preferred to ignore some of the contradictory data. Broca's decision to hold on to his social attitudes in the face of conflicting scientific evidence is a clear example of the influence of social attitudes on science.

Nose shape and size was another characteristic measured across human groups perceived as races. Indeed, this variable is of particular interest because it was taken up by some scientists who defended equality and were later called cultural relativists. They argued that nose size and shape was influenced by climatic conditions, temperature, and humidity in order to optimize breathing and minimize water loss (this idea was still maintained by J. S. Weiner, writing in 1954). The theory of environmental influence on the shape of the nose, however admirable at the time, was always discussed in terms of measurements that set the white, male nose as a standard. For example, the naturalist O. Beccari, who spent time in Borneo at the turn of the century, made frequent references which described the Malays as lacking a prominent nose and described the women as having even flatter noses than the men (Beccari 1904, 22, 24). The smaller, flatter nose was seen as more childlike and even more apelike. It was a feature considered to illustrate the inferiority of the "lower races." Interestingly, somewhere along the line in European culture a small nose became associated with beauty and femininity. Even today a small nose is considered by some to be more beautiful in women, presumably because it makes the face more childlike, and, therefore, it is seen as more female (rather than more apelike!).

Beccari paid credence to "the opinion that the races of Man are climatic productions" (216) and accepted that this is not inconsistent with the theory of evolution. He then discussed in some detail the possibility that "Man" may have evolved from the orangutan. After failing to find any remains of an anthropoid form in Borneo, he concluded that Man must have evolved in Africa or "an ancient dependency of that continent." The chief basis of this premise was that Africans have black skins, and thus "it may be surmised that the first men were black" (220). By implication, despite their flat small noses, the Malays have whiter skin and, therefore, cannot be closely related to the earliest humans. Skin color, therefore, dominates over other characteristics. There is, of course, no fossil evidence of the skin color of early humanoid forms.

Most of the measurement nonsense was later abandoned, but the link between the brain as a measure of inferior status of women and blacks did anything but disappear. For example, the introduction of brain surgery, notably the introduction of prefrontal lobotomies by Ergas Moniz, for which he won the Nobel Prize in medicine in 1949, simply put the arguments in a different context. Walter Freeman, who introduced prefrontal lobotomies to the United States in 1936 and practiced these until his retirement in 1970, found that in these operations "women respond better than men, Negroes better than whites and syphilitics better than nonsyphilitics." He added that, of course, "to limit lobotomy to syphilitic Negro women would be the height of absurdity" (cited in Chorover 1979, 156). At about the same time an English physician in Kenya, J. C. Carothers, stated that the normal behavior of leucotomized or lobotomized European whites resembled the normal behavior of East African blacks. Such behaviors included talkativeness, poor judgment, and a "tendency to be content with inferior performance socially and intellectually" (Carothers 1950, 38; cf. Chorover 1979, 156).

THE "JUSTIFICATION" OF RACISM

The alleged European superiority, seemingly so evident because of its technological advances, by a giant leap somehow incorporated morality and relegated other cultures to a status of contempt (Worsley 1972). Technological, including military, progress was seen to go hand in hand with moral progress. To the confident postindustrial Europeans and their descendants in "new world" and colonialized countries, the indices of attainment of capitalist success were a clear sign of the march of humanity toward some kind of perfection, or heaven on earth. The Europeans saw themselves as taking the lead in world civilization. Theirs was the "steady material and moral improvement of mankind from crude stone implements and sexual promiscuity to the steam engines and monogamous marriage" (Radcliffe-Brown 1952, 203).

This supposed moral superiority, in turn, gave those who were less inclined to be persuaded by mystical explanations a different, and supposedly benign, weapon of control over other peoples. Advocates of this view saw that European (i.e., white) moral superiority imposed grave responsibilities on the "developed" nation-states to instruct the "savages and natives" in the art and fruits of modern civilization. If actions were taken in the light of the latest scientific findings on racial matters, governments could be seen as acting in good faith and even with a degree of magnanimity. English Parliament had the interest "to fulfill the mission of the Anglo-Saxon race, in spreading intelligence, freedom, and Christian faith wherever Providence gives us the dominion of the soil" (cited in Banton 1977, 26).

Hand in hand with the idea of racial superiority came the idea of racial purity and the fear of "miscegenation," which Bloom called "quasi-magical" (Bloom 1972, 119). Gobineau, in his typically oblique ways, had already warned that "blood mixture" and "blood impurities" were the beginning of the downfall of even the best race, which was then condemned to become "human herds, no longer nations, weighed down by the mournful somnolence, [which] will henceforth be benumbed in their nullity, like buffalo ruminating in the stagnant meres of the Pontine marshes" (Gobineau 1855). Chamberlain, echoing a similar sentiment, suggested that, "where the struggle [for race purity] is not waged with cannon-balls, it goes on silently in the heart of society by marriages, by the annihilation of distances which further intercourse" (cited in Bloom 1972, 38).

Perhaps the most direct link between philosophy, biological determinism, the fear of racial pollution, and Nazi biopolicies is provided by Ernst Haeckel, whose most successful work, *The Riddles of the Universe* (1899), was translated into twenty-five languages and by 1933 had sold more than one million copies in Germany alone (Stein 1988). Here social Darwinism obtained a new twist by a new branch of eugenics. Independently of Gobineau and Chamberlain, Haeckel came to the same conclusion that lower races "such as the Vedahs or Australian Negroes—are psychologically nearer to the mammals—apes and dogs—than to the civilized European" and that "therefore [we must] assign a totally different value to their lives" (cited in Stein 1988, 55). The important idea that held together his work was that humans are not distinct from the biological world but, rather, are part of nature and, therefore, represent part of a natural continuum. Natural selection occurs, or should occur, among humans in the same manner as among animals or plants. Obviously, neither liberalism, democracy, nor the ideas of the Enlightenment fitted his scheme. And indeed, he regarded these political and humanistic proposals as quite false because they were based on an assumption of free will and individual autonomy. He dismissed both as an illusion and as the consequence of dogma of the French Enlightenment *philosophes.*

For Haeckel the *only* morality lay in the process of natural selection. According to him, this "morality" of natural selection in human society now required positive intervention in order to correct the errors humans had already brought upon themselves. He advocated the extermination of anybody with any failings—racial, physical, social, or otherwise—because such an artificial process of selection would make "the struggle for life among the better portion of mankind . . . easier." Those he believed should be exterminated included "hundreds of thousands of incurables—lunatics, lepers, people with cancer etc.—who are artificially kept alive . . . without the slightest profit to themselves or the general body." Moreover, he said they polluted the breeding pool and so did "incorrigible and degraded criminals" (cited in Stein 1988, 55). Anthropologists of the time and the Society for Racial Hygiene supported Haeckel and often pronounced very similar views. By the 1920s these various groups, all regarded as consisting of respectable scholars, were proposing concrete programs of euthanasia, sterilization, and other methods of artificial selection in order to "revitalize the genepool." In 1935 H. F. K. Günther was awarded the prestigious Prize for Science for his less than scientific work *Racial Knowledge of the German People.*

THE NEW ERA OF BRAIN MEASUREMENT

Over the past two decades there has been renewed interest in measuring parts of the brain to see if there are sex differences. Once found, as with the early brain measuring studies of the nineteenth century, these differences are seen to provide evidence for the biological basis of a wide range of sex differences in behavior. The reappearance of brain measuring in a search for explanations for sex differences began in the 1960s and 1970s, and this interest has continued to gain impetus (see the later section on brain lateralization). The timing of its emergence coincided with the focus on "proving" sex and race differences in IQ. Although it is clearly part of the same resurgence of biological determinism, it has received much less debate and criticism in the public arena. Part of the reason for this may be that the new measurements of brain size and structure are looking mainly at sex differences, not black-white differences, and that the present-day public may be more prepared to confront racism than sexism. Another reason may be that most of the researchers in this area have generated their data by applying new technology to the study of animal brains (mainly rats) rather than human brains. The implications are there, reported in the scientific literature, but *so far* relatively little of it has leaked out or been taken up by the wider media to be used for social policymaking. Its use for political purpose to curtail the progress of women toward equal rights has, however, begun (see Moir and Jessel 1989).

It should also be noted that there has been a recent report of a study by J. Klekamp et al. (1991) in which the size and development rate of the hippocampus was measured in Australian Aborigines and Caucasians. Slower growth of this brain region was reported to occur in Aboriginal women, and the authors hypothesized this to be a result of either genetic differences, by implication sex linked, or poor diet or both. Are we about to see a resurgence of racist science?

SOCIOBIOLOGY

During the 1970s genetic determinism led to the formation of a new discipline called "sociobiology," demarcated in particular by the publication of E. O. Wilson's book, *Sociobiology: A New Synthesis,* in 1975. The existence of genes for aggression, territoriality, and intelligence was claimed. As these behaviors are all characteristic of the stereotypical male of Western capitalist society, sociobiology reinforces the "naturalness" of patriarchy. It also "explains," and so condones, the existence of violence in society. The latter, coupled with belief in genetically determined race differences in IQ, allows sociobiology to sanction racism as well as sexism. It provides apparent scientific rationale for the existing social order. Put another way, it offers a genetic, and therefore fixed, explanation for social difference and justifies the continued domination of one group by another.

Mating strategies and sex differences in behavior are said to be genetically determined, and the genes are seen as "replicator" units, which are adorned with the sole purpose of replicating and getting into the next generation (see Dawkins 1976). Gene replication is seen as the sole purpose of life, and genes are given personality characteristics, such as "selfishness." All the complexities of animal behavior, the richness of human achievement and endeavor, are mere trappings that spin off from the basic purpose of the replicator units. Thus, analysis of mating strategies and reproduction becomes the main area of study. This burgeoning area of research in sociobiology analyzes data using cost-benefit models. The cost of a certain mating and reproductive strategy is weighed against the benefit for the individual (not the group), and so the biological fitness ("rightness") of the particular mating strategy is determined. The terminology of capitalism is commonly used, and the ideology of individualism is clearly apparent. It offers capitalism feedback in the form biological justification. To this end sociobiological theories have been readily taken up by the media and also incorporated into a range of other disciplines, including sociology and economics. They have also been taken up by the National Front in the United Kingdom and other neofascist organizations elsewhere.

There has been much disagreement over the existence of a gene for altruism (cf. de Lepervanche 1984). Most sociobiologists agree that no such gene could exist for long in a population as it would soon be lost because it would not compete successfully against the "selfish" genes. Yet according to Wilson (1975), the gene for homosexuality, which he hypothesizes to exist, must be linked to a gene for altruism, or it too would have been lost from the population. Wilson's idea is that the gene for homosexuality persists only because homosexual individuals also carry a gene for altruism, and this leads them to assist in the raising of their siblings and their siblings' offspring; that is, they assist the reproduction of individuals who carry a certain percentage of their own genetic material. Thus, "the gene" for homosexuality, so Wilson believes, is an aberration that persists only as a consequence of the coexistence of a protector gene, and the altruism, helping behavior, determined by this protector gene is confined to individuals with whom there is shared genetic material (see also Ridely and Dawkins 1981).

Sociobiologists take into account no aspect of sociology or developmental biology. Had Wilson turned to some sociological records, he might have been surprised to discover that a large percentage of homosexuals do reproduce. Perhaps a more important criticism of the sociobiological approach is its utter disregard for the biological processes of development. Organisms develop in constant interaction with their environment. Genes do indeed influence development, but through each step of the developmental process the expression of the genes interacts with environmental factors in an inseparable, intertwined manner so that, finally, the separate contributions of the genes and environment cannot be determined (Rose et al. 1973). Genes function in an environment, and they cannot be discussed without considering that environment (see Tobach 1972). That environment is not a unitary or easily defined thing. For example, there is the biochemical environment in the immediate vicinity of the gene; there is the environment surrounding the organism itself; and so on. No clear distinction can be made between the environment within and outside the organism (Hambley 1973). Furthermore, genes and environment are not discrete opposites (Tobach 1972); they are both entirely integrated aspects of the developmental process.

Genes cannot behave or be "selfish." By the same token behavior is not in the genome. Behavior is at an entirely different level of organization than the genes; many steps and functions separate the two. Genes are expressed as biochemical processes; behavior is expressed by the whole organism. This is not to say that genes play no part in behavior. Rather, it is not possible to ignore the processes of development, to ignore environmental influences on the expression of genes, and to extrapolate directly from genes to behavior as do the sociobiologists. Again, we see the selective use of information to use (pseudo)science to bolster sociopolitical causes.

GENES, HORMONES, HOMOSEXUALITY, AND SEX DIFFERENCES IN BEHAVIOR

Biological determinism can be applied to a wide range of social phenomena, and the model can shift and move to any subject in which the transgression between biological basis and social reality is seen as a possibility. We suggest that the "scientific" writing on homosexuality, rekindled by Alfred Kinsey's findings of 1948, took a very similar turn to the discussions on race and gender. Kinsey's findings showed to an astounded audience that a very high percentage of males and a much higher than expected percentage of females at one time or another had engaged in homosexual activity (Kinsey 1948). This was morally and socially so unacceptable that studies were undertaken to show that homosexuality was not the behavior of "normal," well-adapted people but, rather, the consequence of a biological abnormality or a congenital defect (although the evidence should have invited some to regard it as far less of an aberration than it was seen to be). In psychiatry homosexuality was treated as a disease. In the 1950s and 1960s the assumed abnormality of homosexuality allowed for biopolicies in the medical field. Under Hitler homosexuals went to concentration camps and were killed; under Mussolini celibacy and being unmarried as an adult were punishable by a prison sentence (Kaplan 1992).

In the postwar Western world the punitive legal procedure was changed into an invasive, even mutilating "treatment" model. In Australia and the United States, as well as in other countries, psychosurgery has been used to "treat" and/or "cure" homosexuality. Frontal lobotomies, which involve surgical severing of connection between parts of the frontal lobes and deeper regions of the brain, became fashionable in the 1940s and 1950s. They were performed enthusiastically in the United States, and, even though the operation was approached with greater caution in the United Kingdom, over ten thousand patients in the United Kingdom were lobotomized between 1942 and 1954 (Whitlock 1979).

Although the discoveries (by Western medicine) of psychoactive drugs in the 1950s led to a decline in the number of lobotomies performed, throughout the following two decades the operation was still performed on a large number of psychiatric patients and also political dissidents. During the 1970s other forms of psychosurgery, such as the cingulotracheotomy operation (lesioning of the cingulate gyrus, part of the limbic system), were developed and to some extent replaced lobotomies. Although these were carried out using more sophisticated techniques and involved the placement of more discrete brain lesions, they were in essence just as crude as the lobotomies, as they involved lesioning areas of the brain not fully understood in terms of their function. They were, in fact, based on no better theoretical background than the older lobotomies (Blakemore 1977). In Australia during the 1970s cingulotracheotomies were given as "treatment" for homosexual behavior, and some homosexuals agreed to undergo psychosurgery in exchange for shortened prison sentences (Watson 1979). Other parts of the brain have also been destroyed as a means of treating homosexuality; for example, lesions have been placed in the hypothalamus (a most risky area of the brain to lesion) to treat a symptom called "latent homosexuality" (Blakemore 1977).

Aversion therapy with electric shock and hot plate treatment were not uncommon forms of treatment for homosexuality in the 1950s to the 1970s. In addition, chemical castration by application of antiandrogen therapy or estrogen treatment has been known to be used in West Germany, South Africa, and Australia (Kaplan and Rogers 1987). In a publication entitled *Sex Variants* (Henry 1948), Dickinson, the writer of "The Gynecology of Homosexuality," concerned himself with lesbians and measured the "erectility" of breast and nipples, the labia majora and minora, pubic hair, clitoris erectility and size, uterus, etc. One needs to note that, as in the nineteenth century, measurement of physical features once again became the guiding procedure for establishing difference (i.e., inferiority or "abnormality"). Because of the sexual focus, however, the customary measurement of brain size had been dropped in favor of measuring the size of genitalia. From these measurements of a total of thirty-one women he claimed to have found significant differences in size and behavior of the sexual organs of lesbians in comparison to, as he calls it, his experience in "office practice." Of course, we do not see any data of his daily experiences, that is, his office practice. Variation of anatomical difference on an extremely small sample is read as abnormality for all lesbians and thus confirms the medical model of homosexuality as a disease. D. J. West's study, first published under the title *Homosexuality* in 1955, has gone through four editions and seven reprints in all, the latest in 1977, revised as *Homosexuality Re-Examined.* West worked as a psychiatrist and reader in clinical criminology at Cambridge, and his book was very influential. Even in the 1977 revised version he argues that "the possibility that homosexual behaviour in humans is caused by some glandular deficiency cannot be dismissed out of hand" (West 1977, 65). According to him, androgen levels influence the strength of sexual desire, and an excess of prepubertal androgen in girls "may masculinise certain aspects of their social attitude and temperament." He quotes lowered sperm count and "relative infertility" as another relationship between male homosexuality and biology (69).

In the psychomedical field there is a huge literature on the determination of sex differences in behavior by the sex hormones, these in turn determined by the genes (X and Y chromosomes). This form of biological determinism was particularly popularized by the studies and writings, in both the scientific and popular press, of J. Money and his coworkers in the 1970s and 1980s (Money and Ehrhardt 1972; Money and Tucker 1975; Dörner 1976).

There are serious flaws in the theoretical basis to the hypotheses of Money and Dörner, and this is best demonstrated by looking more closely at some of their work. Money and Ehrhardt (1972) conducted a study that has had much influence on thought in this area. They scored a range of behaviors and attitudes considered to be gender related in a group of girls who had been exposed to either androgens (adrenogenital syndrome) or the drug progestin (which their mothers took to prevent miscarriage and which has androgenic action) during their fetal development. Compared to controls (the choice of which was rather dubious; see Rogers and Walsh 1980), the girls exposed to androgens during fetal development were said to be more like males in that they scored higher in "tomboyishness," chose boys' clothes and toys, chose career over marriage (note that they were all only teenagers), and, of special note, scored higher IQs. In addition, they were said to have confused gender identity and were late to reach the "romantic age of dating and boy friends." There were numerous faults with the design of these experiments, let alone the premise on which they were based, but we will not elaborate on them here, as they have been covered previously in some detail (see Rogers and Walsh 1980; Rogers 1981; Rosoff 1991). Suffice it to say that much of the data were collected retrospectively by telephone interviews with the mothers (a method most open to error of recall and distortion due to expectations), the format of the questions used in the interviews has never been revealed, the selection of controls was dubious (in one study they were girls suffering from Turner's Syndrome, genetically XO with reduced levels of sex hormones), and no other members of the subjects' families were investigated for possible similar behavior patterns. The assumption made was that the male sex hormones had acted on the developing brain to switch it into being more masculine.

Perhaps the main danger of this work is that it has been widely taken up in popular writings (e.g., Durden-Smith and de Simone 1983) and extrapolated to explain sex differences between women and men. Beyond that it has been used to explain the so-called biological determination of homosexuality, transvestism, and transsexualism. Money has placed the latter three categories on a continuum of increasing disturbance of androgen levels during development (Money 1974, 1976), the male transsexual, for example, being seen as having a "female brain trapped in a male body." There is no evidence that any of these groups has abnormal hormonal levels during development. Yet the thesis persists, and indeed it has been further propagated by Dörner, who asserts that homosexuality should be prevented by treating pregnant women with the sex steroid hormones (Dörner 1976, 1979). To Dörner male homosexuality is caused by insufficient levels of testosterone during fetal life and lesbianism by an oversupply of testosterone. He advocates that stress of the mother during pregnancy may lead to the fetus being exposed to lowered levels of testosterone, and that is why, according to him, more homosexuals were born in Germany during the war years. Thus, that which he sees as abnormal sexual behavior is to be explained as being biologically caused, even though here the ultimate influence is from the stressful environment, as it were, impeding the "proper" cause of nature (i.e., genetic expression). To take his hypothesis literally, he can only mean that more male homosexuals were born during this time, as by extrapolation stress during pregnancy should lower the chance of a lesbian being born, although his focus of attention never extends to the sexuality of women.

BRAIN LATERALIZATION

Most of this recent research has focused on differences in lateralization between male and female brains. Sex differences in lateralization of brain structure and function have now been found in a range of human species, including humans (see Bradshaw 1989; Corballis 1983). Lateralization refers to the left and right sides of the brain processing information differently and controlling different behavioral functions. Structures on the left and right sides of the brain may also differ in size or shape, although lateralization of brain function can occur without there being any obvious lateralization, or asymmetry, in structure.

It is worth diverging somewhat to note that left and right, sinistral and dextral, carry a long history of cultural associations, which are not irrelevant to us here. Left has been characterized as bad, dark, black, unclean, weak, female, and homosexual, whereas right has been characterized as good, light, clean, sacred, strong, white, male, and heterosexual (Star 1979). Left-handed people have been associated with evil, weakness, and all manner of detrimental characteristics throughout history. As we will see, these connotations are still with us today.

In humans, in most cases, language is processed in a site situated in the left hemisphere, and speech production is controlled from another site also in the left hemisphere. Women, however, appear to have an extra site for language in the right hemisphere (Bradshaw and Nettleton 1983; see also Obler and Novoa 1988). Sex differences in structure and function are increasingly being reported for nonhuman species, particularly rats (Denenberg 1981; Diamond 1984) and birds (Andrew and Brennan 1984; Rogers 1986). In rats there are, for example, left-right asymmetries in the thickness of various regions of the cortex and the direction and magnitude of these differs with age and sex (Diamond 1984). Additionally, there are sex differences in lateralization of brain neurochemistry (Denenberg and Rosen 1983).

In mammals the large neural tract, called the corpus callosum, which connects the left and right hemispheres, is considered to be important in generating and maintaining brain lateralization (Denenberg 1981; Gazzaniga and LeDoux 1978; Selnes 1974). Recently, there have been reports that in rats the corpus callosum differs in size between females and males (Denenberg, Berrebi, and Fitch 1989). Although similar data for humans are still in dispute, one group of researchers have reported a sex difference in the size of the corpus callosum (Holloway and de Lacoste 1986; de Lacoste-Utamsing and Holloway 1982; de Lacoste, Holloway, and Woodward 1986). It is important to contest and debate the significance of the data reported for humans, particularly given the difficulty in having adequate controls in the studies of human brains and the low sample sizes. In the light of the data for animal species, however, it is perhaps even more important to ask how sex differences in the brain may be generated. Are they biologically determined by the action of the genes and sex hormones, or are they imposed on the brain by the differential cultural learning that occurs in women and men?

All too readily, many of the researchers opt for biological determinist explanations, even though they may not have attempted to test specifically for such an explanation. For example, de Lacoste et al. (1986) are convinced that their reported sex difference in the size of the corpus callosum is biologically caused, as is most evident from the following statement:

"We believe that our data provide further indirect evidence that the gonadal steroids and/or genetic sex play a role in the development of neural structures, linked with 'cognitive functions,' in the human brain" (95). This is a rather remarkable (or foolhardy) statement given that their study did not investigate the role of hormones in the development of the corpus callosum or any other structure or function. This is yet another case of overstating the data and extrapolating to reinforce social norms.

Nevertheless, sex hormones can indeed influence the development of brain structures, including the cortex (Diamond 1984) and the corpus callosum (Berrebi et al. 1988; Fitch et al. 1990). But experience (environment) and age also influence these forms of lateralization. Lateralization in the developing chicken brain has also been demonstrated to depend on the interaction of sex hormones and environmental input in the form of light stimulation (Rogers 1986). The final form that lateralization takes in a given brain, be it human or nonhuman, has been shown clearly to depend on the interaction of the genes/hormones, environmental experience, and age. Just as it is impossible to separate the relative contributions of genes and environment in determining IQ, so too is it impossible to separate the effects of genes, hormones, and environmental factors in determining brain lateralization.

There are two opposing views on possible differences in lateralization in women and men. One of the theories suggests that because females are more emotional than males they must be right hemisphere dominant (see Starr 1979). This theory ignores the fact that women, for whatever reason, are superior in language ability compared to men and that language ability is a function of the left hemisphere. It is obviously not acceptable that women have left hemisphere dominance, as analytical ability is a property of the left hemisphere (Bleier 1984). Another theory argues that the brains of women are less lateralized than those of men (Levy 1977), the premise being that more lateralized brains (male) are better at visuospatial tasks. As left-handed men are said to be less lateralized than right-handed men, this theory suggests that women are more like left-handed men. Women and left-handed men are said to have more interhemispheric cross-talk and a greater degree of language processing in the right hemisphere. It is the latter that is said to interfere with spatial ability of the left hemisphere. While there is some evidence that women, compared to men in general, have an extra center for processing language in the right hemisphere, as far as we know this has not been investigated in left-handed men. Moreover, the claims of this theory are inconsistent with evidence that there is a higher than average representation of left-handed men among architects (Geschwind and Galaburda 1985).

A contrary theory suggests that the brains of women are more lateralized than those of men (Buffery 1981). Thus, the circular reasoning goes, women are inferior on visuospatial tasks because this ability requires use of both hemispheres and women cannot do this so well because their brains are more lateralized. Human females may be more or less lateralized than males, but this tells us only that lateralization in the brain reflects the different hormonal and environmental inputs to which female and male brains are exposed. It does not tell us something essential and unitary about the biological determination of sex differences in cognitive function, as de Lacoste et al. and others would want to believe.

N. Geschwind and A. M. Galaburda (1987) are influential researchers in the area of brain lateralization who have also opted for a unitary biological explanation for sex differences in lateralization. They have hypothesized that "normal" brain lateralization in males comes about as a result of testosterone influencing the development of the left hemisphere. Environmental and cultural influences are ignored. They claim that low levels of testosterone disturb development of the left hemisphere and that this is why left-handedness (the left hand being controlled by the right hemisphere) is more common in males than females. It is, they claim, also the reason why mental retardation is more common in males. They also suggest that abnormally high levels of testosterone during fetal development cause "giftedness" in males. Since males on average have higher levels of testosterone than females, this apparently would leave females with little chance of being gifted. Females rate little direct mention in the writings of Geschwind and Galaburda.

This was not actually a very original hypothesis of Geschwind and Galaburda. A very similar hypothesis for male "superiority" had been put forward earlier by J. Money and A. A. Ehrhardt (1972). Geschwind and Galaburda therefore appear to have resurrected a rather dubious hypothesis, with no further evidence to substantiate it, and they were prepared to extend their hypothesis to offer some biologically determined associations of homosexuality (Geschwind and Galaburda 1987). Here they displayed the often tortuous path of reasoning and tenuous assumptions so often used for biological explanations of difference. They were keen to explain some anecdotal, and definitely not proven, indication that homosexuals have a higher rate of "nonrighthandedness" (175). First, they adopted a former study showing that stressing rats during pregnancy initially causes testosterone levels in the male fetus to rise and later, after birth, results in permanently lower levels of this hormone. Next they linked this finding to one of Dörner and his coworkers which reported higher levels of "homosexual" behavior in rats stressed in this manner. By extrapolation Geschwind and Galaburda concluded that stress in pregnancy in humans raises the level of testosterone in the male fetus and so disrupts the development of the left hemisphere and leads to more nonrighthandedness, and it also causes homosexuality—hence, there are more left-handed homosexuals. Now they were prepared to go one step further. An elevated level of testosterone in the fetus also suppresses the development of the immune system. Thus, homosexuals may have impaired immune systems and this may be why they are more susceptible to AIDS. By adopting a unitary, biological cause for homosexuality, they were able, in one neat parcel, to suggest an explanation for the epidemiology of AIDS; thus, reductionist explanations subsume other sciences and social sciences.

This convoluted reasoning has taken us far from the original discussion of the new focus on sex differences in brain measurements. If this detour exemplifies anything, it is to show the nature of dead-end roads. They distract and mislead. Some of them have been hailed as new insights and as roads of knowledge for the future. Often this is doubly ironic. The very reason why some deterministic theories acquire publicity and are hailed as new exciting knowledge is precisely because they do not offer anything new but at times confirm even the worst prejudices held in a society at the time—and they are produced by people who themselves commenced their research with a view of, implicitly or explicitly, confirming their own prejudices.

CONCLUSION

We have made it our particular concern to choose for discussion examples of reductionism, biological determinism, and biologisms by well-known and often well-respected works by scholars in the field. The impression should not be gained that the prejudices somehow belong to minor writers or outsiders. The problem is precisely that academic activity in this field has spawned so much that is socially highly approved, albeit scientifically most questionable. On the surface some of the research findings seem quite sophisticated, but in reality some of these tremendous constructs (e.g., modern sociobiology) rest on very shaky and simplistic premises.

The premise is that one biological fact—such as a gene, the size of a bone, weight of a skull, length of a forearm, or the absence or presence of one specific hormone—has explanatory power and can offer *singly* insight into social behaviors of individuals. Yet monocausal explanations in any field of scholarship rarely stand up under scrutiny. For the study and explanation of human behavior it is logially and scientifically impossible for one small facet to explain all when there are a multitude of variables which make up the human environment and human behavior. That is, of course, both the challenge and the difficulty in studying human behavior. In terms of experimentation human behavior is less accessible than is the equivalent in studies using animals, and when a theory comes along that makes the complexities disappear there may be a sense of relief by the general community that finally manageable answers to our searching questions are at hand.

The theories we have proposed here, which we have claimed represent examples of pseudoscience, have created and kept alive the modern monster of social Darwinism. Social Darwinism works back into the biological roots and therefore seeks to find the answers for differences in behavior via biological channels. In this way there hardly seems any difference between the explanations (and solutions) provided by Haeckel in pre-Nazi Germany and those of Wilson in 1975. If aggression and territoriality are biologically given traits and genes are selfish, then Haeckel has a point that free will and individual autonomy do not exist other than as a fictitious account of the French *philosophes.* The only morality, as he concluded then, would be a morality of natural selection, of the survival of the fittest. Whatever is "given" by the genes presumably has a right to exist—a neat biological justification for wars, territoriality, and male aggression against women (see Hunter 1991).

We have shown that the ideas and the "proofs" in pseudoscience serve to state, confirm, and propagate a social or political belief rather than to advance science and knowledge. There are countless examples of poor experimental designs, omission of presenting data, and even falsified data to substantiate this point. We have given some examples of these in this chapter. Another method is to ignore a substantial body of data in order to arrive at the conclusion that the writer has wanted to reach in the first place rather than to work with the data (cf. the stories of Broca and Hutt).

One key element in the psychology of racism and sexism is the apparent need by some to identify a group of people as being inferior to themselves. Of course, the "pay-offs" may be very high, socially, economically, or politically (territorial gains, gains in powers, income, loss of guilt, etc.). Scientists are not free from racism and sexism, and biology has had more than a share in upholding or creating new myths of inequality. The psychology of those needing paradigms in which the world can be divided into inferior and superior can extend anywhere. If it were not racism or sexism, it might be homophobia or ageism; a whole range of items could usefully fill the "inferiority" niche. Racists and sexists may confine their biological determinist arguments to one category at a time, to single out and label a single group. Notwithstanding this, the designated inferior groups are, to them, interchangeable. The construct of biological determinism is general and refers at one time to race, another to sex, and still another to class, sexual preference, or whatever identified inferior group is the flavor of the day. As the argument goes, any one of these groups may be made a substitute for the others (Gould 1981, 103). The crux of the matter, according to the proponents of these views, is to understand the biological basis of inferiority, no matter on what basis that inferiority may be seen to rest. In other words, the approach is to interpret scientific data (measurements) for political and social purpose.

While these relationships of power and control with sexism and racism have been common knowledge at least since the civil rights movements and the new feminist movements all over the world, we need to be wary of the fact that they are not a thing of the past. Forms of control, strictures, and curtailments of equality may change form and argument. Affirmative action programs may be here, but they may be undermined today and tomorrow. Indeed, there is evidence that it is already happening. Backlashes with outbreaks of virulent attacks on difference of any kind (gender, ethnicity, color, sexual preference, etc.) are making headline news in the early 1990s in the very countries that pride themselves on their own democratization and egalitarianism.

REFERENCES

Andrew, R. J., and A. Brennan. 1984. "Sex Differences in Lateralization in the Domestic Chick: A Developmental Study." *Neuropsychologia* 22: 503–9.

Banton, M. 1977. *The Idea of Race.* London: Tavistock Publications.

Beccari, O. 1904. *Wanderings in the Great Forests of Borneo.* London: Archibald Constable.

Berrebi, A. S., R. H. Fitch, J. O. Denenberg, V. L. Friedrich, and V. H. Denenberg. 1988. "Corpus Callosum: Region-Specific Effects of Sex, Early Experience and Age." *Brain Research* 438; 216–24.

Blakemore, C. 1977. *Mechanics of the Mind.* London: Cambridge University Press.

Bleier, R. 1984. *Science and Gender.* New York: Pergamon.

Bloom, L. 1972. *The Social Psychology of Race Relations.* London: Allen and Unwin.

Bradshaw, J. L. 1989. *Hemispheric Specialization and Psychological Function.* New York: John Wiley and Sons.

Bradshaw, J. L., and N. C. Nettleton. 1983. *Human Cerebral Asymmetry.* New York: Prentice-Hall.

Broca, P. 1862. "Sur les proportions relatives du bras, de l'avant bras et de la clavicule chez les nègres et les européens." *Bulletin Société d'Anthropologie Paris* 3, no. 2: 1–13.

———. 1873. "Sur les crânes de la caverne de l'Homme-Mort (Lozère)." *Revue d'Anthropologie* 2: 1–53.

Buffery, A. W. H. 1981. "Male and Female Brain Structure." In *Australian Women: Feminist Perspectives,* ed. N. Grieve and P. Grimshaw, 58–66. Melbourne: Oxford University Press.

Carothers, J. C. 1950. "Frontal Lobe Function in the African." *British Journal of Mental Science.*

Chorover, S. L. 1979. *From Genesis to Genocide: The Meaning of Human Nature and the Power of Behavior Control.* Cambridge, Mass.: MIT Press.

Corballis, M. C. 1983. *Human Laterality.* New York: Academic Press.

Darwin, C. 1871. *The Descent of Man.* London: John Murray.

Dawkins, R. 1976. *The Selfish Gene.* Oxford: Oxford University Press.

de Lacoste, M.-C., R. L. Holloway, and D. J. Woodward. 1986. "Sex Difference in the Fetal Human Corpus Callosum." *Human Neurobiology* 5: 93–96.

de Lacoste-Utamsing, C., and R. L. Holloway. 1982. "Sexual Dimorphism in the Human Corpus Callosum." *Science* 216: 1431–32.

de Lepervanche, M. M. 1984. "The 'Naturalness' of Inequality." In *Ethnicity, Class and Gender in Australia,* G. Bottomley and M. M. de Lepervanche, 49–71. Sydney: Allen and Unwin.

Denenberg, V. H. 1981. "Hemispheric Laterality in Animals and the Effects of Early Experience." *Behavioral Brain Sciences* 4: 1–49.

Denenberg, V. H., and G. D. Rosen. 1983. "Interhemispheric Coupling Coefficients: Sex Differences in Brain Neurochemistry. *American Physiological Society* R151–R153.

Denenberg, V. H., A. S. Berrebi, and R. H. Fitch. 1989. "A Factor Analysis of the Rat's Corpus Callosum." *Brain Research* 497: 271–79.

Diamond, M. C. 1984. "Age, Sex, and Environmental Influences." In *Cerebral Dominance: The Biological Foundations,* ed. N. Geschwind and A. M. Galaburda, 134–46. Cambridge, Mass.: Harvard University Press.

Dickinson, R. L. 1948. "The Gynecology of Homosexuality." In *Sex Variants: A Study of Homosexual Patterns,* ed. G. W. Henry, 1069–129. New York and London: Paul B. Hoeber.

Dörner, G. 1979. "Hormones and Sexual Differentiation of the Brain." *Sex, Hormones and Behaviour* (Ciba Foundation Symposium) 62: 81–112.

———. 1976. "Hormone-Dependent Brain Development and Behaviour." In *Hormones and Behaviour in Higher Vertebrates,* J. Baltharzart, E. Prove, and R. Gilles. Berlin: Springer.

Durden-Smith, J., and D. de Simone 1983. *Sex and the Brain.* London: Pan Books.

Fitch, R. H., P. E. Cowell, L. M. Schrott, and V. H. Denenberg 1991. "Corpus Callosum: Ovarian Hormones and Feminization." *Brain Research* 542: 313–17.

Gazzaniga, M. S., and J. E. LeDoux. 1978. *The Integrated Mind.* New York: Plenum Press.

Geschwind, N., and A. M. Galaburda 1985. "Cerebral Lateralization: Biological Mechanisms, Associations, and Pathology," *Archives of Neurology* 42, 428–653.

———. 1987. *Cerebral Lateralization: Biological Mechanisms, Associations, and Pathology.* Cambridge, Mass.: MIT Press.

Gobineau, J. A. 1855. *Essai sur l'inegalité des races humaines.* Trans. and ed. A. Collins. 1915. *The Inequality of Human Races.* New York: Putnam.

Gould, S. J. 1981. *The Mismeasure of Man.* New York and London: W. W. Norton.

Hambley, J. 1973. "Diversity: A Developmental Perspective." In *Race, Culture and Intelligence,* ed. K. Richardson and D. Spears, 114–27. Harmondsworth: Penguin.

Henry, G. W. 1948. *Sex Variants: A Study of Homosexual Patterns.* New York and London: Paul B. Hoeber.

Holloway, R. L., and M. C. de Lacoste. 1986. "Sexual Dimorphism in the Human Corpus Callosum: An Extension and Replication Study." *Human Neurobiology* 5: 87–91.

Hunter, A. E., ed. 1991. *Genes and Gender VI: On Peace, War and Gender.* New York: The Feminist Press.

Kaplan, G. 1992. *Contemporary Western European Feminism.* Sydney and London: Allen and Unwin. New York: New York University Press.

Kaplan, G., and L. J. Rogers. 1987. "Biology and the Oppression of Women." In *Feminist Knowledge as Critique,* ed. Women's Studies Collective, 175–95. Geelong and Victoria: Deakin University Press.

Kinsey, A. C., W. B. Pomeroy, and C. E. Martin. 1948. *Sexual Behavior in the Human Male.* Philadelphia and London: W. B. Saunders.

Klekamp, J., A. Riedel, C. Harper, and H. J. Kretschmann. 1991. "Morphometric Study on the Postnatal Growth of the Hippocampus in Australian Aborigines and Caucasians. *Brain Research* 549: 90–94.

Levy, J. 1977. "The Mammalian Brain and the Adaptive Advantage of Cerebral Asymmetry." *Annals of the New York Academy of Science* 229: 265–72.

Lewontin, R. C., S. Rose, and L. J. Kamin. 1984. *Not in Our Genes.* New York: Pantheon Books.

Moir, A., and D. Jessel. 1989. *Brain Sex: The Real Difference between Men and Women.* London: Mandarin.

Money, J. 1974. "Prenatal Hormones and Post-Natal Socialisation in Gender Identity Differentiation." In *Nebraska Symposium on Motivation,* ed. J. K. Cole and R. Dienstbeir. Lincoln: University of Nebraska Press.

———. 1976. "Two Names, Two Wardrobes, Two Personalities." *Journal of Homosexuality* 1: 65–70.

Money, J., and A. A. Ehrhardt. 1972. *Man and Woman: Boy and Girl.* Baltimore: John Hopkins University Press.

Money, J., and P. Tucker. 1975. *Sexual Signatures.* Boston and Toronto: Little, Brown.

Mosse, G. L. 1978. *Towards the Final Solution: A History of European Racism.* New York: Howard Fertig.

Obler, L. K., and L. M. Novoa. 1988. "Gender Similarities and Differences in Brain Lateralization." In *Genes and Gender V: Women at Work,* ed. G. M. Vroman, D. Burnham, S. G. Gordon, 37–51. New York: Gordian Press.

Pruner, F. 1866. Article in *Transactions of the Ethnological Society* 4: 13–33. Quoted by E. Fee. 1979. "Nineteenth Century Craniology: The Study of the Female Skull." *Bulletin of the History of Medicine* 53: 415–33.

Radcliffe-Browne, A. R. 1952. *Structure and Function in Primitive Society.* London: Cohen and West.

Richards, E. 1983. "Darwin and the Descent of Woman." In *The Wider Domain of Evolutionary Thought,* ed. D. Olroyd and I. Langham. Boston and London: Reidl.

Richardson, J., and J. Lambert. 1986. *The Sociology of Race.* Ormskirk, Lancashire: Causeway Press.

Ridley, M., and R. Dawkins. 1981. "The Natural Selection of Altruism." In *Altruism and Helping Behavior: Social, Personality and Developmental Perspectives,* ed. J. Philippe Rushton, 19–39. New Jersey: Lawrence Erlbaum Associates.

Rogers, L. J. 1981. "Biology: Gender Differentiation and Sexual Variation." In *Australian Women: Feminist Perspectives,* ed. N. Grieve and P. Grimshaw, 44–57. Melbourne: Oxford University Press.

———. 1986. "Lateralization of Learning in Chicks." *Advances in the Study of Behavior* 16: 147–89.

Rogers, L. J., and J. Walsh. 1982. "Short-comings of the Psychomedical Research into Sex Differences in Behaviour: Social and Political Implications." *Sex Roles* 8: 269–81.

Rose, S. 1988. "Reflections on Reductionism." *Trends in Biological Sciences* 13 (May): 160–62.

Rosoff, B. 1991. "Genes, Hormones and War." In *On Peace, War and Gender,* ed. A. E. Hunter, 39–49. New York: The Feminist Press.

Schwartz, J. H. 1987. *The Red Ape, Orang-utans and Human Origins.* Boston: Houghton Miffin.

Selnes, O. A. 1974. "The Corpus Callosum: Some Anatomical and Functional Considerations, with Special Reference to Language." *Brain and Language* 1: 111–39.

Star, S. L. 1979. "The Politics of Left and Right." In *Women Look at Biology Looking at Women,* ed. R. Hubbard, M. S. Henifin, and B. Fried, 61–74. Cambridge, Mass.: Schenkman.

Stein, G. J. 1988. "Biological Science and the Roots of Nazism." *American Scientist* (January–February): 50–57.

Tobach, E. 1972. "The Meaning of the Cryptanthroparion." In *Genetics,*

Environment and Behavior, ed. L. Ehrman, G. Omenn, and E. Caspari, 219–39. New York: Academic Press.

Watson, L. 1979. "Homosexuals." In *Mental Disorder or Madness?* ed. E. M. Bates and P. R. Wilson, 134–61. Brisbane: Queensland University Press.

Weiner, J. S. 1954. "Nose Shape and Climate." Reprinted in *Race and Social Difference,* ed. P. Baxter and B. Sanson, 44–47. 1972. Harmondsworth: Penguin.

West, D. J. 1977. *Homosexuality Re-Examined.* London: Duckworth.

Whitlock, F. A. 1979. "Psychsurgery." In *Mental Disorder or Madness?,* ed. E. M. Bates and P. R. Wilson, 181–201. Brisbane: Queensland University Press.

Wilson, E. O. 1975. *Sociobiology: A New Synthesis.* Cambridge, Mass.: Harvard University Press.

Worsley, P. 1972. "Colonialism and Categories." In *Race and Social Difference,* ed. P. Baxter and B. Sanson, 98–101. Harmondsworth: Penguin.

◆ PAMELA TROTMAN REID ◆

Racism and Sexism:
Comparisons and Conflicts

Are racism and sexism parallel or separate processes? Can we apply findings from one area of research to the other? Obviously, any response to such questions must be conditional, subject to definitions of the terms themselves as well as to the specific circumstances under which the questions are answered. These questions are necessarily asked, however, in light of this society's long-standing interest in racial prejudice and its increased awareness of discrimination based on gender. For this reason there is a need to understand the extent to which the biased treatment of women may be legitimately compared to that of blacks. In other words, can it be determined whether racism and sexism are parts of a generalized response set or if they are two different behaviors? In this essay, the analysis has two components. In the first part an examination of racism and sexism is presented with respect to a variety of dimensions relative to the assessment of the existence of parallelism: the definitions, the causes, and the scope of the problems. This review emphasizes social-psychological perspectives, although it is recognized that many other disciplines—such as economics, history, and political science—have contributed to the literature on racism and sexism. The second part of the essay deals with the impact of both processes on black women, who have dual identi-

This essay was originally published in *Eliminating Racism: Profiles in Controversy*, edited by Phyllis Katz and Dalmas A. Taylor. It is reprinted here by permission of Plenum Publishing Corporation.

ties and are oppressed under each. In addition, the possibility that these processes may have an additive effect is explored. Specifically, in the second part of the essay, the conflicts arising from the racism and sexism that are presented to black women are examined. It is suggested that black women may need special consideration because of their unique position relative to the movements both for women's equity and for black civil rights.

COMPARISONS OF SEXISM AND RACISM

Definitions of Racism and Sexism

The terms *racism* and *sexism* are frequently used without definition in research literature and in discussion. Indeed, the terms may have such widespread usage that most people believe that they are aware of what is meant. It seems necessary, however, to examine carefully the various ways in which the terms are described so that we may determine whether the concepts described in various situations are actually similar.

Consideration of the terms *racism* and *sexism* may begin with the definitions in the 1975 edition of *Webster's New Collegiate Dictionary. Racism* was defined first as "a belief that race is a primary determinant of human traits and capacities and that racial differences produce an inherent superiority of a particular race." In the second definition, provided by the synonym *racialism,* there is reference to prejudice or discrimination. The same dictionary defined *sexism* as "prejudice or discrimination against women." There is obviously some imbalance in the development of the two concepts based on this common source. In defining *racism,* there is the assumption of a belief system that can support or, at least, explain any discriminatory attitudes or behavior. For *sexism,* no such system is explicitly presented in the definition. The lack of any explanation for sexism may result either from an assumption of a common experience that does not need explication, or from the fact that the concept of sexism does not yet have the history of examination and research which racism has.

Another definition of *racism* is the classic in social psychology from the preface to the 1954 edition of *The Nature of Prejudice* (Allport 1979): "an antipathy based upon a faulty and inflexible generalization. It may be felt or expressed. It may be directed toward a group as a whole, or toward an individual because he is a member of that group" (9). This description of racism—or, more accurately, of "negative ethnic prejudice"—appears to be as easily applicable to the concept of sexism as it is to racism. The definition includes the mode of racist expression, covert or overt; sexist attitudes and behavior may also take these forms. The definition indicates the process involved in racism (faulty generalization), a process identical to the stereotyping that occurs in sexism. Finally, the affective dimension described by Allport (antipathy) and the object of the negative expression (an individual or a group) are both common to racism and sexism. In fact, Allport recognized that sex was the basis of certain discriminatory behavior. He pointed out examples of antifeminism, which, he stated, clearly demonstrated the basic characteristics of prejudice (33–34).

Parallelism between racism and sexism may also be inferred from an examination of the definition developed more recently by Chesler (1976). In his review of contemporary theories of racism Chesler focused on "institutional white racism," describing it in this way: "acts or institutional procedures which help create or perpetuate sets of advantages or privileges for whites and exclusions or deprivations for minority groups" (22). Important to this definition is Chesler's assumption of "an ideology of explicit or implicit superiority or advantage of one racial group over another, plus the institutional power to implement that ideology in social operations" (22). The picture of blacks as powerless with respect to social institutions is also reflected in the discrimination experienced by women. Both groups have had to deal with the expectation and assumption that white men were better suited to certain positions, such as supervisory and managerial positions (Kanter 1977). Both groups have a history of exclusion from prestigious community organizations and clubs (e.g., the Jaycees for the first time accepted women as members in 1986). In addition, both groups have faced limitations on their acceptance to schools and universities. As defined in this research, then, institutional racism appears to have strong parallels with institutional sexism. Although the similarities of sexism to racism are evident for the mode of expression and the process in both the Allport and the Chesler definitions, neither addresses the root or the cause of the negative feelings that exist. The causes of racism and sexism have, however, been offered as an explanation in a number of other theories.

Causes of Racism and Sexism

Ashmore and Del Boca (1976) distinguished between explanations of prejudice that focus on intrapersonal factors and those that emphasize interpersonal relations. The intrapersonal theories have frequently been applied to racist behavior, especially by black researchers. When racism is attributed to intrapersonal factors, personality or cognitive processes are proposed. For example, Biassey (1972) stated that "much of prejudice and racism in America is paranoid in origin and developed by the self-serving, defensive maneuvers of the majority" (353). Comer (1980) similarly defined *racism* as "a low-level defense and adjustment mechanism utilized by groups to deal with psychological and social insecurities" (363). Delaney (1980) also described racism as being the result of a disturbed personality. He called it a "classic pathology with the usual destructive behavior" and as a sickness that "runs deep in the history of this nation" (368). Research on cognitive causes of racism has typically examined the role of perception, cognitive consistency, and belief system congruency. For example, Mezei (1971) found that race was more important than belief congruency in determining social intimacy. Katz (1976) also demonstrated the existence of cognitive components in the development of racism. She found that, in children, the perception of racial differences in physical appearance was accompanied by an awareness of racial status.

The intrapersonal factors are not typically used to describe the roots of sexism. Instead of being labeled as pathological, individuals with sexist attitudes are considered either misinformed, uninformed, or obtuse. Although some writers have suggested that sexists experience anxiety about changing roles or that liberated women are perceived as a threat to the male ego, sexists are more frequently viewed as lacking sensitivity to women's perspectives than as having a deep-seated personality problem. In fact, although most researchers support explanations of racism which focus on the individual level (Ashmore and Del Boca 1976), feminist theorists emphasize societal level and political causes of sexism (Hyde 1985).

Among the interpersonal factors in racial prejudice acquisition which have been investigated are socialization processes, conformity to societal norms, and attribution theory. Researchers have shown how parents, peers, schools, and mass media have instructed the individual directly and indirectly in the dominant cultural belief patterns (Ashmore and Del Boca 1976). Studies of attitudes toward women have also demonstrated the importance of socialization and the agents of that process (Shaffer 1985). In addition to the pressures of family and society, racist belief systems are supported by the type of information available through the media concerning blacks and other underrepresented groups. The image of these groups is distorted; thus, the media actually encourage faulty attributions about the roots of social problems relevant to the specific group (Ashmore and Del Boca 1976). This distortion of image, as well as the other interpersonal factors, appears to be equally applicable to women and to blacks.

The problems of racism and sexism are most accurately described as having multiple causes. Intrapersonal, interpersonal, and societal factors must be recognized as contributors having summative, as well as interactive, effects. Early childhood experiences, familial attitudes, media influences, and peer and social group standards—all play a role in the final pattern of attitudes and behaviors that are adopted by white individuals toward blacks and by males toward females. In a comprehensive review of the early developmental precursors of racial and gender attitudes Katz (1983) underscored the complexity of the issues involved. She noted that explanations rooted in biological, cognitive, and learning theories have been proposed to explain children's responses to gender and racial differences. Although Katz suggested the existence of several similarities in the developmental processes underlying race and sex discrimination, she also indicated that there are differences. One important difference is that gender role expectations change with age, whereas racial attitudes seem to be more fixed. It appears, then, that racism and sexism must be understood in terms of a number of dimensions. Therefore, an evaluation of the scope of the problems of racism and sexism may be a starting point in pursuing an understanding of these concepts and the extent to which each affects American social behavior.

Scope of Racism and Sexism

"Racism is as American as apple pie" was a favorite saying of H. Rap Brown, a civil rights activist of the late 1960s. Although racist attitudes and practices certainly exist in many societies, there appears to be a uniqueness in the present form and function of racism as practiced toward blacks in the United States in comparison with the racism practiced in some other countries. Indeed, several researchers have noted that the type of racism directed at blacks in the United States has resulted from a combination of economic, historic, political, religious, and social conditions that are peculiar to this society (Comer 1980; Delaney 1980). Blackwell (1985) suggested that the resulting U.S. brand of racism may be seen in the adaptations that the black community has made by forming an amalgamation of African and American cultures. The adaptations made by the black people, he suggested, emanated from the segregation and exclusion from mainstream social institutions which both forced and allowed the establishment of parallel black institutions. Black people, rejected by the white community, developed their own sets of community standards and goals. In addition to the lack of social status, the minority position of blacks in a society controlled by majority rights contributes to keeping black people on the fringes of power.

The dimensions of sexism seem to have little parallelism with those of racism. First of all, the sexism practiced in the United States is not considered uniquely American. In fact, the universality of sexist practices, assumptions, and policy have been proclaimed by feminist writers from diverse disciplines (Rogers 1981). Although a few feminist anthropologists argue that, through the domestic sphere, women have the ability to wield great social power, most research has focused on demonstrating that all women are oppressed whether they realize it or not. With respect to social standing in public areas, it can be argued that women have long been on the fringes. They have been excluded and discriminated against in many segments of the labor force and in the political arena. Yet, although women, like blacks, have been grossly underrepresented in positions of power and authority, *women are not a minority group,* despite an attempt to claim that underdog status for them (e.g., Hacker 1981).

Hacker and Weisstein (cited in Cox 1981) have both used the term *minority group* to demonstrate the similarity of the status of women and blacks in the United States. They have identified similarities in the stereotyped behaviors ascribed to each, in the rationalizations of status for each, and in discrimination against and the adaptive behaviors of each. By minimizing the issue of numbers, however, Hacker and Weisstein have failed to recognize the differences in the scope of each problem and the prognosis for improvement. The problem of racism toward blacks as a uniquely American issue is very much related to the minority (meaning few in numbers) position of blacks. One reason is that the elimination of racism may be viewed as benefiting a group of "outsiders" (nonwhites), who constitute only a small proportion of the population. For the most part white people do not believe that the elimination of racism will actually provide any personal gain for them (Pence 1982). Contributing to the notion that racism impacts only negatively on the victims is the isolation that may often be found to exist between the racial groups. It is completely within the realm of possibility for a white person to live all of his or her life without ever engaging in a personal relationship with a black person. The fact that many white people are unacquainted with any black person makes racism almost a theoretical issue for them. It also contributes to the belief that the elimination of racism would help only blacks. On the other hand, sexism is, at the same time, both a personal issue and a universal problem. Even a white man (the traditional embodiment of sexual oppression) may become concerned about discrimination directed at his mother, his wife, his daughter, or a female friend. The socialization of men and women is intertwined intimately at a level that different ethnic groups will probably never attain. Although whites and blacks may be socialized without being aware of each other, this is not likely for girls and boys.

The issue of numbers also makes it clear that, even at their most effective, the most blacks may hope to achieve is some level of proportional representation. It is, at least theoretically, possible for white women to become the dominant force in the society. The possibilities may be illustrated by the dramatic gains of women in a variety of areas since only the mid-1970s. For example, the percentage of women in managerial and administrator positions increased from 17.6 percent in 1972 to 27.5 percent in 1982; women employed as lawyers and judges increased from 3.8 percent to 14.1 percent during the same period; those in personnel and labor relations, from 31 percent to 49.95 percent (Blackwell 1985, 39–40). It should be noted that these data do not distinguish between the gains of white women and black women. Although black men and women have also made gains since the mid-1970s, it often appears that the ceiling may have been reached and that some advantages are slipping away. Support for the claims that blacks are in a worse economic position now than they were in the mid-1970s is found in the *Current Population Reports* (cited in Blackwell 1985, 55). The downward shifting of economic conditions for blacks, who are historically bound to the lower classes, has also been found to have had a deleterious effect on their educational advances. Poverty levels among women are also more common. In examining the data on the feminization of poverty, it should be noted that blacks and other minority women contribute disproportionately to this problem. As we will discuss in the second section of this essay, black women experience double discrimination.

Methodological Issues

Researchers frequently suggest that the solution to many social problems lies in a better understanding of the issues involved. To facilitate understanding, then, they propose to do more research, ignoring the fact that the research methods themselves may interfere with progress toward the goal of understanding. The assumption is that the more research available, the clearer the problem and its solution will become. Yet analyses of research on racism and sexism indicate that, in many instances, methodological bias may obfuscate rather than clarify the issues under investigation. In fact, it may be demonstrated that bias in research not only exacerbates some aspects of the racism and sexism problems but actually represents a subtle manifestation of the researchers' biases. Examination of some of the assumptions, biases, foci, and goals of research on women has identified some of the areas that are a problem. Many of these areas seem similarly relevant to studies of blacks (and to studies of other ethnic minority groups).

In her review of feminist criticism of methodology Grady (1981) demonstrated that bias exists at every stage of the research process. She found that the traditional (i.e., white male as norm) perspective dominates the selection of topics for research, the subject selection, the operationalization of variables, the conceptualization preceding tests of sex differences, and the interpretation of the results. Additionally, it appeared that there was a male bias in the determination of whether an investigation would be published. The bias evidenced in the research on women may also be seen in research on ethnic minorities. In the selection of topics scientists have obviously been influenced by gender role stereotypes. Some research questions frequently studied in women have not, until recently, been investigated among men—for example, the relationship of moods to hormonal cycles and the effect of parental age on offspring. Williams (1980) assessed the work of white researchers in the black community with respect to topic selection. He concluded that, in many studies, researchers "looked for and found pathology" while ignoring strengths and adaptive capacities. According to Williams, the majority of problems researched in black communities are system induced (e.g., health, education, and penal), yet the researchers continue to investigate the black victims as the root of the problems. In research women, too, have been cast as problems, not victims. Hare-Mustin (1983) examined sex bias in psychotherapy and concluded that psychological problems of women reflect societal conditions and attitudes. She noted, however, that the solutions offered deal with the individual and actually combine with other sexist forces affecting women's lives. Unger (1979) also noted that psychological research is designed to focus on internal causes as the source of problems. In studies on both women and black men the issues are typically "how these people are different" (from white men) and "how that difference can be minimized."

Feminists have also claimed bias in research studies on the grounds that there is often no conceptual justification for the many instances of all-male samples. It has been shown that even in comparative behavioral investigations animal samples are typically limited to males (Hyde and Rosenberg 1976). On the other hand, until recently the selection of female-only samples has been rare (Hyde 1985). Research on females was considered valid only if a comparison male group existed.

The problem of sample selection in race research has two aspects. First, as in research on women, there is a tendency to accept only studies that compare blacks with whites. Korchin (1980) revealed his experience of a rejection comment from a journal reviewer who assessed his research as "fatally flawed" because there was no comparison of his black sample with a white group. His anecdote is not at all unique. The value of studying diverse groups as an end in itself has not yet been fully appreciated. Additionally, in race research there appears to be an assumption that greater homogeneity exists among blacks (and other ethnic minorities) than among whites. For this reason very little attention has been paid to socioeconomic differences, to cultural background differences, or even to sex and age differences (Jackson 1980). In fact, Gary (1980) noted that there is a tendency for white researchers "to focus on the lowest income groups of black subjects, and to concentrate on captive subjects (prisoners, mental patients, school children)" (448–49).

The selection of subjects, then, clearly shapes the outcome of findings and represents scientists' implicit assumptions. There are obvious parallels for racism and sexism in how scientists approach investigations in each area because blacks and white women continue to be seen as deviants or as deficient in comparison to a white male norm. Sue (1983) stressed the importance of bicultural research that would "emphasize understanding of ethnic minority groups in their own terms" (588). Sue believes that psychologists err in allowing the "etic" approach (an acceptance of core similarities in all humans) to dominate their thinking and research. Although he recognized that the assumption of "universals" has some validity, he suggested that the recognition of cultural variance is also a valid and necessary objective.

Wallston (1981) observed that the socialization of researchers is another important part of the bias problem. She argued that professors have "the tendency to train people in our own image" (607). Because most professors are white men, traditional training often amounts to educating people to evaluate problems using the standards and norms of white men. Sue (1983) pointed out that, although the past notion of Anglo-Saxon cultural superiority is not accepted by most, training, testing, and other practices in education proceed as if it were. Many professional women and black men will admit that it is difficult for them to analyze their black and/or female experiences without the traditional perspectives they have adopted from their professors. They cannot easily develop theoretical frameworks that do not use terms and assumptions previously defined by white men. It may be even more difficult, however, for experienced white male researchers to accept new concepts, refutations of theoretical principles, or reinterpretations of longstanding data. Parlee (1981) believes that new theoretical perspectives will need powerful proponents. She suggested that women will have to become reviewers and editors if they wish to "determine what research is 'methodologically sound' enough and 'interesting' enough to publish" (641). The same suggestion has been made with respect to black scientists. In the field of psychology, however, whereas white women have made some strides toward increasing their numbers among publishing decision makers, the success of blacks in gaining access to the publication network has been relatively slight.

The analysis and interpretation of research data from a biased perspective has been demonstrated in studies of race differences as well as of sex differences. The most insidious aspect of this problem is that the bias may not be apparent, even to careful observers, because the researchers appear to follow sound methodological practice. For example, Jones (1983) was able to reveal the bias in published research comparing black and white children only by a complete reanalysis of the data. In his analysis, contrary to the published findings, black children were not more aggressive than white children. The actual difference was in his assumption that same-race, not cross-race, interactions should be used as the basis for the statistical comparisons. An example of research interpretation suggesting deviance in the black community is the labeling of black female assertiveness as "black matriarchy" and dominance. Similarly, interpretation bias has been found in the analysis of female behavior when expectations of inferiority are built into the variable labels. Unger (1979) cited the example of the terminology used in perception research, that is, "field-dependent versus field-independent." She pointed out that the value-laden term *dependent,* given to behavior that is more often female, promotes the conclusion that one perceptual type is better than the other. She suggested that an alternative term—for example, *field-sensitive*—would have very different connotations. Another example of sex bias has been noted in researchers' interpretation of parental behavior. When a child does not have the benefit of regular paternal influence, the circumstance is termed *father absence;* if it is the mother's influence that is missing, the term is *maternal deprivation.* The implication is that maternal deprivation is a worse condition, and the unproven assumption is that mothers are more necessary to a child's well-being. A more extensive analysis of methodological concerns from a feminist perspective is provided by Wallston and Grady (1985).

Current Perceptions of Racism and Sexism

White racism has been a topic of continuing concern to blacks in recent years. The concern is due to the reemergence of white hostility in subtle, as well as blatant, ways, after an apparent decline during the heyday of the civil rights movement. The reappearance of overt racist behavior has been attributed to the belief on the part of many whites, and even some blacks, that racism is no longer an issue to which our society need attend. The fact that blacks have entered many areas of public and private employment, that political awareness among blacks has increased, and that admission to educational institutions and to public accommodations seems assured by law appears to many as prima facie evidence that racial discrimination is a thing of the past. There is actually little research support for the claim that racism has disappeared (Sue 1983).

Articles about the "new racism" have appeared with some regularity over the past few years in periodicals and newspapers, such as the *Washington Post* and the *New Republic*. Despite many counterclaims that racism in the United States is now different, there is a growing recognition that behaviors that were unacceptable and defined as racist a decade ago are now increasingly apparent. Barker (1981) explained that past emphasis on explanations of racism in terms of inferiority and superiority simply concealed some of the other reasons for racial prejudice. He hypothesized a link between race and national unity, suggesting that racism exists because certain groups are perceived as "outsiders." McConahay and Hough (1976) theorized that racism is now more complex than in the past. They suggested that symbolic issues associated with blacks (e.g., busing and welfare) offer the opportunity for hostile expression while direct antiblack sentiments are suppressed. This *symbolic racism* has been defined as the feeling by whites that blacks are making illegitimate demands for changes (Sears and McConahay 1973). Although the concept of out-groups and the use of symbolic codes are not really new, the fact that research still attempts to define *racism* indicates that important questions still have not been satisfactorily resolved.

Concurrent with the surges and declines of attentiveness to racism have been changes in the amount of significance attached to instances of sexism in our society. Today sexual harassment, violence toward women, pornography, and rape are among the topics subjected to public scrutiny. A number of programs have been instituted to encourage equity in the education of women in nontraditional areas. Women are slowly gaining acceptance in formerly all-male occupations. Attention to training male personnel in the avoidance of overt discrimination is an important component in the management of many large companies. Widely adopted editorial policies exist that recommend nonsexist language in books and articles. Yet only a few decades ago sexism was little more than a joke. An example of the disregard of sexist attitudes fifty years ago is found in a 1945 research study on prejudice (Dyer, cited in Allport 1979). In the experiment the researcher disregarded boys' negative statements about girls while recording expressions of prejudice against other groups. Not only were the hostile comments about girls rejected as examples of prejudice, they were, in fact, believed to be normal responses of adolescent boys. Researchers today are consistently reminded to guard against obviously sexist hypotheses and to investigate their previously conceived assumptions regarding sex role behavior. In fact, concern about sex roles appears to have overtaken attention to race relations, as indicated easily by the number of articles, books, journals, and magazines devoted to each subject.

In examining the parallels between racism and sexism, one must wonder whether one set of data may be sufficient to explain most dimensions of discrimination. Although many commonalities exist, the number of differences suggests that problem solving in one area may not be facilitated by the practice of too quickly generalizing to the other. On the surface, it appears that types of discriminatory behavior, psychological effects, and even social responses to discrimination are similar for blacks and white women. The tendency of social scientists to discuss racism and sexism on an abstract level, however, limits the applicability of research to real-world conditions. In fact, although scientists appear to consider racism and sexism discrete problems, under several conditions the processes may be interacting. What impact might result from this interaction? What conflicts occur for the victims? To investigate some of the issues we must go beyond abstractions and consider some specifics. Black women provide an example of those who are influenced by both racism and sexism. Although there are other women of color who are also influenced by both processes, there is more research available on black women than on other groups of women of color.

RACE AND SEX CONFLICTS: THE CASE OF BLACK WOMEN

The possibility that race and sex prejudice may have interactive, or even additive, results has seldom been considered by social scientists. Psychological research and theory have typically ignored the possibility that gender differences may mediate reactions to racial characteristics. Similarly, studies of discrimination based on sex often fail to recognize the existence of race as a factor. In this section, therefore, consideration is given to the problems of dual identity for women of color, that is, an examination is made of their identification as members of an ethnic minority group and as women. Specifically, the case of black women is considered because of their greater numbers among people of color and because of the long history of discrimination against blacks in the United States. This section also explores the conflicts that black women experience as the result of their dual allegiance to the civil rights movement and the women's movement. Race and gender stereotypes, as well as the available research data, are examined for their impact on present behavior and attitudes.

Gender Differences in the Treatment of Blacks

Historically, the sexual attractiveness of black women was vigorously denied by white women and even by white men, despite evidence of many sexual liaisons between black female slaves and their white male masters. The denials and distortions of the relationship of white men and black women during slavery have helped to erase the image of black women as victims; instead, a stereotype of black women as licentious and promiscuous has developed. hooks (1981) suggested that white men were able to act out their misogynistic attitudes through their treatment of black women. She cited documentary evidence that colonial white men terrorized black women through rape and sexual torture. White women, hooks hypothesized, either were convinced that black women deserved such treatment or accepted them as scapegoats. Other researchers (Ashmore and Del Boca 1976; Simpson and Yinger 1953) have used the defense mechanism concepts, repression and guilt, and projection theory to make a similar point about the sexual exploitation of black women during slavery. These researchers have described a theory of antiblack prejudice in which whites projected their tabooed sexual drives onto blacks.

This apparent early recognition of sexual differences among blacks, however, was considered only when it served the purposes of the oppressors. The idea that black women or men were eligible for any privileges or power because of gender was certainly a notion treated as absurd and impractical. Both black women and black men were treated in the past as children with no rights to respect, no power, and no authority because of their adulthood. In social status and in discrimination, therefore, it has been assumed that black men and black women are social equals. Although many of the attitudes and prejudices of the past have been disgarded, this assumption of "equality under oppression" appears to remain. The volumes of books devoted to the study of racism attest to this assumption by their failure to discuss the relationship of gender or sexual status to the facets and forms of racial discrimination which existed in the past or have developed over the years (e.g., Barker 1981; Dorn 1979; Katz 1978; Willie 1983). In fact, the consequences of racism have not been gender blind. The reality of the masculinity or femininity of black persons has often been integrally related to the reactions of white men and white women. Furthermore, the domains of maleness and femaleness have also been defined as important by black men and women for themselves as they have struggled to be accepted into the mainstream of U.S. society. There has even developed an idealization of the mainstream model of gender roles in the black community, even when the likelihood of maintaining the ideal was considered low (Hannerz 1969).

Sexism: Conflict with Black Men

White behavioral and social scientists note with much interest the efforts of past and present-day European immigrants to become acculturated and accepted into the U.S. mainstream. Similar efforts by black families have, on the other hand, often been derided and misinterpreted. One aspect of black family life which has received this treatment in research and popular media is black family relationships. The well-accepted myth is that the black woman is the head of a matriarchal structure. The stereotype of the controlling black woman has gained such strength, despite refuting empirical evidence and denials by black researchers (Jackson 1973; Willie 1983), that the actual relationship between black women and black men has not been fully recognized. For this reason, it has been a surprise to some that the patriarchal philosophy is alive and strong in the black community and that some black men have fully adopted a sexist perspective.

It is increasingly obvious that many black men strongly desire the recognition and control that they believe is due to all *men*. In fact, some black men, in the effort to enhance male power, suggest that black women should restrict their thrust for opportunities and self-determination. Hare (1978), for example, in discussing the inequities of full-time earnings based on race and sex, complained that black women's gains have severely limited "the black male's ability to prevail and compete in a perpetually patriarchal society" (4). His unquestioning acceptance of men's rights and power is also evident in his statement that "the black man will be able to *bring the woman along* in our common struggle, so we will not need a black women's liberation movement" (Hare 1971, 34; emphasis added). Hare has not been alone in his desire for black women to stand aside while black men take leadership positions or in his predictions of disaffection between black men and black women if they do not. Staples (1981), in fact, blamed the economic independence of black women, past and present, for dissolved marriages and suggested that educational and economic success "detracts" from a woman's desirability as a mate.

There are also black men who, rather than proclaim their sexism, appear to ignore the importance of gender differences in determining the black experience. Jenkins (1982) and Pugh (1972), for example, both discussed the black experience from a psychological perspective and yet almost completely excluded any mention of issues related to sex. The denial of the gender factor by black men, in effect, suggests the strategy advocated by Staples (1981), that is, attack racism first and, afterward, consider what to do about the problem of sexism. This approach, however, requires women to relinquish their needs as women and to postpone their liberation.

Black women have recognized for many years that "sexism could serve black men as well as it has whites if they too could manage to get ahead at the expense of their women" (Torrey 1979, 47). Even during the abolitionist era Sojourner Truth, a black suffragist, warned, "If colored men get their rights, and not colored women theirs, you see the colored men will be masters over the women, and it will be just as bad as before" (cited in Hood 1978, 48). Although some black men believe that the civil rights movement's main goal has been to establish a black male power structure, many others agree with black women who view the freedom of black men as inextricably tied to that of black women (e.g., Casenave 1981). Research has shown that these beliefs are backed by actions—for example, egalitarian decision-making characterizes black husband-wife relationships (Mack 1974)—and that black men participate in child care more often than white men (Daneal 1975). Black men are not alone, however, in their divisions with respect to race and sex allegiance. Black women have also made claims and counterclaims regarding the side that they should take. Often an adversarial position is drawn which has black men on one side and white women on the other; black women are left to decide where they should stand.

Dual Identity: Conflict for Black Women

The double bind in which black women find themselves consists of the conflicting demands of racial identity and gender identity. For most black women there is a clear solution to this dilemma: end racism *and* sexism. The consensus is strong. Black women who castigate white women for their role in the oppression of blacks (e.g., LaRue 1970), together with those who view black men as "absorbing the dominant white male disease" (Lorde 1979), recognize the need to respect all human potential. Yet black women seriously question the notion that they have the power to effect such social changes, and they wonder who does and who will. Taking sides with white women is critically assessed by some. For example, LaRue (1970) asked, "If white women remained silent while white men kept the better positions and opportunities, can we really expect them to be more open-minded when placed in direct competition for jobs?" (19). Additionally, few black women expect that white women will rectify the injustices of the society. In fact, black women who work in white organizations have often learned to be wary of whites who wish to act as interpreters of their experience (Gilkes 1983). With respect to their positive or negative influence on black men both Sojourner (1979) and ya Salaam (1979) contended that black women do not have the power to affect black men outside the sphere of home and family.

Although black women may view their power as limited, many are socialized to accept the responsibility of working toward the "betterment of their race." The women who seem to have a commitment to serving their community through active involvement cope with their frustrations, in part, by giving high value to their own experiences. One woman described the situation this way: "If I could change anything in my life, I don't think I would. . . . You really do grow; you learn a lot from life; it makes you very strong; you have to be strong; you don't have much choice; you learn responsibility at a very early age, because you have to" (quoted in Gilkes 1983, 135). The goals toward which black women apply themselves are varied and often conflicting. Yet the poignancy of the effort must be recognized in the articles, books, and speeches given day after day. Perhaps the spirit of many is captured in the words of a black woman, a mother, a community organizer, and a women's rights activist: "In black women's liberation . . . we're fighting for the right to be different and not be punished for it. . . . I want the right to be black and me"(Wright 1972, 608). Frequently, however, black women are judged against standards constructed for white women.

Race Differences in the Treatment of Women

The race difference most often cited in demographic and research literature is the employment participation rate of black and of white women. Black women are the second highest in the percentage employed of any female labor group (Asian-American women are highest). Black women contribute more income and share more family power with their spouses than do women in comparable white families (Richmond-Abbott 1983). Additionally, McAdoo (1980) found no differences in the types of jobs held by black middle-class mothers who were married and by those who were single parents. Obviously, however, the single-parent families were more vulnerable to economic stress because of differences in overall income (Walker and Wallston 1985).

Along with the expectation of their economic contributions black women are also called on by their families to fulfill traditional duties and to give emotional support (McAdoo 1978). In response to the demands for energy, resources, and time, black women have developed a life-style of involvement in an extended kin network that appears to characterize them more than it does white women. Regardless of social class status, the majority of black women remain connected to relatives and "fictive kin" through their adult lives, participating in an exchange of child care and emotional and financial help (McAdoo 1980). Although the network of relatives and friends is regarded as a valuable cultural pattern that supports black women, it is a double-edged sword. Those who get assistance must also give. Belle (1982) noted that for women struggling in poverty the assistance received does not always compensate for the additional stress placed on them by the responsibility to reciprocate the aid.

The importance of family and work notwithstanding, we must also consider, as part of the treatment of women, the public and private standards that society establishes to judge feminine value. All children, boys and girls, develop feelings of self-respect and self-esteem based in large part on society's reactions to them. Society sets standards not only for appropriate behavior but also for physical attractiveness. The standard set for the ideal American woman is unambiguously white. In fact, the black woman is the antithesis of the American standard. This point is repeated in the print, film, and television images of black women. In their rare appearances in children's books black female characters were found to be presented in stereotypical female roles (e.g., mother or maid) and to be depicted as unattractive (Dickerson 1980). Black female characters on television programs were high in dominance, high in nurturance, and low in achievement behavior; they were portrayed as significantly different from white women (Reid 1979). Based on her analysis of media images, Rawles (1978) emphatically stated that "identifying with the image of white femininity is an exercise in self-hate for black women" (245). Although white women also decry the stereotyping and the limited images of white women's roles, they are not, as black women are, subjected to the consistent and virtually unrelenting representation of themselves on television as castrating, immoral, and ugly.

Racism: Conflict with White Women

The notion that black women hold values that differ from those of white women has been successfully dispelled by the results of a large-scale survey conducted in 1974 and 1979 under the sponsorship of Virginia Slims cigarettes. Heiss (1981) analyzed these survey data on motivation for marrying, acceptance of nontraditional family forms, and acceptance of reasons for divorce. Race commonalities were more evident than differences. Yet, although many values of black and white women are the same, the social and economic conditions under which they live their lives are, in the main, widely disparate. Bernard (1981) described the world of white women as "primarily a middle-class, if not a wholly egalitarian, world" (254). This middle-class classification has also been given to the women's movement by others (Bardwick 1979; Frieze, Parsons, Johnson, Ruble, and Zellman 1978). The world of black women, however, is best typified as lower class and poor, although it is the middle-class and professional black women who are more likely to have the education and opportunity to give voice to black concerns.

Despite differences in economic levels, black women are at least as likely as white women to advocate female liberation (Hemmons 1980) and are even twice as likely to approve the women's movement goals (Harris poll, cited in Torrey 1979). Therefore, a question often arises about the lack of the noticeable participation of black and other women of color in national and local women's organizations. Although black and white women share a common oppressor—white men—there are many differences in life experiences which suggest to some black women the need for separate paths (Hood 1978). Among the differences between white women and black women are the conflicting allegiance to race versus sex which black women often experience but which white women do not; the greater level of social acceptability that white women receive compared with black women; and finally, the fact that white women are necessary to the existence of white men, whereas black women are not necessary. Although the differences in life-styles and expectations may explain, to some extent, the absence of black women from women's movement activities, the presence of racism is also part of the answer.

From the earliest days of the suffragist movement there has been a recognition by white women that black women and black men were both their allies and their competitors in the struggle for political power. There were, of course, among the women's movement, staunch abolitionists. hooks (1981) claimed, however, that there is "little historical evidence to document the assertion that white women as a collective group or white women's rights advocates are part of an anti-racist tradition. . . . They attacked slavery, not racism" (125). The fact that some white women are clearly racist has not escaped the notice of black women who have attempted to align themselves with feminist organizations. Although Alice Walker (1982) declared it is "inherently an impossibility" to be both truly feminist and racist, the late civil rights activist Fannie Lou Hamer described the conflict with white women this way: "The white woman felt like she was more than us . . . you know the white male, didn't go and brainwash the black man and the black woman, he brainwashed his wife too. He made her think that she was an angel" (quoted in Hood 1978, 50).

Just as some black men have ignored the needs of black women as women and have rejected the notion that sexism is an important problem for them, white women have frequently ignored the unique needs of black women as blacks. This omission has been interpreted as rejection and racism. It is evident in many of the growing number of scholarly books in fields such as psychology, sociology, and history that *women* means white women and that other women are treated as afterthoughts, if included at all. Just as white men have overlooked the attitudes, contributions, and perspectives of white women, black women have been similarly treated. For example, in Strasser's history (1982) of American housework only one paragraph was devoted to black women's plight; their importance was seen as being the new servant class, as Irish and other immigrant workers moved up in social status. Greenspan (1983) did not give any consideration to racial factors in her book on women's therapy; neither did Scarf (1980) in hers on depression, nor did Notman and Nadelson (1978) in theirs on health care. One explanation for these omissions is that the authors did not believe that any racial differences existed among white women and women of color. This seems highly unlikely. A more plausible explanation is probably that consideration of ethnic differences remains unimportant to many white researchers, whether they are male or female. Gaertner's explication (1976) of liberal racist behavior includes the definition of the aversive racist as one who "tries to avoid contact with blacks." This concept supports the notion that the exclusion of ethnic concerns may be interpreted as racism, whether conscious or not.

Even when the concerns of black women are incorporated into the feminist discussion, the problem of racism is not often considered in much depth. A review of psychology of women textbooks showed that most offered token or no references to African-American women (Brown, Goodwin, Hall, and Jackson-Lowman 1985). Admittedly, some white women are uncomfortable about dealing with this problem (Pence 1982). One example of this discomfort is the discourse on black women and racism found in Bernard (1981). She began her exploration of racism toward blacks by focusing on the hatred it engendered among black women for whites and ended by claiming that black women hate white women for taking black men. No discussion of the detrimental effect of racism on black women was included. A brief reference to white women's racism during the suffragist era was explained by the fact that it "made more sense to have [southern congressmen] as allies than as enemies of the women's [sic] cause" (340). Increasingly, however, the realization of the impact of racism as a daily event in the lives of black women has become evident, as many recent women's studies textbooks and courses have attempted to include issues affecting people of color and to present relevant research on these issues (e.g., Hyde 1985; Richmond-Abbott 1983).

Conflicts in Research

The paradox of the black woman's situation is, to paraphrase de Beauvoir (cited in Bernard 1981), "that they belong at one and the same time to the white world, to the male world and to the other spheres in which those worlds are challenged; shut up in their world, surrounded by the others, they can settle down nowhere in peace" (20). Compounding the double conflict of racism and sexism for black women is the fact that few others understand the pressures endured. The extent of the divisions with black men because of sexism and with white women because of racism are infrequently assessed; the comparisons most often made treat sex and race as separate phenomena. Gurin and Pruitt (1978) pointed out the effect of assessing race and sex discrimination separately. For example, economic comparisons that examine the relative position of black men to white men and black women to white women result in the conclusion that black men experience greater discrimination, despite evidence indicating that black women have the lowest salaries of any race-sex group. The comparison that would indicate the results of black women's experiencing both sex and race discrimination is typically neglected. This was the case in a study of the relationship of racism and sexism in the job market (Szymanski 1976). The indicator of sexual discrimination was the ratio of white female to white male median earnings. The indicator of racial discrimination was the ratio of black male to white male median earnings. Black females were alternately considered

"Third World people" and "women," as the need of the study dictated.

Similarly distorted assessments have been made of comparisons that purport to demonstrate both race and sex effects for educational attainment (Gump and Rivers 1975) and occupational aspirations (Gurin and Epps 1975). One negative example was found in a recent book on the psychology of sex roles. Richmond-Abbott (1983) reviewed the research on early-school sex role socialization and found agreement on the fact that teachers give less attention to girls and that school materials are not relevant to blacks. She then concluded, however, that black girls were considered less deviant in the class than black boys and that the likelihood of some black female teachers meant that the school experience "probably doesn't hurt their [black girls'] self-image as much as it might hurt their female white classmates" (136). This conclusion, drawn from research that did not compare the sex-race groups, is not unusual. In effect, it underscores the observation that there exists a dearth of research and documentation on the effects of discrimination specifically directed at the black girl or the black woman.

In assessments of research in the area of sexism and racism it has become apparent that the analysis of these processes as independent functions is inadequate. Instead, racism and sexism should be examined in relationship to each other (Smith and Stewart 1983). It has been suggested, therefore, that researchers adopt a model of research that incorporates a contextual and an interactive framework, that is, a model in which the experiences of black women are compared with those of the other three sex-race groups within specific social situations, rather than the continued use of sex and race as independent status characteristics.

The need for an understanding of the interactive process of racism and sexism has been demonstrated in only a few studies. For example, an investigation of high school students' career development suggested that for black female adolescents, the effects of racism and sexism are combined as well as independent (Chester 1983). Adams's analysis (1983) of sex and race status characteristics on dominance behavior in college students indicated the need to consider context in social situations. Adams found that black women did not respond as predicted by their sex or race group. In fact, she concluded that the statuses associated with sex and race were not constant across situations and did not combine by any simple averaging process. Lykes (1983) concurred in the assessment of context as an important factor in determining behavior in situations of discrimination. An exploration of the effects of institutional oppression and individual prejudice on black women indicated that highly successful black women depend on contextual cues and use them to respond differently to the sexism and the racism that they encounter. Specifically, Lykes found that situational factors, such as the racial composition of the workplace, affected both the degree of directness and the flexibility of coping in black women.

The investigators who recommended the interactive and contextual approach presumed this methodological strategy capable of affecting the integration of the disparate views of black women which have emanated from society and the social sciences. The question that must also be considered, however, is whether an accurate description of black women's behavior will in any way resolve or ameliorate the conflicts of gender and race identity which will be encountered. Although investigations into the forms and purposes of discrimination could be developed further, at some point the focus of research should be shifted to illuminate the means by which discrimination and its effects can be minimized.

Diversity versus Divisions

The Hunter College Women's Studies Collective (1983) admitted that "women are divided not only by race and class but also by age and sexual orientation" (12). They argued, however, that any resistance to one type of discrimination is resistance to all. Although in theory this seems to be sound reasoning, the argument is unconvincing in light of the evidence that many workers committed to one cause exhibit much less concern about other inequities. Bardwick (1979) appeared to concur in this assessment. She stated that "divisiveness within the women's movement came about in the first place because of the diversity of women. . . . Divisiveness between women is increased when a commitment to women seems to require less commitment to men and to children" (151). It would appear, therefore, almost unnatural to expect that black women (or white women) could or would totally divorce themselves from the policies and practices of their fathers, brothers, sons, and husbands.

Nevertheless, the increased effort by many feminist groups to integrate the concerns, problems, and positions of black women and other women of color with those of white women is a positive step toward eliminating some of the racial divisions and conflicts now existing. We can continue to seek our commonalities in addition to recognizing our differences. Yet the difficulty in avoiding racist traps in interpreting data and making assumptions is greater than many realize. We have all been socialized into the same society, although with different perspectives on it. Both sexism and racism are ingrained in our society's expectations, and they operate together in ways that we are trained to accept. The admission of this condition may allow us to examine more realistically the possibilities for positive social change.

SUMMARY AND CONCLUSIONS

A review of the social-psychological literature reveals many similarities between the processes of racism and sexism. The definitions of each indicate the operation of a basic belief system that describes the objects of the discrimination, either women or minorities, as inferior to white men. Multiple causes—interpersonal, intrapersonal, and societal—appear to be necessary to explain the development and manifestation of each process. Analyses of methodological strategies demonstrated that bias exists in research on race and sex discrimination based on assumptions, samples, procedures, and interpretations. The commonalities found between the two processes, however, are not sufficient cause to ignore the many differences. The differences, in fact, lead to the conclusion that racism and sexism must be studied and understood as they operate separately in society.

Among the differences between racism and sexism the difference of scope appears to have the most far-reaching implications for social power. The manifestation of racism in the United States is described as resulting from some uniquely American situations, whereas sexism is viewed as more universal in form and practice. The significance of the numerical minority status of ethnic group members contrasts with the proportions of women in society. The notion is that women have, at least theoretically, the potential for equal status through numbers. In current perspectives on the progress of women versus people of color in the drive toward equity with white men, although the retreat from affirmative action goals is viewed as having affected both civil rights and women's movements, the concerns of race relations are believed to be overshadowed by interest in women's issues.

Although racism and sexism are distinct processes, these forms of discrimination may combine or interact for some women, specifically in the case of black women, whose dual identification impacts on their experiences. Conflicts for black women arising from their interactions with white women, white men, and black men present unique sets of issues and problems. Although the race and sex equity movements both claim that black women should join their ranks, each group has exhibited some extent of discrimination against them. The results indicate that black women have been most disadvantaged, economically and socially, when compared to the other race-sex groups.

Although some efforts have been made to incorporate the concerns of women of color into predominantly white women's organizations, the dilemmas that arise from their diversity are not expected to be resolved quickly or easily. Ultimately, the problem of discrimination has societal, as well as individual, solutions. Research is needed to address the concerns of race and sex bias by increasing the information base available on women of all backgrounds. Richardson (1982) underscored this point when she asked: "What body of knowledge is one left with when any generalization or abstraction about women as a group is subject to what seems to be an unending series of qualifications. As opposed to the *reductio ad absurdum* argument . . . this sensitivity to the interacting forces of other social statuses and roles with that of gender demands new conceptual tools and a constant critical revision of what is known" (48). The use of diversity in research and theory development must be used, as Richardson suggested, not only to prevent divisiveness, but also to promote social equity for various race and gender groups.

NOTE

In preparing this chapter, I benefited greatly from the comments of Irvin D. Reid. Barbara S. Wallston also provided helpful assistance and comments.

REFERENCES

Adams, K. A. 1983. Aspects of social context as determinants of black women's resistance to challenges. *Journal of Social Issues* 39(3): 69–78.

Allport, G. W. 1979. *The nature of prejudice. Twenty-fifth Anniversary Edition.* Reading, Mass.: Addison-Wesley.

Ashmore, R. D., and F. K. Del Boca. 1976. Psychological approaches to understanding intergroup conflicts. In P. A. Katz (Ed.), *Towards the elimination of racism.* New York: Pergamon Press.

Bardwick, J. 1979. *In transition.* New York: Holt, Rinehart & Winston.

Barker, M. 1981. *The new racism.* Frederick, Md.: Aletheia.

Belle, D. 1982. Social ties and social supports. In D. Belle (Ed.), *Lives in stress: Women and depression.* Beverly Hills, Calif.: Sage.

Bernard, J. 1981. *The female world.* New York: Free Press.

Biassey, E. L. 1972. Paranoia and racism in the Unites States. *Journal of National Medical Association* 64: 353–58.

Blackwell, J. E. 1985. *The black community: diversity and unity,* 2d ed. New York: Harper and Row.

Brown, A., B. J. Goodwin, B. A. Hall, and H. Jackson-Lowman. 1985. A review of psychology of women textbooks: Focus on the Afro-American woman. *Psychology of Women Quarterly* 9(1): 29–38.

Casenave, N. 1981. Black men in America: The quest for manhood. In H. P. McAdoo (Ed.), *Black families.* Beverly Hills, Calif.: Sage.

Chesler, M. A. 1976. Contemporary sociological theories of racism. In P. A. Katz (Ed.), *Towards the elimination of racism.* New York: Pergamon Press.

Chester, N. L. 1983. Sex differentiation in two high school environments: Implications for career development among black adolescent females. *Journal of Social Issues* 39(3): 29–40.

Comer, J. P. 1980. White racism: Its root, form, and function. In R. L. Jones (Ed.), *Black psychology,* 2d ed. New York: Harper and Row.

Cox, S. 1981. *Female psychology: The emerging self,* 2d ed. New York: St. Martin's Press.

Daneal, J. 1975. *A definition of fatherhood as expressed by black fathers.* Unpublished doctoral dissertation, University of Pittsburgh.

Delany, L. T. 1980. The other bodies in the river. In R. L. Jones (Ed.), *Black psychology,* 2d ed. New York: Harper and Row.

Dickerson, D. P. 1980. *The role of black females in selected children's fiction.* Ms., Howard University.

Dorn, E. 1979. *Rules and racial equality.* New Haven, Conn.: Yale University Press.

Frieze, I. H., J. E. Parsons, P. B. Johnson, D. N. Ruble, and G. L. Zellman. 1978. *Women and sex roles.* New York: Norton.

Gaertner, S. L. 1976. Nonreactive measures in racial attitude research: A focus on "liberal." In P. A. Katz (Ed.), *Towards the elimination of racism.* New York: Pergamon Press.

Gary, L. E. 1980. A mental health research agenda for the black community. In R. L. Jones (Ed.), *Black psychology,* 2d ed. New York: Harper and Row.

Gilkes, C. T. 1983. Going up for the oppressed: the career mobility of black women community workers. *Journal of Social Issues* 39(3): 115–39.

Grady, K. 1981. Sex bias in research design. *Psychology of Women Quarterly* 5(4): 628–36.

Greenspan, M. 1983. *A new approach to women and therapy.* New York: McGraw-Hill.

Gump, J. P., and L. W. Rivers 1975. A consideration of race in efforts to end sex bias. In E. E. Diamond (Ed.), *Issues of sex bias and sex fairness in career interest measurement.* Washington, D.C.: Department of Health, Education and Welfare, National Institute of Education.

Gurin, P., and E. Epps. 1975. *Black consciousness, identity, and achievement.* New York: Wiley.

Gurin, P., and A. Pruitt. 1978. Counseling implications of black women's market position, aspirations and expectancies. In *Conference on the educational and occupational needs of black women,* vol. 2. Washington, D.C.: National Institute of Education.

Hacker, H. M. 1981. Women as a minority group. In S. Cox (Ed.), *Female psychology: The emerging self,* 2d ed. New York: St. Martin's Press.

Hannerz, U. 1969. *Soulside: Inquiries into ghetto culture and community.* New York: Columbia University Press.

Hare, N. 1971, June. Will the real black man please stand up? *The Black Scholar* 2: 32–35.

————. 1978, April. Revolution without a revolution: the psychology of sex and race. *The Black Scholar* 9: 2–7.

Hare-Mustin, R. T. 1983. An appraisal of the relationship between women and psychotherapy: Eighty years after the case of Dora. *American Psychologist* 38: 593–601.

Heiss, J. 1981. Women's values regarding marriage and the family. In H. P. McAdoo (Ed.), *Black families.* Beverly Hills, Calif.: Sage.

Hemmons, W. M. 1980. The women's liberation movement. In L. Rodgers-Rose. *The black woman.* Beverly Hills, Calif.: Sage.

Hood, E. F. 1978, April. Black women, white women: Separate paths to liberation. *The Black Scholar* 9: 45–56.

hooks, b. 1981. *Ain't I a woman: Black women and feminism.* Boston: South End Press.

Hunter College Women's Studies Collective. 1983. *Women's realities, women's choices.* New York: Oxford University Press.

Hyde, J. S. 1985. *Half the human experience: the psychology of women,* 3d ed. Lexington, Mass.: Heath.

Hyde, J. S., and B. G. Rosenberg. 1976. *Half the human experience: the psychology of women.* Lexington, Mass.: Heath.

Jackson, J. J. 1973. Black women in a racist society. In C. Willie, B. Kramer, and B. Brown (Eds.), *Racism and mental health.* Pittsburgh: University of Pittsburgh Press.

————. 1980. *Minorities and aging.* Belmont, Calif.: Wadsworth.

Jenkins, A. H. 1982. *The psychology of the Afro-American.* New York: Pergamon Press.

Jones, J. M. 1983. The concept of race in social psychology: from color to culture. In L. Wheeler and P. Shaver (Eds.), *Review of personality and social psychology,* vol. 4. Beverly Hills, Calif.: Sage.

Kanter, R. M. 1977. Women in organizations: Sex roles, group dynamics, and change strategies. In A. Sargent (Ed.), *Beyond sex roles*. St. Paul, Minn.: West.

Katz, J. H. 1978. *White awareness: Handbook for anti-racism training.* Norman: University of Oklahoma Press.

Katz, P. A. 1976. The acquisition of racial attitudes in children. In P. A. Katz (Ed.), *Towards the elimination of racism.* New York: Pergamon.

———. 1983. Developmental foundations of gender and racial attitudes. In R. Leahy (Ed.), *The child's construction of social inequality.* New York: Academic Press.

Korchin, S. J. 1980. Clinical psychology and minority problems. *American Psychologist* 35: 262–69.

LaRue, L. 1970. The black movement and women's liberation. *Black Scholar* 1(7): 36–42.

Lorde, A. 1979. Feminism and black liberation: the great American disease. *Black Scholar* 10(8): 17–20.

Lykes, M. B. 1983. Discrimination and coping in the lives of black women: Analyses of oral history data. *Journal of Social Issues* 39(3): 79–100.

Mack, D. 1974. The power relationship in black and white families. *Journal of Personality and Social Psychology* 30: 409–13.

McAdoo, H. P. 1978, November. Factors related to stability in upwardly mobile black families. *Journal of Marriage and the Family,* 761–76.

———. 1980. Black mothers and the extended family support network. In H. P. McAdoo (Ed.), *The black woman.* Beverly Hills, Calif.: Sage.

McConahay, J. B., and J. C. Hough. 1976. Symbolic racism. *Journal of Social Issues* 32(2): 23–45.

Mezei, L. 1971. Perceived social pressure as an explanation of shifts in the relative influence of race and belief on prejudice across social interactions. *Journal of Personality and Social Psychology* 19: 69–81.

Notman, M. T., and C. C. Nadelson. 1978. *The woman patient.* New York: Plenum Press.

Parlee, M. B. 1981. Appropriate control groups in feminist research. *Psychology of Women Quarterly* 5(4): 637–44.

Pence, E. 1982. Racism—A white issue. In G. T. Hull, P. B. Scott, and B. Smith (Eds.), *All the women are white, all the blacks are men, but some of us are brave.* New York: The Feminist Press.

Pugh, R. W. 1972. *Psychology and the black experience.* Monterey, Calif.: Brooks/Cole.

Rawles, B. 1978. The media and their effect on black images. In Lipman-Blumen (Ed.), *Conference on the educational and occupational needs of black women,* vol. 2. Washington, D.C.: National Institute of Education.

Reid, P. T. 1979. Racial stereotyping on television: A comparison of the behavior of both black and white television characters. *Journal of Applied Psychology* 64: 465–71.

Richardson, M. S. 1982. Sources of tension in teaching the psychology of women. *Psychology of Women Quarterly* 7(1): 45–54.

Richmond-Abbott, M. 1983. *Masculine and feminine: Sex roles over the life cycle.* Reading, Mass.: Addison-Wesley.

Rogers, S. C. 1981. Woman's place: a critical review of anthropological theory. In S. Cox (Ed.), *Female psychology: The emerging self,* 2d ed. New York: St. Martin's Press.

Scarf, M. 1980. *Unfinished business: Pressure points in the lives of women.* New York: Ballantine.

Sears, D. O., and J. B. McConahay. 1973. *The politics of violence: The new urban blacks and the Watts riot.* Boston: Houghton Mifflin.

Shaffer, D. R. 1985. *Developmental psychology: Theory, research and applications.* Belmont, Calif.: Brooks/Cole.

Simpson, G. E., and J. M. Yinger. 1953. *Racial and cultural minorities: An analysis of prejudice and discrimination.* New York: Harper and Row.

Smith, A., and A. Stewart. 1983. Approaches to studying racism and sexism in black women's lives. *Journal of Social Issues* 39(3): 1–15.

Sojourner, S. 1979. The perpetuation of myths. *Black Scholar* 10(8): 31–32.

Staples, R. 1981. Race and marital status: An overview. In H. P. McAdoo (Ed.), *Black families.* Beverly Hills, Calif: Sage.

Strasser, S. 1982. *Never done: The history of American housework.* New York: Pantheon Books.

Sue, S. 1983. Ethnic minority issues in psychology: A reexamination. *American Psychologist* 38(5): 583–92.

Szymanski, A. 1976. Racism and sexism as functional substitutes in the labor market. *The Sociological Quarterly* 17: 65–73.

Torrey, J. W. 1979. Racism and feminism: Is women's liberation for whites only? *Psychology of Women Quarterly* 4(2): 281–93.

Unger, R. K. 1979. *Female and male.* New York: Harper and Row.

Walker, A. 1982. One child of one's own. In G. T. Hull, P. B. Scott, and B. Smith (Eds.), *All the women are white, all the men are black, but some of us are brave.* New York: The Feminist Press.

Walker, L. S., and B. S. Wallston. 1985. Social adaptation: A review of dual earner family literature. In L. LaAbate (Ed.), *Handbook of family psychology.* Homewood, Ill.: Dow Jones Ervin.

Wallston, B. S. 1981. What are the questions in psychology of women? A feminist approach to research. *Psychology of Women Quarterly* 5(4): 597–617.

Wallston, B. S., and K. E. Grady. 1985. Feminist methodology and the crisis in social psychology. In V. E. O'Leary and R. K. Unger (Eds.), *Women, gender and social psychology.* Hillsdale, N.J.: Erlbaum.

Williams, R. L. 1980. The death of white research in the black community. In R. L. Jones (Ed.), *Black psychology,* 2d ed. New York: Harper and Row.

Willie, C. V. 1983. *Race, ethnicity, and socioeconomic status.* Bayside, N.Y.: General Hall.

Wright, M. 1972. I want the right to be black and me. In G. Lerner (Ed.), *Black women in white America.* New York: Pantheon Books.

ya Salaam, K. 1979. Women's rights are human rights! *Black Scholar* 10(6): 9–16.

◆ BEVERLY GREENE ◆

African-American Women: Derivatives of Racism and Sexism in Psychotherapy

African-American women are socialized and develop in a society in which racial, gender, and sexual orientation oppression are pervasive. These interrelated realities and the discriminatory practices that accompany them create a unique range of psychological demands and stressors, which African-American women must learn to address. Similarly, clinicians who treat African-American women must be aware of these realities and their effects if effective treatment is to take place. In addition to the extreme demands of racism, sexism, and heterosexism, African-American women must manage the routine and mundane developmental tasks and life stressors that most other persons face. The potential for negative effects on the psychological well-being of African-American women in this scenario is high. This essay reviews the salient factors that must be considered in psychotherapy with African-American women, in the context of discriminatory systems and institutions, in ways that are sensitive to the complex psychological and cultural realities of African-American women.

AFRICAN-AMERICAN WOMEN

African-American women, with some Native American and European ethnic admixture, are descendants of the tribes of western Africa and were the primary objects of the United States slave trade. African-American women are perhaps the only group of U.S. women of color whose members were unwilling participants in their immigration. Clinical significance is assigned to inquiries about the nature and circumstances surrounding the entry of members of immigrant groups into the United States. It is presumed that the reasons for immigration and the differences between the life-style in a person's country of origin and in the United States will bear on how they view their current circumstances as well as their relative optimism or pessimism about the possibility of altering current situations for the better. The struggles of African Americans are simplistically viewed as if they ended with emancipation, ignoring over a century more of legal racial discrimination and disenfranchisement. Furthermore, comparisons between the conditions African Americans and members of other immigrant groups find themselves in are often invoked with the notion that all immigrants were the targets of discrimination at some time or another. It is then suggested that the history of racial oppression does not account for the disparaged conditions in which African Americans find themselves.

In a subtle manner the denial of the impact of slavery and institutional racism on African Americans fuels old assertions of innate, biological inferiority. Biology is conveniently used in such instances to explain the sequelae of societal phenomena. While it is obvious that such arguments buttress political agendas, they are not infrequently invoked in therapy as one rationale for viewing all members of immigrant groups as "the same."

Comparing the discrimination confronting African Americans and members of other groups as if it were the same can be demeaning and insulting to the African-American woman in treatment. It is likely that she has heard this before, in contexts in which it was used to minimize her experience, deny aspects of the uniqueness of that experience, and minimize the anxiety evoked in its user by avoiding realities of racism. Clinicians are urged to be wary of such inclinations. The minimization of the relevance of their involuntary immigration and subsequent treatment to the current perceptions of African-American men and women stands in stark contrast to the appropriate importance accorded to remembering the Holocaust and exploring the impact of the losses and other sequelae associated with it on its survivors and their descendants. Toni Morrison challenges her listener to attempt to understand the impact of slavery on African Americans by imagining what it would be like to experience World War II for two hundred years.

While sexism devalues all women compared to men, the interaction between sexism, the history of racism, and involuntary immigrant status combines to affect African-American women differently than the history of sexism affects their white counterparts. Similarly, the history of involuntary immigrant status and institutional racism may affect African-American women in ways that are phenomenologically different than for other women of color. It should be noted that, while women's experiences of oppression may differ phenomenologically, such differences do not warrant the assumption that differences in experience are hierarchical.

African-American women entered the United States as pieces of property whose purpose was to provide free labor, to be sold as any commodity, and to produce offspring who would become salable commodities as well. A poignant symbol of their dehumanized status as merchandise is reflected in the practice of entering the birth, death, and sale records of slaves in the financial ledgers and business records of plantations (Brice-Baker, pers. comm. 1992). For many African Americans the most tangible piece of evidence of an ancestor's existence may be found in a financial ledger, listed with the farm animals under the category "livestock."

African-American women's roles in American society from the very outset have been synonymous with work, labor outside the home, and legitimized sexual victimization (B. Greene 1993 and 1993b). One of the features that distinguished African-American women from their white counterparts was their role as workers. In these roles they did not differ greatly from the roles assumed by African-American men (Collins 1990; Fox-Genovese 1988; B. Greene 1992b, 1993b, and 1994). Notably, conventions of femininity made many forms of labor, which were deemed routine for white males, inappropriate for white females. These courtesies have never been extended to African-American women as a group, as Elizabeth Fox-Genovese (1988) notes in her discourse on life within plantation households. She contends that slavery had, in fact, deprived slave women of the traditional roles and status that were accorded to other American females.

African-American women continued to be a significant presence in the U.S. workplace after the end of slavery and well into contemporary environments. Therefore, the dominant cultural norm of women remaining in the home, while men worked outside the home to support the family, was never practically obtainable, although it was desired by many African-American women. Racism in the workplace often discriminated against African-American men, limiting their ability to support their families in the ways that their white counterparts were able to do. Johnnetta Cole (1989) writes:

Black women ain't been put on no pedestals . . . nine out of every ten worked in the fields alongside black men. But everytime we have this image of slavery, there she is either setting the table for master or getting in his bed . . . the myth of the black woman profiting at the expense of black men is the oldest rap around . . . it's been unbelievably important to keep it going, to divide black men from women.

African-American women were and still are often required to bring essential and not supplementary income to the family. When they assume this role, out of necessity, they are pathologized for having done so successfully. The assumption of a working role was and is currently done in many creative ways, from establishing child care systems within their homes to engaging in all kinds of work, frequently for low wages, outside the home. Work outside the home has often been touted as the key to "women's liberation." While this may be more the case for white women, for African-American women it is important to make a distinction between having the opportunity to work and having to work. Work for many African-American women is seen as a burdensome necessity, without the glamor of "career status," for which they realistically expect to be paid less than their white counterparts. African-American women in the domestic work arena were, and may still be, found in the employ of their white counterparts, being treated as inferiors and not as "sisters."

Despite differences in roles and treatment, African-American women are nonetheless held accountable to standards based on idealized depictions of their white counterparts. Included in such depictions are cultural beauty standards based on the white female ideal. Since physical attractiveness serves, for women, a functional role analogous to social power among men, what any female client believes to be true about the relative attractiveness of her physical characteristics and what extremes must be taken to alter them is an important aspect of therapeutic inquiry. When compared to the white female ideal as the norm, traditional African physical features—darker skin colors, broad or thick facial features, and kinky hair textures—are generally deemed by the dominant culture to be unattractive and inferior (Collins 1990; B. Greene 1992b and 1993a; Neal and Wilson 1989; Okazawa-Rey, Robinson, and Ward 1987).

African-American women are encouraged to imitate and are rewarded for approaching the white female ideal. Responding to this injunction from the dominant culture inevitably entails attempting to eradicate the very physical characteristics that define African-American women racially and ethnically. A review of media images reveals advertisements for products that hold the fallacious promise of delivering, for most African-American women, an unrealistic fantasy of approaching the ideal. The fact that these products do a flourishing business suggests that the old messages that devalued African physical characteristics are not a thing of the past. Rather, they are consistently infused with new life, despite assertions of racial pride. Many of the elements of those old messages continue to linger, albeit unconsciously, in the minds of many African-American women (B. Greene 1993a).

For many African-American women there is a sense of shame about their physical characteristics. This sense of shame is often reinforced by the preoccupations and perceptions of family members about the relative "goodness" of physical characteristics of white women and the "badness" of those characteristics found in Americans of African descent (Boyd-Franklin 1991; B. Greene 1992b and 1994). James Baldwin (1964) wrote:

> One's hair was always being attacked with hard brushes and combs and Vaseline: it was shameful to have nappy hair. One's legs were always greased so that one would not look "ashy" in the wintertime. One was always being scrubbed and polished, as though in the hope that a stain could thus be washed away ... the women were forever straightening and curling their hair ... and using bleaching creams ... yet it was clear that none of this effort would release one from the stigma and danger of being Negro; it merely increased the shame and rage.

Although Baldwin wrote this passage almost thirty years ago, many of these same sentiments are expressed by African-American women in group and individual therapies today. These concerns are manifested in the expression of negative feelings about the color of their skin—particularly, but not exclusively, if their skin colors are dark—the size and shape of their facial features, their body shapes and sizes, and their hair textures (Boyd-Franklin 1991; B. Greene 1993a and 1994; Neal and Wilson 1989; Okazawa-Rey, Robinson, and Ward 1987). The negative associations with these images represent the convergence of one of the cruel elements of both racism and sexism for African-American women in their objectification as African Americans and as women. It is incumbent upon African-American mothers and parenting figures to provide to their daughters more positive messages and alternatives to the white female ideal in order to mitigate the negative reflections they see of themselves in the eyes of the dominant culture (B. Greene 1992c). The failure to do so or the tendency to reinforce such attitudes can be associated with poor self-images in many African-American women.

While not all African-American women are negatively affected by this legacy, the history of negative perceptions about the adequacy of their physical appearance continues to have a demonstrable effect on many African-American women in terms of their perceptions of their femininity and worth as women, as did the compulsory breeding and sexual exploitation of African-American women during slavery. Such practices were used to construct images of African-American women as morally loose, sexually promiscuous, and immune to sexual victimization, which was rampant. This was in stark contrast to the view of white women, elevated to a pedestal of purity, sexual chastity, and virtue. Rather than acknowledge their realistic role as victims, the dominant culture often depicted African-American women as sexual aggressors who conveniently served as the repositories of sexual propensities found in all persons but deemed negative by the dominant culture. Having been depicted in this manner over time, and thus deemed unworthy of protection, they were not only vulnerable to the sexual and aggressive urges of the dominant culture's males, and subsequently other males, they were blamed for this victimization as well (Collins 1990; B. Greene 1992b, 1993a, 1993b, and 1994).

This form of objectification of African-American women, as African Americans and as women, served to justify their victimization, but it also did more. Hazel Carby (1987) asserts that the purpose of stereotypes is not to reflect reality accurately but, rather, to function as a disguise of societal reality. Stereotypes of African-American women served as a reflection of a larger schema used to justify discriminatory treatment of members of disparaged groups to the benefit of idealized and privileged groups. Such rationales are also intended to convince members of disparaged groups that their lot in life is a part of the natural, normal order of things, the work of "mother nature," rather than the result of unfair social practices deliberately designed to keep institutional power in the hands of the already powerful and privileged (Carby 1987; Kamin 1974; Karier 1972). Members of disparaged groups, in this case African-American women, who accept such premises are more likely to blame themselves when they encounter discriminatory barriers than to question the political underpinnings of the policies that serve as rationales for those barriers.

In traditional Western thought differences between males and females and blacks and whites have been defined in oppositional terms; in these dichotomous frameworks, that is, members of one group are defined as the opposite of the other. Therefore, that which is not the preferred, or norm—the idealized depiction of the white, heterosexual, able-bodied male—is defined as "other." This other can then be readily objectified, and when the objectification is accomplished views of the other can be easily manipulated and controlled by the use of negative images such as those represented in many racial and gender stereotypes (Collins 1990, 68; B. Greene 1993a; L. Greene, pers. comm. 1992).

Cheryl Clarke (1983, 199) describes the atmosphere of the dominant culture as one that is "sexually repressive" and claims that it leaves African-American women with a predisposed need to "debunk the racist mythology which says our sexuality is depraved." In this schema African-American lesbians are viewed as other to the other, that is, defined in opposition to heterosexual African-American women, who are already defined in opposition to heterosexual white women (Collins 1990). African-American lesbians then take on an additional set of negative images, which results in their being relegated to the lowest rung of the hierarchical ladder of women. As a consequence of this status, African-American lesbians face an additional set of psychological and environmental demands. They are forced to manage the racism, sexism, and heterosexism of the dominant culture; the heterosexism, sexism, and the internalized racism of individuals within the African-American community; the racism found within the lesbian community; the sexism found within the gay community; for many, a sense of conflicting loyalties between lesbian and African-American communities as well as African-American lesbian and white lesbian communities; and a heightened sense of awareness of devalued multiple identities. There is in this scenario the potential for negative effects on the health and psychological well-being of African-American lesbians (B. Greene 1992c, 1993a, and in press).

This discussion has reviewed some of the differences between African-American women and their white counterparts' social and psychological realities, despite their shared history of gender oppression. The history of racism experienced by African-American women "colors" their experience of sexism and other oppressions and may transcend and intensify many other aspects of their experience. In psychotherapy the effects of oppression based on race, gender, and sexual orientation are interrelated and cannot be separated from one another, in any individual client, without losing a sense of the interactive phenomenological effects of the two. Hence, African-American women are left with a range of interrelated internal psychological and external societal realities that may challenge, facilitate, or undermine key aspects of their development (B. Greene 1992b and 1993a; Jones 1985). These psychological realities may be viewed as spheres that overlap at different points and converge in a unique way in the client's presenting problem. The extent to which they overlap, where the overlap occurs, and the relative importance of each sphere will vary from client to client and will vary at different times in the individual client's life. This variance is an expression of the uniqueness of each client, of her particular dilemma, and, most important, of her experience of that dilemma (B. Greene 1993a; Jones 1985).

One component of the psychological reality of African-American women involves integrating the role of African cultural derivatives into their lives, when African people have been depicted as inferior, savage, impulsive, and less intelligent than their white counterparts (Thomas and Sillen 1972). Furthermore, accurate depictions of precolonial African cultures and the exploitation of Africa's people, land, and rich mineral resources by more "civilized" nations have been obscured and distorted by the institutions of the dominant culture. Given that African culture has been defined as the negative opposite of Western cultures, it may be difficult for some African-American women to form a positive identification with their African heritage. Pride in one's ethnic background and cultural heritage can, however, be a rich source of psychological resilience, group identification, and support. The need to deny, establish distance from, or experience shame or conflict about one's racial or ethnic identity can be associated with less than optimal psychological outcomes, which may negatively affect self-esteem and the ability to cope (B. Greene 1993a). Conflict in this area may also interfere with the ability to seek and utilize appropriate group support. African-American women share many constellations of characteristics that have their origins in African cultures. (For a more detailed review of cultural practices that derive from African cultures, see Boyd-Franklin 1989 and B. Greene 1990.)

Another major piece of psychological reality for African-American women involves the integration and often the mitigation of the influence of certain aspects of the dominant culture. The racism and sexism inherent in the dominant culture and its accompanying negative images of African-American women are communicated to all Americans. This leaves African Americans with the task of developing coping mechanisms in response to racism and negotiating the discriminatory barriers that result from institutional racism in addition to the normal range of life's routine and catastrophic stressors. To do this successfully African-American women must make careful choices about which aspects of dominant culture they identify with, as many of its values include an insidious devaluation of persons of color. Internalized racism may result when, unconsciously and without censor, both the negative stereotypes about African Americans and the idealized stereotypes of white Americans are internalized and negatively affect the African American's sense of self. This is, of course, complicated for African-American women, who also bear the mantle of negative gender stereotypes, and for African-American lesbians, who bear negative stereotypes associated with their sexual orientation in addition to all others. (In my 1992 essay entitled "Still Here" I detail clinical manifestations of this phenomena, which, when observed, must be addressed as a part of the therapeutic work.) Problematic adjustments to racism and sexism are prevalent, yet they tell only a part of the story.

Each generation of African Americans, usually but not exclusively within the family, prepares the next generation for the challenge of being African American in a society that devalues them. Mary Frances Berry and John Blassingame (1982, x) describe the heart of this process in their rationale for the title chosen for their book on the black experience in America:

> The title we chose for this book, *Long Memory,* symbolizes our rejection of the view of Afro Americans as an atomized, rootless people who begin each generation without any sense of what preceded them. Whatever they do, black people talk to each other. They have always done so. The searing vignettes passed on by old sages to youth made memory itself an instrument of survival.

Eloquently summarized, this "long memory" is and has been an important survival tool that has helped African Americans make psychological sense out of their often demoralizing predicament.

A major task in this endeavor is to communicate to African-American children the racial dangers and realities of the world, how to recognize and cope with them, and, perhaps of greatest importance, whether or not the demeaning messages of the broader culture are true. African-American mothers and fathers face a unique challenge in socializing their daughters with regard to the demeaning messages that confront them both as African Americans and women (B. Greene 1992c). Despite the fact that they are required to function in a ubiquitously hostile environment that opposes their optimal development, African-American women have made healthy adjustments that are both undeniable and not accidental. Their psychological flexibility is often a reflection of an active socialization process that takes place within African-American families and communities which prepares its members to make psychological sense out of a hostile environment and to negotiate its institutional barriers without internalizing the demeaning messages that often accompany those barriers.

Adaptive responses to the demand to cope with racism may be

observed in the processes of armoring (Faulkner 1983; Sears 1987), healthy cultural paranoia (Grier and Cobbs 1968), and racial socialization (B. Greene 1994). These maneuvers reflect the need of African Americans to make psychological sense out of their institutionally disadvantaged position and the requirement to negotiate and deflect a hostile environment in healthy and adaptive ways. What is noteworthy is the paucity of information in the psychological literature which explores how these adaptive phenomena work and how they might be utilized to assist persons who experience difficulty coping with both personal and institutional barriers. Perhaps that is another story as well.

PSYCHOTHERAPY AND AFRICAN-AMERICAN WOMEN: ADDRESSING THE VICISSITUDES OF RACISM AND SEXISM

It is important in psychotherapy with African-American women to explore the derivatives of their personal histories, racism, and gender role traditions in an integrated fashion. African-American womenare invariably shaped and affected by the institutions and systems that surround them and of which they are a part. They are capable, however, of developing a subjective understanding of both their inner worlds and external social realities and of using their understanding to make changes in themselves and their circumstances. Facilitating this process is one of the ultimate goals of therapy.

It is important in this process for therapists to be aware of their feelings and attitudes about the similarities and differences between themselves and their clients. Just as interpersonal and institutional racism and sexism affect clients, they affect therapists as well. It is often assumed that clinical training purges therapists of stereotypes about gender and race, despite the fact that many of those stereotypes are often reinforced by professional literature that fails to challenge them. Gender and race constitute two major dimensions around which most people organize themselves and which influence both their understanding of the world and of their relative place in it (B. Greene 1992c). Because mental health practitioners develop as a part of this culture and not apart from it, like clients, they will have feelings about stereotypes, whether or not they agree with them. It is incumbent on therapists to be aware of the realistic and not fantasied power differentials in our culture between men and women and between African Americans and white Americans and also what they mean in the life of the client. In this regard an appreciation of the complexity of race and gender in the socialization and therapy process and its reflection in the legacy of racism and sexism in African-American women's lives is essential if treatment is to be successful. No therapist comes to the process of psychotherapy race or gender blind, nor would this be desirable. It is important to recognize that people may be of equal worth without being the same.

Therapists who treat African-American women must understand and be able to make distinctions between internal psychological conflicts that partially or completely obstruct self-actualizing behaviors and realistic external forces that oppose or obstruct an individual's efforts to meet his or her needs. In addition, the complex interplay between these two overlapping phenomena must be appreciated. When fears or obstacles have a realistic basis, it is important to be aware of the reality-based circumstances in the client's life which evoke his or her concerns and fears as well as the realistic, not fantasied, obstacles that must be overcome in addressing them. In the case of African-American women the barriers of institutional racism, sexism, and heterosexism and the extent of their impact must be acknowledged. Once acknowledged strategies to address these barriers must evolve out of an understanding of the realistic dangers they pose, the client's cultural and social framework, and actions congruent with the client's resources and values.

Therapists who work with African-American women must be careful not to dismiss prematurely their complaints about racial and gender discrimination. Such a response serves only to minimize the reality of the client's distress and the justifiable anger evoked in encounters with racism and sexism. It is equally important, however, that the therapist not be too quick to accept, before carefully exploring other areas, that racial or gender discrimination is the central issue in therapy or the only issue that should be addressed. Furthermore, racial and gender oppressions should not be used by the therapist to avoid setting appropriate limits or interpreting the client's acting out, as it is not ultimately helpful. Rather, it may serve as the therapist's collusion with the client in unhealthy behavior as well as the therapist's avoidance of a realistic confrontation with the client. Rarely is racial or gender bias the sole source of all of a client's problems. For some clients race or gender discrimination may be less painful to address or acknowledge than other problems, particularly their experiences of rejection or abuse by loved and trusted figures. In addition to maintaining an awareness of social barriers, simultaneously, the therapist must be aware of significant figures, relationships and their patterns, and events in the client's life. It is important to understand the extent to which those previous relationships and events bear on the development of the client's self-esteem, current actions, and perception of solutions and alternatives in addressing current realistic problems.

While there are realistic racist and sexist barriers in the world that African-American women share as a group, each individual has her own unique experience and understanding of that reality, which is what the therapist seeks ultimately to understand. The therapist must avoid romanticizing the strengths forged from African-American women's struggles with institutional barriers by neglecting to appreciate the often debilitating effects of those struggles. Furthermore, the temptation to use these struggles as an explanation for all of a client's problems must also be avoided. To expose or explore the parameters of characterological difficulty or psychopathology in a client does not mean that she is to "blame" for everything that happens to her or that racism and sexism are just excuses for internal deficiencies. Many clients have little interest in or desire to change institutional barriers. Whether or not this is a part of the therapeutic agenda should always be the client's choice. Many others may not have the option of doing so. Therapy offers African-American women the opportunity of having their accurate perceptions validated, identifying and understanding the conscious and unconscious methods they employ in confronting and negotiating systemic and personal barriers, analyzing the effectiveness of their methods, and developing a wider range of personally compatible options (B. Greene 1992c). Personal problems do not minimize the legitimacy of the realistic experience of racial and gender discrimination, or vice versa. Psychological difficulty must not be seen dichotomously or in discrete pieces but, rather, as a puzzle with many interrelated pieces in which no one piece tells the whole story.

SUMMARY

Effective psychotherapy with African-American women explicitly requires cultural literacy of its practitioners. This cultural literacy includes understanding the collective social plight of African-American women and the individual client in the context of the prevailing reality of race, gender, and sexual orientation bias and the interpersonal and institutional barriers that result from that bias. Cultural literacy presumes a willingness on the part of the therapist to educate him- or herself about the client's cultural background and milieu and to validate the client's accurate perceptions of discrimination and bias and

their impact on the client's life (B. Greene 1992a). The culturally literate practitioner will acknowledge and appreciate the wide range of
diversity within African-American women as a group. No client
should feel forced to fit a preconceived stereotype of what African-
American women are supposed to be. The individual client's intrapsychic and familial endowments and personal relationship history
as they are embedded in the aforementioned context should be carefully explored and understood as well as all relevant social factors.
Finally, the therapist must be willing to scrutinize his or her feelings
and motivations for working with African-American women. What
should follow is a careful analysis of the developmental interactions
of these variables and how they promote an individual's view of the
world, her perceptions of her options, her strategies for negotiating institutional barriers, her relationships with other persons, as well as
any contributions she makes, consciously or unconsciously, to her
own dilemma (B. Greene 1992a and 1992c).

Discussions advocating cultural literacy and explorations of potential countertransference issues in interracial psychotherapy
dyads, such as my 1985 essay in *Psychotherapy,* have been presumed by C. M. Brody (1987), for example, to imply that only
African-American therapists can effectively treat African-American
women who are clients. Such an interpretation erroneously assumes
that, if cultural literacy is required, only African-American therapists can be culturally literate and sensitive to African-American
cultural norms. While such an assumption is troubling enough, it is
often followed by expressions of concern that clinical skill is more
important than cultural sensitivity, as if they were mutually exclusive, with the implication that this skill would be harder to find in
African-American therapists or, for that matter, other therapists of
color. The insidious presence of racism, whether intended or not, is
clear in such statements and concerns. There is no reason to assume,
even if cultural similarity were deemed most important in the therapy dyad, and it is not, that African-American or other therapists
who are persons of color would be any less skilled than their white
counterparts. The notion that quality must suffer when persons of
color are sought out to perform this task is dangerous and serves little purpose other than to perpetuate racist stereotypes of the inferiority of persons of color.

When a member of a dominant group treats a member of a
dominated group, it is reasonable to assume that tensions and feelings
attached to racial and gender issues that exist in the culture will not
remain outside the therapy process. This observation is valid even if
the therapist and client are both members of dominated groups. In

this case each may harbor feelings about their status or group membership, and each may experience their oppression differently from the other. The presence of a white therapist as an authority figure provides fertile ground for the recapitulation of the normative power relationship between African Americans and white Americans, just as the male therapist as an authority figure may recapitulate our culture's imbalance of power between men and women (B. Greene 1993a; Owens 1984). What is important is not that the client and therapist be the same but, rather, that the therapist be aware of the realistic power differentials in society and the ways in which they may affect the therapy process and the client's day-to-day life. Presuming that a discussion of such material is a plea for homogeneity in the therapy process is a distortion of this position and can often serve to discourage discussion about a topic most Americans are socialized to avoid, racial tension.

Advocacy for cultural literacy in psychotherapy is not synonymous with a plea for cultural similarity between the therapist and client. Cultural literacy alone will not foster a helpful alliance if the therapist harbors unresolved or poorly understood feelings about his or her own ethnic background and its meaning or the client's ethnic background and its meaning to the therapist or if the therapist is poorly trained. Conversely, the best intentions in the traditionally trained therapist can be hampered by the absence of cultural literacy. Appropriate interpretations of behavior cannot be made without some understanding of the client's culturally proscribed way of viewing and experiencing the world.

Similarly, for African-American women gender oppression is not unimportant; its meaning and primacy, however, may not be the same as it is for their white counterparts. The presumption that it must be so or that alliances between African-American women and white women are stronger than alliances between African American women and men ignores the impact of racism and its interrelationship with sexism. In this context the question of whether gender or cultural similarity in the therapist is most important is moot. The question that should logically evolve from this is: Most important to whom? For some African-American women cultural similarity in the initial stages of therapy may help facilitate the process; for others it will make no difference. The same is true for gender similarity. For some African-American women, depending on their own characterological issues and their reasons for entering therapy, greater levels of comfort will be established sooner if the therapist is female; for others it will not matter.

The dimension of sexual orientation adds yet another significant variable. For some African-American lesbian clients the therapist's sexual orientation is deemed by the client to be more important than race or ethnicity, while still other clients prefer that the therapist be a lesbian of color or a woman of color.

Generally, no single dimension is inherently better than any other. Rather, the importance of race, gender, or sexual orientation of the therapist and its effect on the therapy process will vary from client to client. The client's preference should be respected but should also be understood in keeping with the need to explore the potential wish for or need to avoid certain kinds of relationships or material as well as its transference significance. Generally, the range of preferences in this area will vary in ways that reflect the wide range of healthy diversity among African-American women as a group.

The tendency to avoid explorations of social, cultural, and institutional barriers and variables in a client's life in many traditional psychotherapies has been attributed to the idea that intrapsychic phenomena are structured universally and are of greater import in shaping individual personality than environmental factors. Cheryl Thompson (1987), however, articulately defines this avoidance on the therapist's part as a manifestation of countertransference resistance and not as an appropriate interpretation of psychodynamic theory.

Psychological science and theories of human behavior have been used historically to defend the practice of slavery, notions of the intellectual inferiority of African Americans and females, forced sterilization of "mental defectives," immigration quotas, racial and gender oppression, and other forms of social discrimination and control (Guthrie 1976; Kamin 1974; Karier 1972; Mays 1985; Thomas and Sillen 1972). Such explanations for social inequities have been used in the service of blaming institutionally disparaged persons for their lots in life while simultaneously supporting and defending the dominant culture's notion of white supremacy and white cultural superiority. This is consistent with theories that are based on biological determinism. When it does not support the prevailing political agendas or practices or else contradicts them, knowledge derived from psychological research and practice is simply overlooked or ignored. The political reality of this trend is represented in the myth of the meritocracy in America. Acceptance of this myth leads to the conclusion that people who do not succeed have always themselves to blame, failing to appropriately acknowledge and explore the tenacity of institutional barriers. Psychological theories, particularly psychodynamic theories, are among the many solicited and selectively used when there is a need to marshal support for genetic explanations of social inequities and what would be otherwise unacceptable contentions and practices (B. Greene 1993a; Thomas and Sillen 1972; Thompson 1989).

REFERENCES

Baldwin, J. 1964. *Nobody Knows My Name.* London: Michael Joseph.

Berry, M. F., and J. Blassingame. 1982. *Long Memory: The Black Experience in America.* New York: Oxford University Press.

Boyd-Franklin, N. 1989. *Black Families in Therapy: A Multisystems Approach.* New York: Guilford.

———. 1991. "Recurrent Themes in the Treatment of African-American Women in Group Psychotherapy." *Women and Therapy* 11, no. 2: 25–40.

Brice-Baker, J. 1992. Personal communication.

Brody, C. M. 1987. "White Therapist and Female Minority Client: Gender and Culture Issues." *Psychotherapy* 24, no. 1: 108–13.

Carby, H. 1987. *Reconstructing Womanhood: The Emergence of the African-American Woman Novelist.* New York: Oxford University Press.

Clarke, C. 1983. "The Failure to Transform: Homophobia in the Black Community." In *Home Girls: A Black Feminist Anthology,* ed. B. Smith, 197–208. New York: Kitchen Table–Women of Color Press.

Cole, J. 1989. "Johnnetta Cole." In *I Dream a World: Portraits of Black Women Who Changed America,* ed. B. Lanker, 38. New York: Stewart, Tabori, and Chang.

Collins, P. H. 1990. *Black Feminist Thought.* Boston: Unwin Hyman.

Faulkner, J. 1983. "Women in Interracial Relationships." *Women and Therapy* 2, nos. 2–3: 193–203.

Fox-Genovese, E. 1988. *Within the Plantation Household: Black and White Women of the Old South.* Chapel Hill: University of North Carolina Press.

Greene, B. 1985. "Considerations in the Treatment of Black Patients by White Therapists." *Psychotherapy* 22, 2d ser.: 389–93.

———. 1990. "Sturdy Bridges: The Role of African-American Mothers in the Socialization of African-American Children." *Women and Therapy* 10, nos. 1–2: 205–25.

———. 1992a. "Black Feminist Psychotherapy." In *Psychoanalysis and Feminism: A Critical Dictionary,* ed. E. Wright, 34–5. Oxford: Basil Blackwell.

———. 1992b. "Still Here: A Perspective on Psychotherapy with African-American Women." In *New Directions in Feminist Psychology: Practice,*

Theory, and Research, ed. J. Chrisler and D. Howard, 13–25. New York: Springer.

———. 1992c. "African-American Women: The Burden of Racism and Sexism." *American Family Therapy Association Newsletter* 48, (Summer): 20–23.

———. 1993a. "Psychotherapy with African-American Women: Integrating Feminist and Psychodynamic Models." *Journal of Training and Practice in Professional Psychology* 7, no. 1 (Spring): 49–66.

———. 1993b. "Stereotypes of African-American Sexuality: A Commentary." In *Human Sexuality,* ed. S. Rathus, J. Nevid, and L. Rathus-Fichner. Boston: Allyn and Bacon.

———. 1994. "African-American Women." In *Women of Color: Integrating Ethnic and Gender Identities in Psychotherapy,* ed. L. Comas-Diaz and B. Greene. New York: Guilford.

———. In press. "African-American Lesbians: Triple Jeopardy." In *The Psychology of African-American Women,* ed. A. B. Collins. New York: Guilford.

Greene, L. W. 1992. Personal communication.

Grier, W., and P. Cobbs. 1968. *Black Rage.* New York: Basic Books.

Guthrie, R. V. 1976. *Even the Rat Was White: A Historical View of Psychology.* New York: Harper and Row.

Jones, A. 1985. "Psychological Functioning in Black Americans: A Conceptual Guide for Use in Psychotherapy." *Psychotherapy* 22, 2d ser.: 363–69.

Kamin, L. J. 1974. *The Science and Politics of I.Q.* New York: Lawrence Erlbaum and Associates.

Karier, C. 1972. "Testing for Order and Control in the Corporate Liberal State." *Educational Theory* 22, no. 2: 154–80.

Mays, V. M. 1985. "The Black American and Psychotherapy: The Dilemma." *Psychotherapy* 22, 2d ser.: 379–88.

Neal, A., and M. Wilson. 1989. "The Role of Skin Color and Features in the Black Community: Implications for Black Women and Therapy." *Clinical Psychology Review* 9, no. 3: 323–33.

Okazawa-Rey, M., T. Robinson, and J. V. Ward. 1987. "Black Women and the Politics of Skin Color and Hair." *Women and Therapy* 6, nos. 1–2: 89–102.

Owens, M. 1984. "Racial Issues in Interracial Supervision Triads: When the Supervisor Is Black, the Therapist Is White and the Patient Is Black." MS.

Sears, V. L. 1987. "Cross Cultural Ethnic Relationships." MS.

Thomas, A., and S. Sillen. 1972. *Racism and Psychiatry.* New York: Brunner Mazel.

Thompson, C. 1987. "Racism or Neuroticism: An Entangled Dilemma for the

Black Middle Class Patient." *Journal of the American Academy of Psychoanalysis* 15, no. 3: 395–405.

———. 1989. "Psychoanalytic Psychotherapy with Inner City Patients." *Journal of Contemporary Psychotherapy* 19, no. 2: 137–48.

· II ·

Philosophical and Historical Issues in Racism and Sexism

◆ LINDA BURNHAM ◆

Race and Gender:
The Limits of Analogy

INTRODUCTION

Facile analogies between racism and sexism have long irked women
of color who are active in the feminist and antiracist movements.
Such analogies were a staple of the women's movement of the late
1960s and 1970s.[1] Thankfully, in recent years the impulse to analogize race and class has abated for at least two reasons. First, there has
been an accumulation of work by feminists of color which exposes
the limitations of comparing racism and sexism, including stinging
critiques of the tendency of the analogizing vantage point to "lose
sight" of women of color.[2] Second, over the years white feminists
have become far more aware of the particularity of their vantage point
and less inclined to speak for "women in general."[3] This is all to the
good.

Yet the issue of how to analyze and express the interconnection
between relations of oppression and privilege associated with race,
class, and gender will not die. It has been a dominant theme of feminist theory for many years and no doubt will continue to be for many
years to come. The question has been addressed in the form of the exploration of theoretical models that are capable of taking into account
the racial and class dimensions of women's lives; the application of
feminist scholarship to the history and present-day realities of women
of color and women of the working class; critiques of the race and

class bias of much of early feminism; and the ideological and theoretical elaboration of racially or ethnically defined feminisms: Black feminism, Latina feminism, Asian feminism, etc. This vibrant outpouring of work has taken us far beyond the crudities of early feminism in which the perspective and interests of white women of the middle classes dominated the terrain.

Models, paradigms, and metaphors have multiplied as feminists have struggled to articulate an interconnectedness that, precisely because it is experienced in an infinite number of ways in daily life, has proven extremely difficult to capture as an abstraction. The substantial body of work on these issues is testament both to the perceived centrality, complexity, and intractibility of the problem and to the persistence of feminist theorists. Among Black feminists alone a lively dialogue is under way concerning additive models versus those that take into account the compounding effects of race, class, and sex; Afrocentricity as a theoretical stance for Black feminism; and the relevance of postmodernist theory to illuminating the condition of Black women.

Submerged in these dialogues, given its ignoble and unproductive past, is the issue of what, if anything, is similar about race and gender—in what ways may they be productively compared, and what are the limits of analogy? Rather than giving these comparisons one last good riddance, it is the intent of the remainder of this essay to resurrect the analogy to explore what made it so compelling in the first place, whether there are theoretically legitimate comparisons to be made, and the basis for the strong negative reaction to comparisons of race and gender oppression. In examining these issues, significantly more attention will be given to the explication of relations based on race. This is a reflection of my particular bias: that a deepened theoretical and historical grasp of race and racism will immeasurably enrich all strains of U.S. feminism; that a feminist understanding of the interconnection between race and gender is dependent upon this work; and that the women's movement has a tremendous amount to lose from the failure to develop a more intelligent comprehension of the dynamics of U.S. racism.

THE ATTRACTION OF ANALOGY AND ITS CRITIQUE

Analogizing racism and sexism was one of the recurrent themes of 1970s feminism. The conclusions drawn from such comparisons were varied, but they all were based on the same presumption: there was something to be learned or demonstrated about women's oppression and the struggle against it by comparing it to oppression and discrimination based on race.[4]

There is, of course, a centuries-long history of drawing analogies between race and sex in science and popular culture. Women and Blacks, for example, have been deemed comparable on the grounds that both groups are instinctual, emotional, irrational, childish, of lesser intelligence, and altogether less fully evolved than white men. This use of analogy served to confirm the inferiority of both women and Blacks by "proving" that they held certain lower-order character traits in common. The "natural" dominance of white men was viewed as the inevitable outgrowth of their dissimilarity from those being so compared.[5]

But when the white feminists of the 1970s took up the analogy of race and gender they had a very different project in mind than the confirmation of gender and racial hierarchy. Indeed, their intent was to make visible and comprehensible a form of oppression which was largely unrecognized—sexism—by comparing it to racism, a form that was well recognized; to demonstrate the unjustness of one by way of comparison to the unjustness of the other; to understand the modes and mechanisms of domination and the nature of the political and ideological opposition; to borrow lessons, power, and rhetoric for a then-fledgling movement from one that was more mature. In sum, the intent was to strengthen the hand of those engaged in the struggle against sexism.

The comparison of racism and sexism met with immediate resistance and criticism for a number of complex reasons. First, white feminists were viewed as drawing off the power and legitimacy of the racial justice movements for a project that was not fundamentally, or even peripherally, antiracist. There was also the perception that these feminists had no intrinsic interest in understanding racism per se but only focused on racism insofar as it could illuminate something about sexism. Second, most feminists were viewed as white, middle class, and relatively privileged in comparison to the materially disadvantaged people of color to whom they were comparing themselves. Third, white feminists were perceived as conveniently writing themselves out of the drama of racial oppression, in which they were part of the oppressor group, by writing themselves in as victims in the drama of gender domination. And fourth, sexism within the racial justice movements impeded the recognition that sexism was a pervasive form of oppression that affected not only white women of the middle class but women of color and poor and working-class women as well. This same sexism—and a certain resentment—also forestalled awareness that there might be lessons to be shared with or learned from the women's movement.

This is not the place to assess the negative impact of racism in the women's movement and sexism in the racial justice movements on understanding the commonalities and differences between these forms of oppression. Suffice it to say that the analogizing of racism and sexism was promoted and elaborated by feminists not adversely affected by racial oppression and almost universally rejected by those who experienced discrimination on account of race or on account of both race and gender. Feminists of color, in particular, have criticized the race/sex, racism/sexism, analogy as a model that has made the experience of women of color "theoretically invisible."[6]

White feminists finally heard this critique or, for reasons of their own, have retreated from superficial comparisons of racism and sexism.[7] But why was the tendency to compare race and gender so compelling in the first place? In large part its prevalence was clearly due to the fact that it conferred a powerful sense of political righteousness. It is also true, however, that the analogy is theoretically apt—at a certain level of abstraction. The nineteenth-century hat trick of pretending that the "essential character" of woman could better be fathomed by way of reference to the essential character of the "lesser, non-white races" (and vice versa) was analogizing at its worst. The 1970s version, though fired by the spirit of liberation, was tainted with political opportunism and slovenly methodology. Yet there is something to be learned about the workings of our society by examining the parallelism, the similarities, the concordances, between these two systems of oppression.

Just as important is the examination of the limits of comparison, because, when the racism/sexism analogy is strained beyond its limits, it becomes not only theoretically insupportable but ideologically biased and politically divisive as well. As we shall explore in the last section of this essay, the limits of analogy have much to do with the issues of (1) the level of abstraction at which the analogy is being drawn and (2) the degree to which the realities of class stratification and oppression are or are not integrated into the analysis.

SEMBLANCE AND RESEMBLANCE

In the most elementary and obvious sense race and sex are comparable in that each forms the basis for complex relations of dominance and subordination, privilege and exploitation, power and oppression. Sex and race both serve as sorters. That is, in a gross and general way, people are socially sorted onto one or another pole of these power oppositions on the basis of their position within socially recognized categorical schema of race and sex. The modes of expression of dominance, attributes of privilege, and exercise of power are extremely diverse, as are the forms of discrimination, marginalization, and psychic insult which are the lot of subordinate races and the female sex. And of course, in any given social setting the dynamics of each operates not in isolation but simultaneous with and impinging upon the other, and both are further mediated by class, sexual orientation, and a score of lesser determinants. But the basic point remains: radical inequities of power and privilege are a defining feature of both race relations and gender relations.

The analogy has been persuasive too because both racism and sexism bear similar, though far from identical, relations to the nature/culture and biological/social dichotomies. In this they are distinct from domination and oppression based on class or religion. These dichotomies themselves have been grievously overburdened in the Western intellectual tradition. Duly noting the perils of polarity, however, it is surely significant that both sexism and racism depend upon the production and sustenance of particular social interpretations of naturally occurring differences. The attribution of social meanings to biological differences that do not inhere in the differences themselves is the sine qua non of both racism and sexism.

The mainstream feminist movement has long recognized this process and expressed it in the distinction between sex and gender: one is born female but becomes (is socially and culturally constituted) girl or woman. Perhaps less well recognized, one is born human but becomes "white" or "Black" in the context of a racially polarized and constantly racializing society.[8] For both racism and sexism this becoming entails the social exaggeration of physical and biological differences and dissimilarities and the reification of meanings attached to those differences, along with the suppression, negation, and denial of convergence/similarity/overlap/identity and the denial of meanings that might arise from such convergence.

There is, for example, tremendous overlap in the physical capacities of men and women, yet the differences that do exist have been enormously exaggerated in certain cultural contexts in the service of the cultural icons "strong man" and "frail woman."[9] Just so, the physical features associated with different "races" have been given enormous significances and have been said to account for radical differences in intelligence, psyche, and possession of a soul (or just soul, for that matter). Batteries of scientists have given over their lives to manufacturing physical differences that did not, in fact, exist as the foundation and affirmation of racial differentiation. Meanwhile, it has been shown that the human race shares in common an enormous proportion of its genetic inheritance. That there are any socially significant behavioral or cultural manifestations associated with those elements of genetic material which occur with more frequency in one population group than another is entirely unsubstantiated.[10]

The sociocultural constitution of gendered and racialized subjects are both based on the magnification and distortion of naturally occurring differences together with ideologically biased interpretations of those differences in the service of explaining, "scientizing," "naturalizing," justifying, and consolidating social subordination.

Closely related to the issue of the social elaboration of biological differences is the historicity of gender and race, sexism and racism. That is, implied in the notion of the contemporary production and reproduction of racism and sexism is a historical constitution, both in terms of origins and in terms of historically specific formations of race and gender. For those whose interest extends beyond the theoretical analysis of race and gender to the issue of how racism and sexism will be overcome, historical context is an all-important weapon to be wielded against those who argue for the biologically fixed or historically transcendent character of these forms of oppression. The recognition of sociohistorical origins and historically specific modes of oppression carries with it the potential for nonexploitative interpretations of natural difference and for the historical demise of racism and sexism in changed social circumstances.

While much of early feminism tended to project perspectives and conclusions from the particular experience of white, privileged Western women onto entirely different sociohistorical settings, more recent feminist analysis has recognized the historical specificity of sexism and incorporated or sought to demonstrate this understanding as an element of historical, anthropological, and cross-cultural research. The historically bounded character of sexism has also been reflected in ongoing theoretical speculation about "origin(s)" together with the investigation of relatively transitory models of "woman," as, for example, the nineteenth-century cult of true womanhood and today's do-it-all superwoman.

Less well recognized among many feminists is the historical constitution of racialized subjects. And unlike the origins of sexism, which is the subject of much speculation but no hard data, the original racialization of U.S. society can be located with some historical precision. The conquest of the Americas and the onset of the intercontinental slave trade opened up an era of European and European-American supremacy that has yet to be brought to a close. National, social, economic, cultural, and political domination gave rise to both "popular racism" and "scientific racism"—including the various classificatory schemes that, beginning in the eighteenth century, dressed prejudice and ignorance in the garb of scientific fact.[11]

Racial categorization in the United States developed as a crucial element in the successful attempt to create an unfree and unfreeable labor force. The historical development of slavery as a labor form and class distinction served, at the same time, to constitute a racially differentiated population. The racial categories "white" and "Black," as we in the United States understand and use them with such facility, did not predate the enslavement of Africans but, rather, arose as its result. It took most of the seventeenth century to produce the unambiguous equations Black = subject to enslavement and white = not subject to enslavement *and* able to own other humans as a form of property. The statute books of colonial America reflect the coming into being of specifically racial differentiation. "Negro," as a racial category, came to subsume all the ethnic, language, and religious differences among Africans (including, for that matter, group variation in physical appearance). These differences were of no social significance to Europeans. The social content that *did* "matter" in the racial category "Negro" came to be "the human bearer of unfree labor in the form of lifetime, inheritable slavery." "White" evolved as the ethnic, religious, and nationality distinctions among Europeans receded in relative importance, and the term took on the social content that survives today in our vernacular: to be "free, white, and twenty-one" implies being completely unfettered, both literally and figuratively. U.S. racial slavery has been eliminated, but the origins of U.S. racial categories and a racialized population *in* racial slavery is generally unacknowledged.[12]

In addition to the historical issue of origins there is also the history-in-the-making, daily constitution, adjustment, and reshaping of what it is to be man or woman, white or black. Racism and sexism are mutable, and their reshaping is the source of considerable political and ideological tension. Much of the recent controversy over the concept "underclass," for example, has had to do not so much with whether the phenomena said to characterize this population are or are not "true" as it has concerned what will constitute the image and profile of Black America at the tail end of the twentieth century and who will define that profile. In point of fact, attention to the specificities of historical context—social relations and ideological constructs of race and gender which are passing out of existence, coming into being, or fully emerged and dominant—is the bedrock of both insightful analysis and effective political action.[13]

There are further parallels to be drawn between race and gender in that, once categorically constituted in the context of relations of domination, racism inheres in the categories of racial differentiation, and sexism inheres in gender categories. The historical process of subordination and the concomitant creation of gendered and racialized subjects leaves pronounced traces on the categorical distinctions that define the terrain of gender and race relations. Thus, these categorical distinctions—here principally man/woman, Black/white—are far from a neutral naming of objective things.

The degree of neutrality or objectivity declines dramatically as one moves from the opposition male/female to man/woman to masculine/feminine. In this transition the categories become increasingly freighted with gender inequality and subjectivity. *Man* obviously means far more than a human being who participates in a particular way in the reproductive process, as does *woman*. It has been noted, however, that sexist presumptions can and do invade even the "scientifically objective" description of sexual reproduction at the molecular level, so the struggle to strip these categories of their accretions of sexually biased meanings is formidable.[14]

So, too, racial categories, while being popularly understood to be the simple naming of obviously differentiated groups, are in actuality heavily burdened with racially biased content. It is only partially true that the racial categories "white" and "Black" are a neutral way to name those of European descent or those of African descent. The absence of neutrality is revealed by the fact that, in the United States, children that result from the mixing of subordinate and dominant groups are assigned the name and status of the subordinate group. As in few other countries, the "gray area" of "race mixing" is simply taken care of by denying the existence of shades between the racial poles. The terms for those of mixed African and European ancestry lost their social meaning and fell out of use since they did not denote a qualitative difference in status, at least from the perspective of whites. *Mulatto, quadroon,* and *octoroon* passed out of usage, and *Black* took on its familiar meaning of *all* those with any degree of African ancestry, while white acquired the meaning of only those of "purely" European ancestry. The sociohistorical logic of this, sustained in the way we use these categories to this day, enabled the greatest possible inclusivity in delimiting that portion of the population subject to enslavement. The conceptual (and racist) logic was and is to create as polar opposites the "pure" and exclusive white population on the one hand and the "tainted" and inclusive Black population on the other. Though slavery, the driving social rationale for this exercise in irrationality, has passed from the historical stage, our current usage continues to reflect these origins, and the conceptual hierarchy of pure/tainted is part of the freight carried by the categories themselves.[15]

Relations of gender and racial domination generate, sustain, and are sustained by basic categories that contain within them historical and conceptual material saturated in inequality.

Both gender and racial categories also appear to have a greater measure of fixity and stability than is actually the case. Social relations between the races and between the sexes have the capacity to give rise to new categorical distinctions and to obliterate others. The most conspicuous way in which this has happened vis-à-vis gender relations in the West has to do with the emergence and stabilization of homosexuality as a socially recognized, though still embattled, individual and group identity that has served to challenge, though not yet negate, the presumed and implied heterosexual content of *man* and *woman*. That that content has been shaken but not displaced may be deduced from the fact that, though "lesbian" and "gay man" have surfaced as social beings, the heterosexuality of "man" and "woman" is still assumed, unless otherwise specified. Heterosexist presumptions about the social institutions of marriage and family have been challenged by changing gender relations. Also noteworthy as a spur to disassembling the woman/heterosexual/wife/mother package is the emergence (at the intersection of the lesbian identity and political movements and advances in reproductive technology) of the lesbian mother and, yet more complex, the lesbian nonbiological mother/ coparent as new social figures, claiming social space, defining, asserting, and fighting for civil recognition and civil rights.[16]

Given the conceptual polarity of race distinctions together with the reality of social and sexual intercourse, the space between the poles is a productive field for the generation and dissolution of socially recognized categories. As already noted, racial categories have been established through the submergence of national, ethnic, religious, and class distinctions within each pole in the service of emphasizing the polarity between them and the denial of social or linguistic recognition to breaches of that polarity. More recently, however, there has been an increased usage of the terms *biracial* and *multiple heritage* to denote, among others, those who in previous generations might have been designated "mulatto." There have also been challenges to the rigidity of school districts and the census bureau for failing to provide space for this reality. Whether "biracial" and "multiple heritage" will emerge as full-scale social identities remains to be seen. Working against that eventuality is both the powerful U.S. tradition of either/or bipolar race relations and the fact that the terms encompass extreme heterogeneity in that they can refer to any combination of racial, ethnic, or national groups. Working for it, however, is an increased societal legitimization of the complexities of diversity. In any case, this area is volatile, especially along the Black-white axis, and it will no doubt take some time before there is a categorical settling. And whatever settling does occur will be relative and temporary in light of the likelihood of renewed shiftings of racial identities.[17]

Also interesting to note is the reemergence of ethnicity and nationality as an issue of social consequence among Blacks. Although the voluntary migration of Caribbean Blacks to the United States has been going on for more than a century, the numbers of immigrants have increased enormously in the past several decades, giving the Caribbean Black community social weight and pushing forward cultural, economic, and political distinctions (and sometimes tensions) between Blacks whose racial and national identities were formed in the United States and those whose identities were formed in the nations of the Caribbean. Whether these distinctions will persevere over generations, given the tendency to revitalize racial polarization while submerging ethnic and national differences, is questionable. It may well become another distinction that has some measure of significance within the Black community while being invisible outside of it.

Both race and gender relations have the capacity to generate new social figures that, for whatever set of complex reasons, become insistent on recognition. Changes in these relations may also result in the snuffing out of socially marginalized identities: the maiden aunt and the octoroon are historical relics. In this race and gender are roughly analogous.

Finally, useful comparisons may be drawn in the area of contention over racism and sexism. Both forms of domination produce political movements that aim to challenge the prevailing power relations and the ideological conceptions and stereotypes that denigrate the subordinate group. These movements seek to address social domination, political exclusion, and material inequality through activism on behalf of social reform, the extension of civil rights, democratic principles, and equality of opportunity. In that process both the antiracist and antisexist movements also generate radical, moderate, and conservative wings with differing perspectives on how to pursue contention over relations of inequality, along with separatist and revolutionary tendencies. The political challenge to the racism and sexism of the status quo produces a multitude of issues in which interests, strategies, and tactics are seldom, if ever, identical but often parallel, overlapping, and consonant. And given the biological substrate of gender and racial differentiation, a central element of the ideological challenge to both sexism and racism entails combatting the "scientific" theories and popular notions of natural inferiority which continually arise in new form.

On each of these levels, then—as relations of domination and subordination, as relations that impart complex social meanings to biological difference, as relations that are constituted and transformed in particular historical contexts, as relations whose core categories bear within them the biases of the relations themselves, as relations that create the ground for the production and demise of significant social figures, and as relations that are the source of political and ideological contention—in all these ways and, no doubt, in ways not reflected upon here there are profitable comparisons to be made. Our understanding of one set of dynamics is enhanced by way of its comparison to another, and we comprehend more about hierarchy in society and ideologies of oppression by knowing what is similar about race and gender, racism and sexism.

THE LIMITS OF ANALOGY

Yet analogy has been roundly and righteously criticized, most cogently by feminists of color. The political failure of analogy is perhaps most obvious. In assuming a community of interests of all women vis-à-vis men which is in some way similar to the presumed community of interests of Blacks vis-à-vis whites, feminists have developed perspectives and strategies that neglected to address the fact that all actors were participants in the dramas of race relations, gender relations, and class relations and that all plays were unfolding simultaneously on the same stage. More particularly, it has been insufficiently recognized that the common interest of Black women and men in resistance to racial oppression and the common interest of all too many white women and men in acting together to protect racial privilege might affect whether Black women conceive of themselves as participating in a community of interests with white women and whether they view men as an undifferentiated oppositional force. Generally, white feminists' understanding of themselves as subordinated gendered subjects in a system of sexual inequality has not been matched by an understanding of the meaning of their whiteness in a system of racial oppression. Women of color are afforded no such lapse, and their quality as both gendered *and* racialized beings is an ever-present element of their reality. It is only recently that white feminists have begun to grapple forthrightly with the *particularity* and inherent limitedness of the experiences and worldviews of white, middle-class women.[18]

But the failure of analogy in its corrosive effect on attempts to build political relations of trust among women of different races is rooted in a broader analytical problem. That is, analogy is revealing in the ways addressed above, but only at a high level of abstraction. Once analogy is drawn into service to shed light on the concrete realities of race and sex, racism and sexism, it is far more likely to confuse, mislead, and obscure than it is to clarify.

The level of abstraction at which analogy "works" is that wherein: (a) gendered subjects are stripped of other qualities (such as race, class, nationality, and sexual orientation) in the realm of gender relations; (b) racialized subjects are devoid of other qualities in the realm of race relations; and (c) the two realms do not overlap.[19] It is disappointing but perhaps not surprising that analyses that either were seemingly devoid of racial and class content or that presumed to speak for women of all races and classes "came naturally" to many early feminists. Since white is the norm in U.S. racial ideology in relation to which all other racial groups are, peripherally, "the other" and since the material and ideological culture of the middle classes is the mainstream of U.S. society, much work that focused on gender presumed these elements as "givens." It has taken the work of class-conscious feminists and feminists of color to point out the invisibility of working-class women and women of color in these scenarios and to read class and race back into the script.

The plane of analysis in which one encounters and compares the abstractions "woman" and "Black" has some usefulness analytically, if it is consciously acknowledged that it is from this plane that one's vantage point arises—but this is a very far remove from racism and sexism as they are actually lived and experienced. For the *lived* experiences of racism and sexism are notably dissimilar.[20] One of the principal reasons for that dissimilarity has to do with the profound differences in the ways in which class relations articulate with those of race in contrast to the ways in which they articulate with gender relations.

Probably the central feature of U.S. racism on the Black-white axis is the divergence in the class profiles of the white and Black sectors of the population. The class stratification of Blacks is heavily weighted toward the bottom end of the income and wealth spectrum, with 30 percent of the population living below the government-defined poverty line and another substantial proportion of the population living within a stone's throw of poverty. At the opposite end of the income spectrum only 9.5 percent of blacks earn over $50,000 per year. Thus, to be Black in the United States, whatever one's individual situation may be, is to be identified with a largely impoverished group. The white population, on the other hand, has a much thinner representation at and below the poverty line, with 11 percent below the official poverty mark. The great majority of the white population survives in the broad middle of the income and wealth spectrum, and 24.4 percent earn more than $50,000 per year.[21]

Quite obviously, these differences in the class contours of whites and Blacks are at the root of differences in access to adequate housing, nutrition, education, and services as well as differences in vulnerability to crime, disease, and premature mortality. These differences cross-cut the gender line, providing both white women and men with less vulnerability and greater access than Blacks and accounting for many fundamental dissimilarities in how racism and sexism are experienced as well as significant differences in their ideological construction.[22]

Despite substantial differences in their earnings, white women share a similar class profile with white men. While it is most definitely true that white women who are single, single parents, divorced, or widowed are at a significant economic disadvantage relative to white men, it is still the case that the majority of white women spend the greater part of their lives in households that include men. That is, gender relations still include relations of intimacy (be those relations happy and nurturing or alienated and abusive) across the gender line in the context of the family and/or household. Women's economic status is only partly (and one-sidedly) revealed by way of reference to their earning capacity. Household economy based on pooled earnings and wealth (or lack of same) is at least as important in determining women's class vulnerability or privilege. It is significant, in this regard, that not only is white men's income considerably greater than Black men's and white women's income slightly larger than Black women's, but the marriage and remarriage rate of whites is higher, the divorce rate lower, and the time between marriages briefer. Thus, white women are less likely to be never-married or divorced and have considerably greater access to the economic advantages of pooled income than do Black women.[23] Those Black women who are married share their households with men whose accumulated lifetime earnings are only 56.1 percent that of white men.[24] Furthermore, white households command more than ten times the wealth of Black households, as measured in real property, savings, stocks, etc. In 1988 the median net worth of white households was $43,280. The net worth of Black households was $4,170. The difference between female-headed households was even starker: the median net worth of households headed by white women was $22,100; for households headed by Black women the figure was $760.[25]

Family forms have become much more diverse in recent years, and women have exercised a far wider range of choices in making decisions about whether to enter into or remain in marriages. Yet it should be obvious that, depending on her class and racial background, the decision of a woman to remain single might be an expression of individual autonomy and economic independence, or it might be a sober assessment of the absence of the economic prerequisites for setting up a viable household.

While relations of intimacy and economic interdependence continue to be a prominent feature of gender relations, relations along the racial axis are characterized by separation, segregation, and ghettoization. One of the effects of this active distancing is to concentrate the symptoms and effects of class inequalities within a particular racial group. The concentration of minorities in inner cities with eroding infrastructures and declining tax bases is one of the more recent expressions of this phenomenon. White flight is not white male flight. It is the exodus of white families—men, women, and children—to communities that are often de facto racially exclusive.

There are, clearly, a multitude of other ways in which racism and sexism are more divergent than analogous. Relations of intimacy within the context of male domination subject women to an inequitable burden of household labor, emotional and economic dependence, domestic violence, and date, marital, and acquaintance rape. But it is not these phenomena—which are characteristic of and unique to women's oppression and which distinguish it from racial or class domination—which elude feminists. What has too often escaped them, rather, are the peculiar and unique features of U.S. racism as it affects men, women, and children of all racial groups and classes and the ways in which racial and class subordination compound and amplify the sexism experience by women of color.

The ability of U.S. feminism to come to grips with the racial and class particularity of much of feminist theory and politics, to comprehend the profound differences in racism and sexism as forms of oppression, and to understand the specific experiences of women of color has everything to do with the struggle to understand the distinct and unique historical and operational features of U.S. racism and the degree of attention given to the complexities of U.S. class formation. In the absence of such an approach resorting to analogy does not enhance our understanding of either sexism or racism or the relationship between them. Instead, while appearing to create linkages between those with an interest in the struggle against racism and those with an interest in the struggle against sexism, facile analogies can actually drive them apart by privileging the experience of an already dominant racial group and a relatively advantaged class.

The burgeoning of a sophisticated and diverse body of work by feminists of color together with a growing awareness on the part of many white feminists of the boundedness of their experience and point of view hold considerable promise that both the instructive potential and the limitations of the pursuit of analogy will be recognized, along with the urgent need for analyses that go to the specific conditions and concrete circumstances of women in all their diversity.

NOTES

1. See, for example, Shulamith Firestone's chapter "Racism: The Sexism of the Family of Man," *The Dialectic of Sex* (New York: William Morrow, 1970), 119–41; Helen Mayer Hacker, "Women as a Minority Group," in *Women: A Feminist Perspective,* ed. Jo Freeman (Palo Alto, Calif.: Mayfield, 1979); Kate Millett, *Sexual Politics* (New York: Doubleday, 1969), 24–25. See also Catharine R. Stimpson, "Thy Neighbor's Wife, Thy Neighbor's Servants: Women's Liberation and the Black Civil Rights Movement," in *Woman in Sexist Society: Studies in Power and Powerlessness,* ed. Vivian Gornick and Barbara K. Moran (New York: New American Library, 1972), in which Stimpson makes reference to a women's liberation pamphlet that cites eleven ways in which women's status is similar to that of Blacks.

2. See, for example, Gloria T. Hull, Patricia Bell Scott, and Barbara Smith, eds., *All the Women Are White, All the Blacks Are Men, But Some of Us Are Brave* (New York: The Feminist Press, 1982), which, in its title and introduction, makes clear the exclusion of Black women from the analyses of white feminists; Gloria I. Joseph and Jill Lewis, *Common Differences: Conflicts in Black and White Feminist Perspectives* (Boston: South End Press, 1981); Deborah E. King, "Multiple Jeopardy, Multiple Consciousness: The Context of a Black Feminist Ideology," in *Black Women in America,* ed. Micheline R. Malson, Elisabeth Mudimbe-Boyi, Jean F. O'Barr, and Mary Wyer (Chicago: University of Chicago Press, 1990).

3. For an extended critique of the theoretical stance of much of white feminism, see Elizabeth V. Spelman, *Inessential Woman: Problems of Exclusion in Feminist Thought* (Boston: Beacon Press, 1988).

4. Catharine R. Stimpson details the ways in which first-wave feminism grew out of and learned from the abolitionist movement, the woman/slave analogy that was part of the rhetorical stock-in-trade of nineteenth-century feminism, the sense of mutual betrayal which developed between the two

movements, and the parallel process that evolved a century later between the civil rights movement of the 1950s and 1960s and second-wave feminism: "The [civil rights] movement clarified concepts of oppression, submission, and resistance and offered tactics . . . for others to use to wrest freedom from the jaws of asses. . . . [W]omen use blacks to describe themselves. They draw strenuous analogies between themselves and blacks, between women's civil rights and black civil rights, between women's revolution and the black revolution. The metaphor litters even the most sensible, probing, and sensitive thought of the movement" (Stimpson, "Thy Neighbor's Wife," 648–49).

5. "The analogy . . . linking race to gender . . . occupied a strategic place in scientific theorizing about human variation in the nineteenth and twentieth centuries. . . . [G]ender was found to be remarkably analogous to race, such that the scientist could use racial difference to explain gender difference and vice versa." (Nancy Leys Stepan, "Race and Gender: The Role of Analogy in Science," in *Anatomy of Racism,* ed. David Theo Goldberg [Minneapolis: University of Minnesota Press, 1990], 39).

6. Deborah King briefly summarizes both the history of analogizing and critiques of the practice. King notes that "the race-sex correspondence has been used successfully because the race model was a well-established and effective pedagogical tool for both the theoretical conceptualization of and the political resistance to sexual inequality." It is King's conclusion, however, that "we learn very little about black women from this analogy" ("Multiple Jeopardy," 266, 268).

7. Stimpson, as early as 1971, stated: "I believe that women's liberation would be much stronger, much more honest, and ultimately more secure if it stopped comparing white women to blacks so freely. The analogy exploits the passion, ambition, and vigor of the black movement. It perpetuates the depressing habit white people have of first defining the black experience and then of making it their own. Intellectually sloppy, it implies that both blacks and white women can be seriously discussed as amorphous, classless, blobby masses" ("Thy Neighbor's Wife," 650).

Elizabeth Spelman acknowledges the troublesome comparisons white feminists have drawn between race and gender and between racism and sexism. She also explores at length the point made by many Black feminists that the supposedly generic "woman" of much feminist theory was actually white and middle class all along. Spelman criticizes "attempts to study race and class that do nothing to dislodge white middle-class women as the focus of feminist theory and that take the race and class privilege of such women to be of no theoretical significance" (*Inessential Woman,* 164).

bell hooks notes the "efforts made by women of color to call attention to white racism in the struggle as well as talking about racial identity from a standpoint which deconstructs the category 'woman.' Such discussions were part of the struggle by women of color to come to voice and also to assert new and different feminist narratives. . . . In actuality the theoretical groundwork for all reconsiderations of the category 'woman' which consider race . . . was laid by women of color" (*Yearning: Race, Gender, and Cultural Politics* [Boston: South End Press, 1990], 21).

Angela Harris identifies three contributions Black women make to feminist anti-essentialism: "The recognition of a self that is multiplicitous, not unitary; the recognition that differences are always relational rather than inherent; and the recognition that wholeness and commonality are acts of will and creativity, rather than passive discovery" ("Race and Essentialism in Feminist Legal Theory," *Stanford Law Review* 42 [Feb. 1990]: 608).

8. This essay deals exclusively with the dynamics of racial differentiation and polarization along the Black-white axis. This, obviously, is only a part of the story, since the white racial group in the United States was also forged in contradistinction to Native Americans, Mexicans, and Asians. See Ronald T. Takaki, *Iron Cages* (Oxford: Oxford University Press, 1979), for an account of the development of white racial (and racist) ideology and identity vis-à-vis other nationalities and ethnicities.

9. "Women and men exhibit enormous overlaps in body shape and form, strength, and most other parameters. The diversity within the two groups is often as large as the differences between them" (Ruth Hubbard, "Race and Sex as Biological Categories," in this volume, 15).

10. "A few outstanding traits of external appearance lead to our subjective judgment of important differences. But biologists have recently affirmed—as long suspected—that the overall genetic differences among human races are astonishingly small. Although frequencies for different states of a gene differ among races, we have found no 'race genes'—that is, states fixed in certain races and absent from all others" (Stephen Jay Gould, *The Mismeasure of Man* [New York and London: W. W. Norton, 1981], 323).

11. For a brief review of the history of the concept of race, see Lucius Outlaw, "Toward a Critical Theory of Races," in Goldberg, *Anatomy of Racism,* 61–64. For the history of "scientific racism," see Gould, *Mismeasure of Man.*

12. See Barbara Jeanne Fields, "Slavery, Race and Ideology in the United States of America," *New Left Review* (London) no. 181 (May–June 1990), for a penetrating essay on U.S. "society in the act of inventing race."

13. Paul Gilroy notes that the "analysis of particular local racisms . . . demands that the development of racist discourses must be periodized very carefully and that the fluidity and inherent instability of racial categories is constantly appreciated." He goes on to do a close analysis of contemporary British racial politics and the politics expressed through black popular music ("One Nation under a Groove," in Goldberg, *Anatomy of Racism,* 265).

14. "The active male–passive female dyad has been part of biological dogma and is the metaphor that informs standard descriptions of procreative

biology at every level. . . . Given that fertilization is an active process in which two cells join together and their nuclei fuse, why is it that we say that a sperm *fertilizes* the egg, whereas eggs are fertilized?" (Hubbard, "Race and Sex, 16–17).

15. The ongoing struggle of African Americans to name themselves is, in large part, a response to this fact. Whites have been satisfied to remain designated as whites from relatively early on in U.S. history. Blacks, on the other hand, once they gained some influence over how they were to be designated, have restlessly shifted from negro and colored to Negro to Black to African American. Each shift has represented a renewed assertion of identity and pride as well as an attempt to unload some of the racist burden that inevitably accrues to our name—even, in a society steeped in inequality, to those names we have chosen for ourselves. The African-American colloquial warning not to "call me out of my name" is an indication of the power of derogation and insult contained in naming. A parallel colloquialism in use among whites does not come to mind.

16. The legal battle of lesbian coparents for custody rights is the subject of "Lesbians' Custody Fights Test Family Frontier," *New York Times,* 4 July 1990, sec. 1, 1, 10.

17. An indication of the ongoing confusion, irrationality, and fluidity attached to the space between the poles occurred in an article about interracial romance as depicted in film and television. In describing the child of one such television union, the article begins, "So Molly Dodd has a black baby." In the following paragraphs this same baby is described as a "mixed-race child," a "half-black" child (why not half-white?), and, confusingly, "a child of mixed-race parents." This is not just a matter of editorial variety but evidence of a conceptual and linguistic struggle to name a social character who has had no name for generations.

In that same article Spike Lee, attuned as always to currents in popular culture, resurrects a figure and term buried a century ago: "He cites the impact of an 'enormous population' of people with mixed parentage. 'The mulatto culture and look are highly visible,' he says, mentioning such performers as Prince, Rae Dawn Chong, and Mariah Carey" (Gail Lumet Buckley, "When a Kiss Is Not Just a Kiss," *New York Times,* 31 March 1991, sec. 2, 1, 20).

18. This grappling has been especially ardent among those feminists who have applied themselves to the issue of the relationship between feminism and postmodernism/deconstruction/poststructuralism: The practice of feminist politics in the 1980s has generated a new set of pressures which have worked against metanarratives. In recent years, poor and working-class women, women of color, and lesbians have finally won a wider hearing for their objections to feminist theories which fail to illuminate their lives and address their problems. They have exposed the earlier quasi-metanarratives, with their assumptions of universal female dependence and confinement to

the domestic sphere, as false extrapolations from the experience of the white, middle-class, heterosexual women who dominated the beginnings of the second wave. For example, writers like bell hooks, Gloria Joseph, Audre Lourde, Maria Lugones, and Elizabeth Spelman have unmasked the implicit reference to white Anglo women in many classic feminist texts. Likewise, Adrienne Rich and Marilyn Frye have exposed the heterosexist bias of much mainstream feminist theory. Thus, as the class, sexual, racial, and ethnic awareness of the movement has altered, so has the preferred conception of theory. It has become clear that quasi-metanarratives hamper rather than promote sisterhood, since they elide differences among women and among the forms of sexism to which different women are differentially subject (Nancy Fraser and Linda J. Nicholson, "Social Criticism without Philosophy: An Encounter between Feminism and Postmodernism," in *Feminism/Postmodernism,* ed. Linda J. Nicholson [New York: Routledge, 1990], 33).

19. Feminism has dug itself into a hole more than once in operating from the stripped-down abstraction "woman." The analysis of the family wage, for example, suffered grievously from the unacknowledged fact that this mark of gender oppression for some women was also a mark of their racial and class privilege. Likewise, in maintaining that "women in general" were threatened by the feminization of poverty, feminists failed to confront class differentiation among women or the class dimension of racial oppression. See Linda Burnham, "Has Poverty Been Feminized in Black America?" *Black Scholar* 16, no. 2 (March–April 1985).

20. Elsa Barkley Brown, among others, has pointed out the foolhardiness— particularly when analyzing the experiences of Black women—of treating race and sex as exclusionary isolates. She argues for a "both/and worldview" and "holistic" approach to understanding the intersection and independence of race and sex ("Womanist Consciousness; Maggie Lena Walker and the Independent Order of Saint Luke," in Malson et al., *Black Women in America,* 195). In a similar vein Patricia Hill Collins contends that a "both/and conceptual stance" offers an "inclusive model [which] provides the conceptual space needed for each individual to see that she or he is *both* a member of multiple dominant groups *and* a member of multiple subordinate groups" (*Black Feminist Thought* [Boston: Unwin Hyman, 1990], 230). Clearly, the question posed to Black women, "Are you more oppressed by racism or sexism?" has no sensible answer, as the likelihood of unraveling motivation and intent behind the innumerable instances of discriminatory treatment experienced by Black women is remote indeed. Yet and still, it does not follow from the complex intermingling of racism and sexism in the lives of Black women that the dynamics and effects of the two forms of oppression are the same. The substantially divergent vantage points of those feminist activists and theorists whose life experiences encompass both racism and sexism and those who are subject to sexism but not

racism are one small indicator that, while race and sex may well be intimately interwoven, their effects are not indistinguishable.

21. Gerald David James and Robin M. Williams, Jr., eds., *A Common Destiny: Blacks and American Society* (Washington, D.C.: National Academy Press, 1989), 279. David Swinton, "The Economic Status of Black Americans," in *The State of Black America, 1989* (New York: National Urban League, 1989), 15.

22. The persistence of stereotypes of Blacks as lazy, unmotivated, incapable of setting long-term goals, inclined to criminality, and irretrievably immersed in a culture of poverty is obviously linked to the peculiarities of their class formation.

23. "By 1987 the differences in the marital status distribution of black and white women were much larger than they had been in 1940. Just over one-third of black women were currently married, compared with almost two-thirds of white women. Well over one-third of black women had never married, compared to less than one-fifth of white women. Almost 30 percent of black women were either divorced or widowed, compared with 16 percent of white women" (U.S. Commission on Civil Rights, *The Economic Status of Black Women: An Exploratory Investigation* [Washington, D.C.: 1990], 27–28). See also Mary Corcoran, Greg J. Duncan, and Martha S. Hill, "The Economic Fortunes of Women and Children: Lessons from the Panel Study of Income Dynamics," in Malson et al., *Black Women in America,* 106.

24. James and Williams, *A Common Destiny,* 300.

25. Robert Pear, "Rich Got Richer in 80's; Others Held Even," *New York Times,* 11 January 1991, sec. 1, 1, 13, citing U.S. Census Bureau statistics.

◆ GARLAND E. ALLEN ◆

The Genetic Fix: The Social Origins of Genetic Determinism

INTRODUCTION

Media hype surrounding the human genome project (or "initiative," as it is sometimes called) has increased dramatically in the past few years. Among general readership periodicals *Business Week* (26 May 1990), the *New Republic* (9 July 1990), *Newsweek* (18 May 1990), and *Plain Truth* (September 1990) have all featured cover stories on the marvels of the new genetic engineering. Among professional scientific journals *Science* magazine, organ of the large and highly influential American Association for the Advancement of Science (AAAS), featured an endorsement of the genome project as a cover story in its 11 October 1990 issue.

By now nearly everyone has heard something about the human genome initiative as biology's "Manhattan Project." While there are many reasons to worry about the human genome project—as a way of doing science, for one thing, or for the issues it raises about privacy and legality, for another—the most disturbing features are the promises its supporters are making about it becoming the panacea for all social ills. In his editorial introducing the 11 October issue of *Science,* for example, Daniel Koshland, editor-in-chief, wrote (referring to a gunman in Berkeley, California, who took a number of hostages in a bar, killing one and wounding another) that people exhibiting such sociopathic behavior could be helped better by the findings of the human genome project than by psychology or sociology. To Koshland it seemed clear that antisocial beings operated with miswired nervous systems and brains. Koshland suggests that genetics will ultimately be able to explain and cure such neurological defects with DNA splicing. The naïveté of such a claim is appalling enough, but, if naïveté is all that is involved, I would worry only for the future of *Science* magazine.

The much more serious issue is that the human genome project is becoming the figurehead—the leading edge, as it were—of a strong hereditarian movement that has been growing for the past several years, even before the genome project became big news. The human genome project gives hereditarian arguments the seal of approval from mainstream science, that is, from genetic engineering itself. With the human genome project promising that the tools of base-pair analysis and mapping can be applied to the solution of human social ills, the public is being led to have faith not in human and social solutions but, rather, in technological solutions to persistent, and worsening, social problems. The genome project is being sold as a technological fix—or, more specifically, what Amatai Etzioni (1993) labeled two decades ago as "the genetic fix."

The idea that genetic malfunctions ("bad genes") lie at the heart of many social problems is not new with the human genome project. In modern times it traces back at least to anthropological movements in the mid-nineteenth century, with studies of cranial capacity, facial angles, and skull contours as indicators of social and intellectual capacity. Cesare Lombroso's criminal anthropology movement in the 1890s was one of the first to try to tie physical, biological factors directly to the cause of social problems, but he was quickly followed by eugenics, based on the newly discovered Mendelian genetics, in the early decades of the century. In the 1960s and early 1970s the issue of genetically determined racial differences in IQ saw a revival of the argument that social traits are biologically based, and the mid-1970s saw the rise of the same basic views couched in neo-Darwinian terms.

In the past several years a new onslaught of genetic claims has emerged, focusing on such traits as alcoholism, criminality, manic depression, schizophrenia, shyness, and homosexuality, among others. These claims are receiving widespread popular dissemination through mainline media channels. In 1985 two Harvard professors, James Q. Wilson, a political scientist, and Richard Herrnstein, a psychologist, published *Crime and Human Nature,* arguing that there was a strong genetic component to criminal behavior and that "bad families produce bad children" (215). The authors cite twin and adoption studies as well as research on biological correlates such as body shape and criminal behavior to back up their argument. Following Harvard's lead, in 1986 the *Wall Street Journal* carried a three-part series, "The Genetic Bases of Anti-Social Behavior" (their examples were alcoholism and criminality), and 1987 became a banner year for genetic determinist claims. In March, in a study widely publicized in newspapers and on TV, Daniela Gerhard of Washington University claimed to have found a genetic marker for manic depression on chromosome 11. In April 1987 *Newsweek* magazine carried a cover story entitled "The Gene Factor—How Genes Shape Personality." With references even to the "Baby M" case, a custody battle between biological parents and a surrogate mother who wanted to keep the child she had carried to term, the article opened with the confident statement: "Scientists have speculated for generations that people are the products of their genes, but proof was lacking. Now that has changed. Solid evidence demonstrates that our very character is molded by heredity. If so, how much did Baby M's future hinge on which family got her?" (58).

The answer to the last question was "Not very much," since, as the article tries to show, much of Baby M's personality was already determined at the time of conception. The *Newsweek* article is replete with references to sensational cases from the Minnesota twin study in which, for example, identical twins, separated at birth, found that they hold their beer cans alike, have a passion for John Wayne movies, and may even carry a common "gene for risk-taking." These claims were also extended with reference to data on alcoholism and criminality by the much-publicized Swedish adoption studies. Finally, in their 30 November issues both *Time* and *U.S. News and World Report* carried cover stories on the genetic basis of alcoholism.

Then, in 1988 and 1989, J. Philippe Rushton, a psychologist from the University of Western Ontario, created a major sensation, first at the AAAS annual meeting in February and later in the press, by claiming that among racial groups Asians show the most evolutionary advancement, with whites coming in a close second, and African Americans lagging significantly behind. Rushton has employed a now largely outdated ecological concept (r- and K-selection theory) to suggest that blacks and whites have adopted different life-styles with regard to parenting and reproduction in order to "maximize" their reproductive strategies. Blacks are r-selected, that is, have many children but do not parent them well, while whites are K-selected, that is, have fewer children but invest more parental care in each. The fact that virtually no ecologists today extend r- and K-selection theory as useful beyond the insect groups for which it was originally developed has not bothered Rushton, who applies the theory across not only different species and classes but different phyla as well.

Recent biological determinists have also turned their attention to male-female differences. In its 28 May 1990 issue *Newsweek* ran a cover story entitled "Guns and Dolls: Scientists Explore the Differences between Boys and Girls." The headline for the story itself begins, "Alas, Our Children Don't Exemplify Equality Any Better than We Did. . . ." The thrust of the article is that there are biological reasons (it doesn't say just what but, presumably, genes at some level) why little boys gravitate to guns and little girls to dolls. *U.S. News and World Report* had run a similar cover story on 8 August 1988 entitled "Men *vs.* Women: The New Debate over Sex Differences." Both articles conclude that stereotypical role differences are not culturally but, to a significant degree, biologically determined and that society should learn how to work with these differences rather than try to change them.

All in all, then, in recent years there has been a powerful resurgence of biological explanations for social phenomena—what some critics call biological determinist arguments. Most of this has centered, directly or indirectly, on claims for a genetic basis, or substratum, for our social behavior.

What does it mean that such a rash of media attention has been devoted to the genetics of human behavior—especially what is regarded as socially deviant behavior, such as alcoholism or criminality? I argue that the recent media onslaught is not a result of fundamentally new scientific discoveries but, rather, represents a deeper historical process at work. That process has to do with the confluence of several social and political forces. One is associated with economic crises—in the present case the worsening U.S. balance of trade, manufacturing decline, and fall in the rate of profit for U.S. businesses. The other is the rise of new scientific ideas and/or technologies—in the present case the techniques and concepts of DNA manipulation, or "genetic engineering." At a time of social and economic crises, when people are experiencing cutbacks in employment, health care, and salaries hereditarian arguments serve a special social and political function. By suggesting a genetic cause for persistent or recurrent social dilemmas, hereditarian theories suggest that the victims, not the social system, are the cause of their own problems. This view implies, even if it is not always stated explicitly, a general solution. If it is nature rather than nurture which is the cause of our social problems, then the solution is not to be found in political and social change but, instead, in change in the genetic makeup of the population. Such changes can come about either by programs for selective breeding, sterilization, or, eventually, gene therapy, using the techniques of recombinant DNA. This is the true and ultimate "genetic fix": the belief that many of our social problems are rooted in the genes and can be solved by genetic, rather than social, change. The idea of the genetic fix and the biological determinist arguments on which it is based point to a deeper, and disturbing, historical trend.

In the following essay I will discuss three main points. First, the claims of a genetic basis for criminality, manic depression, or alcoholism are not isolated examples but, instead, represent a trend that has been on the upswing for several years beginning in the late 1960s. Indeed, in various forms such theories have recurred periodically in the West since Plato first articulated the "noble lie" of the metals in the *Timaeus* (Gould 1981) but with increasing frequency since the rise of science in the sixteenth and seventeenth centuries. Second, such theories are too often characterized (even in their respective historical periods) by nonrigorous, sloppy, or sometimes actually dishonest use of information or techniques of analysis. Historically, they appear as one sorry string of half-truths, misrepresentations, or popular biases clothed in scientific garb. Finally, the prominence of theories of biological determinism at any given time closely follows social and economic upheaval; under such social conditions the theories serve to divert attention away from environmental toward biological causes of social problems. Theories of biological determinism usually serve a hidden agenda—namely, the construction of social attitudes and the maintenance of social control by a wealthy elite, who stand to suffer by broad-ranging social and economic changes.

To illustrate these points I will use one historical case study: the U.S. eugenics movement between 1910 and 1940. I am focusing on this example for several reasons. One is that it is my own main area of research in the history of science. Another is that we have enough time lag since the movement's heyday to discern its full impact and to understand the social factors involved in its rise to prominence. Still another reason is that, depressingly, many of the modern claims for a genetic basis of alcoholism or criminality sound almost identical to claims made by eugenicists sixty or seventy-five years ago. I do not, of course, want to suggest that modern hereditarian theories are simply "guilty by association" with tainted theories of the past. What I would like to suggest is that we keep our eyes open to how such theories in the past have come into prominence and what social purposes they served. We may then begin to ask whether such theories might be serving the same social purposes at present. In a word it would be foolish to shut our eyes to parallels and similarities between the past and present and not to try to learn from history. There is no reason to think that we are so sophisticated or knowledgeable today that we are immune to the intellectual and social errors made by our predecessors.

EUGENICS IN AMERICA, 1900–1940: A BRIEF OVERVIEW

Eugenics is a term coined originally by English biometrician Francis Galton (1822–1911) in his book *Inquiries into Human Faculty* in 1883. It meant "truly born" and served as the rallying point for a movement that reached considerable popularity in both England and the United States (also in Scandinavia, Germany, the Soviet Union, and, to a lesser extent, France) in the first four decades of the twentieth century. According to Charles B. Davenport (1866–1944), the intellectual leader of eugenics in the United States, the movement was defined as "the science of the improvement of the human race by better breeding." Buttressed by Mendel's laws of heredity, rediscovered in 1900, eugenicists sought to improve the social as well as the physical nature of humanity by eliminating genetically undesirable traits from the population. At the time genes were postulated to control everything from Huntington's chorea to alkaptonuria, polydactyly, criminality, and pauperism. It was these latter sorts of traits, social and behavioral, which particularly interested eugenicists.

The eugenics movement in the United States involved two basic activities: research into the nature of human heredity and social action, or propaganda, programs, including education, popular lectures, and lobbying in state legislatures and Congress. Research activities were centered at the Eugenics Records Office (ERO) at Cold Spring Harbor, Long Island, under the overall leadership of Davenport, with the day-to-day organization carried out by his deputy, Harry Hamilton Laughlin (1880–1943). A variety of eugenics research projects originated at, or were overseen by, the ERO, including the collection of thousands of family pedigrees, cross-referenced by family name, hereditary conditions, and geographic locality. The ERO became a major repository for eugenic data on inheritance of human physical, mental, and personality traits. Other eugenical research was carried out under the auspices of institutions such as the American Museum of Natural History, whose president, Henry Fairfield Osborn (1857–1935), was a staunch eugenicist, and at various universities, by individual biologists such as Edwin Grant Conklin (1863–1952) at Princeton, William Ernest Castle (1867–1962) at Harvard, and S. J. Holmes (1868–1964) at the University of California at Berkeley.

The eugenicists' social action programs encompassed a wide variety of activities. They wrote popular articles on eugenics for both their own publications such as the *Journal of Heredity* and *Eugenical News* and for major popular magazines such as *Good Housekeeping, Popular Science Monthly, Century Magazine,* and *The Dial;* newspapers such as the *New York Times* regularly carried articles about eugenic conferences and speeches. Eugenicists also sponsored popular lectures, lobbied for inclusion of eugenics material in school and college curricula, wrote textbooks, and mounted exhibits for state fairs and national occasions such as the Philadelphia Sesquicentennial in 1926. Their most long-lasting effect in the social sphere was seen in 1924 in the passage, in the U.S. Congress, of the Johnson Act, which restricted immigration from southern and central Europe and from the Balkans and the Soviet Union, and in compulsory eugenical sterilization laws, which, by 1935, had been passed in over thirty states. Significantly, the basis of such social legislation was claimed to be the high incidence of hereditary "defectives" among the poor, immigrants (from eastern and southern Europe), and ethnic minorities (Jews, blacks, and Native Americans).

The eugenics movement reached its heyday in the mid- to late 1920s, experiencing a slow decline from its ultrahereditarian claims by the time of World War II. The changing public face of eugenics was partly a result of some of its own exaggerated claims about the genetic basis for racial and national differences and partly a result of the bad name given to eugenics by Nazi racial and genetic theories. Contrary to the claims of some historians, such as Mark Haller or Daniel Keveles, however, I will argue that eugenical thinking did not die out but, instead, persisted in several forms after the war, most principally as the newly emerging "population control movement," spearheaded by Frederick Osborn (1888–1983), nephew of Henry Fairfield Osborn, and financed by the Rockefeller-funded Population Council. Just as earlier eugenicists had claimed that the poor, working-class strata of society were outbreeding the wealthy elites at home, the more recent population control advocates warned that the poor nations of the world were outbreeding the wealthy and advanced nations at an alarming rate (Weissman 1970; Commoner 1975). The eugenics ideology itself did not die so much as did the focus on individual family pedigrees and simplistic Mendelian models of inheritance which was popular in the period between World Wars I and II. And today, as I suggested at the outset of this essay, there appears to be a resurgence of such thinking, which ought to give us cause for alarm.

AN EXAMPLE OF EUGENICS RESEARCH PROGRAMS:
THE WORK OF CHARLES B. DAVENPORT

Eugenicists past and present argued that not only were a number of clinically definable human traits such as brachydactyly, polydactyly, and baldness inherited but also a whole host of social traits such as alcoholism, criminality, seafaringness, feeblemindedness, rebelliousness, and artistic sense. On what sort of evidence were their claims based? What was the nature of the research carried out in support of such views? Davenport's research on the inheritance of thalassophilia (literally, "love of the sea," or what he called "sea lust") and criminality will serve as two examples of the research base on which typical eugenical claims were based.

Thalassophilia is a condition that Davenport found commonly expressed in the families of naval officers, traveling salesmen, and truants. In his lengthy (236 pp.) study, *Naval Officers: Their Heredity and Development,* with the help of his wife and an assistant, Mary T. Scudder, Davenport surveyed the family histories of sixty-eight U.S. naval officers. With cautionary notes at the outset that thalassophilia is not a "simple" trait and that it is very much influenced by environment (9), Davenport argued that love of the sea is genetically determined, as a subset of the more general trait known as "nomadism." For the thalassophilic traveling on land will not suffice, however, because "movements are less free and the horizon more restricted" (27).

Evidence of the trait's hereditary nature is revealed in the series of sixty-eight family pedigrees Davenport constructed for his study. He noted that thalassophilia occurred almost exclusively in males and, hence, qualified as either a sex-linked or possibly sex-influenced trait such as rose comb in fowl (male fowl have large combs, whereas females, if they have the trait at all, have much reduced combs). Furthermore, thalassophilia often skips generations or is found in only some of the sons from a thalassophilic father. Davenport's conclusion is illustrative of his approach, in which a trait is assumed to be totally genetic (despite his lip service paid earlier to environment) because it runs in families:

> Thus we see that thalassophilia acts like a [Mendelian] recessive, so that, when the determiner for it (or the absence of a determiner for dislike [of the sea]) is in each germ-cell the resulting male child will have a love of the sea. Sometimes a father who shows no liking for the sea, like Perkins' father, may carry a determiner for sea-lust recessive. It is theoretically probable that some mothers are heterozygous for love of

the sea, so that when married to a thalassophilic man half of their children will show sea-lust and half will not. (29)

Although Davenport explicitly recognized that the recurrence of
seafaringness in males, rather than females, was at least partly a social
trait, he virtually ignored family or social environment in his studies
of the origin of thalassophilia. Consideration of social or environmental influences was purely a formality that played no role in his actual
pedigree analysis.

While Davenport's claims for the genetic nature of thalassophilia
were based on a questionable analysis of family pedigrees, he did at
least collect the data and present it in a systematic form. When it
came to criminality, however, he forsook data altogether, turning to
general impression and anecdote. In his 1928 article "Crime, Heredity, and Environment" Davenport again began with a warning to the
reader that criminality is not a simple trait and is very much condi-
tioned by social context—for example, bigamy is a crime in some
countries and the accepted custom in others (Davenport 1928, 304).
He went on to point out that two opposing schools of thought have
existed over the years on the origin of criminal behavior: the environmental school and the hereditary school, the most extreme form of
the latter being Cesare Lombroso's late-nineteenth-century school of
criminal anthropology. Davenport dismissed as overly simplistic
Lombroso's claim that he could predict criminal behavior from facial
and body anatomy. The only account of the origin of criminality to
comply with modern biology, Davenport asserted, is one that sees it
as a product of both heredity and environment. So far, so good—a
sensible and well-balanced presentation.

Having said this much, however, Davenport goes on to claim that
criminality is in reality an expression of several, more simple behavioral defects, such as "inadequate social instinct" and "feeble self-
control." For a person afflicted with feeble self-control good
environment will no more improve the ability to act altruistically
than "the most assiduous cultivation of the Bantam corn will . . .
make an eight foot stalk" (310). What is the proof for this conclusion?
A number of Davenport's references are to individual cases, real and
hypothetical:

> Thus I have in mind a boy who does well in school, except for inatten-
> tion. He prefers the companionship of older, wild boys; he lies, steals,
> runs away from home. He has two fine studious brothers. His father is
> a strong character and a successful lawyer; his mother is an excellent
> woman, intelligent and firm. But her father's father was erratic and no-

madic; and he preferred to go about in an Indian blanket. He traced
back to Indian ancestry. He has three nomadic descendants. (308)

Other supporting references are simply to general observations. In
claiming, for example, that criminal tendencies must be partly hereditary, Davenport notes that orphan asylums, which expose all children
to the same environment, produce some criminals alongside a large
number of sound citizens. He concludes that defective heredity must
therefore play a role in determining the behavior of the few derelicts.
The data presented, consisting of only one or a few cases, is not documented and is at best merely anecdotal.

Another important form of argument used by Davenport—and
one that is extremely common in all biological determinist claims—is
reasoning by analogy. Many of the analogies derive from agriculture
or practical breeding, as, for example, Davenport's reference to inheritance of comb type in chickens or to Bantam corn. Other analogies
are to simple everyday occurrences—for instance, the claim that criminals cannot learn cause-and-effect and are thus like children who repeatedly play with fire even though they get burned every time. A
rather bizarre analogy is Davenport's recounting the story of a woman
with an insane cat that killed its own kittens and attacked other cats.
The owner wanted to drown the unfortunate animal but was persuaded by what Davenport considered to be a misguided neighbor
that the more humane response would be to keep the cat in a cage for
the rest of its life. Davenport's point is that such advice seems non-
sensical with regard to badly misbehaving cats but that it is routinely
followed in the case of human beings.

With arguments of this kind Davenport built his case for a strong
hereditary component to criminal behavior. The solution to the crime
wave that Davenport saw engulfing the United States in the 1920s,
then, was a combination of tougher laws and penal codes combined
with eugenics. Eugenics is preferable, he states, because it is preventive; it attacks the problem at its roots. As he wrote at the end of
"Crime, Heredity, and Environment": "We are breeding too many people with feeble inhibitions and without proper *social* instincts. . . .
Satisfactory progress will be made only when we understand how
those with congenital criminalistic make-up are bred and try to prevent such breeding. If we permit them to be born, then we must apply
such special treatment as will prevent their behavior from disorganiz-
ing society" (313).

We may legitimately wonder how such reasoning could attain the
status of "scientific research." Charles B. Davenport was not regarded
by his contemporaries as a fool, nor was he a member of the lunatic

fringe. He received his doctorate under E. L. Mark at Harvard in the early 1890s, was a professor of zoology at the University of Chicago before founding the Station for Experimental Evolution and Eugenics Record Office at Cold Spring Harbor, and was a member of both the National Academy of Sciences and the National Research Council. In 1932 he served as secretary-treasurer of the Sixth International Congress of Genetics in Ithaca, New York, and was well-respected by his colleagues for the good work he did on poultry genetics. Although many disagreed with his eugenical "research," and some even went so far as to disassociate themselves from the Eugenics Record Office and its hereditarian pronouncements, Davenport maintained throughout his life a prestigious scientific profile among many segments of the biological community and certainly among the lay public. What seems today to be utterly simplistic and naive research methods and claims were at the time, and especially in the full flush of success of the new Mendelian genetics, considered acceptable forms of investigation.

MODERN METHODS OF RESEARCH IN BIOLOGICAL DETERMINATION

Today's research methods share many characteristics with those of the older, prewar eugenics movement. The work of James Q. Wilson and Richard Herrnstein on the inheritance of criminality, of Thomas J. Bouchard (the Minnesota twin studies) on personality, of C. Robert Cloninger on criminality and alcoholism, and of J. Philippe Rushton on racial differences are all plagued with the same kinds of methodological problems which Davenport and earlier eugenicists encountered but ignored. A few examples will indicate the degree to which these problems exist in the current literature and the degree to which the authors ignore or minimize these problems in drawing their conclusions.

In an attempt to demonstrate that a tendency toward criminal behavior is biologically based (somehow genetically determined), Wilson and Herrnstein (1985) cite a 1950 study by Sheldon and Eleanor Glueck which purports to show a relationship between body shape and criminality. The study compared two groups of adolescent boys based on generalized body types: ectomorphic (vertical, or linear, i.e., thin, lanky), mesomorphic (muscular, square), and endomorphic (round, i.e., fat, stocky). One sample was composed of boys from a Massachusetts correctional facility; while the other, the control group, was drawn from nondelinquents supposedly matched for various possible environmental socioeconomic factors. In both groups the ages ranged from ten to seventeen, with the majority being between four-teen and fifteen (Kamin 1986). The Gluecks found that delinquents had on the average a more mesomorphic body shape than nondelinquents, a feature they took to be a physical, or biological, in-dicator of criminal tendency. Wilson and Herrnstein adopted this con-clusion without question. There were problems with the original study, however, which Wilson and Herrnstein failed either to recog-nize or to report to their unsuspecting readers. First, the whole proce-dure of correlating body types (called "somatotyping") with social or personality traits has proven to be highly unreliable (as an indicator of anything significant) and is virtually discarded by most psycholo-gists today. A follow-up study stimulated by the Glueck's original in-vestigation found, for example, that a sample of Princeton college students was on the average *more* mesomorphic than the Boston de-linquents. Subsequent studies have confirmed that there is little or no correlation between body shape and occupation or any other social or personality characteristics.

Second, the two comparison groups were not well matched for socioeconomic status or age. On the average the delinquents came from families with lower income and less education than the matched sample; moreover, the delinquents were on average six months older (some up to fourteen months older) than the nondelinquents. At what is clearly a critical *growth period* in adolescent life an age difference of six months or more can have a great effect on body shape, in ex-actly the direction noted—toward a more mesomorphic (muscular, square) build. Again Wilson and Herrnstein made no mention of these methodological problems in drawing their conclusion that criminality is related to biological traits such as general body build.

A second example comes from the work of Bouchard and the no-torious Minnesota twin studies. For several years Bouchard has claimed that a biological (genetic) basis exists for homosexuality. He and his coworkers (Eckert et al. 1986) studied the incidence of homo-sexuality in monozygotic twins raised apart. The study consisted of a total of six pairs of twins, two male and four female pairs. Of the two male pairs both members of one pair are homosexual, while in the other pair only one member is homosexual. Of the females only one member of each of two pairs is either homosexual or bisexual, while the members of the other pair are both heterosexual. From this "large" data base the authors conclude that male homosexuality has a strong heritable component, while female homosexuality does not (Dusek 1987). Needless to say, a conclusion based on such a small sample size (really, one case only for the male pairs) represents a considerable lapse of statistical rigor.

I introduce these examples to show how similar methodological problems plague contemporary as well as much older determinist research. It is as if the older literature never existed and that modern researchers proceed blindly ahead, learning nothing from the mistakes of their predecessors. There is in operation either a self-selection process by which people prone to naive, simplistic, and sloppy methodology gravitate to determinist research or a political agenda on the part of researchers and/or their patrons which accounts for the persistence of research plagued by such fundamental methodological flaws. As I suggest in the analysis section of this essay, it is likely to be some combination of all of these factors—but I would argue that the congruence of the political aims of the researchers and the benefactors provides the main driving force for much of this type of research, past and present.

OPPOSITION TO DETERMINIST ARGUMENTS:
THEN AND NOW

It would be incorrect to leave the impression that simpleminded determinist arguments such as those advanced by Davenport and others went unopposed at the time. A number of geneticists reacted to eugenical claims with a range of responses, from considerable skepticism to open rejection. As early as 1915 Thomas Hunt Morgan (1866–1945) of Columbia University resigned from the eugenics committee of the American Breeders' Association because, as he explained in a letter to Davenport, he felt the claims for inheritance of many human traits were not backed up by any significant evidence. In 1925 Herbert Spencer Jennings (1868–1947) of John Hopkins University wrote a scathing attack on the testimony that Harry H. Laughlin had given before the House Committee on Immigration and Naturalization in 1924. In his testimony Laughlin claimed that the majority of immigrants from southern and central Europe were feebleminded and degenerate (Laughlin 1923). While not decrying the principles of eugenics per se, Jennings was highly critical of Laughlin's findings and of his unjustified claims for the inferiority of certain racial and ethnic groups (Jennings 1924).

Another, and in the United States at least one of the most vocal critics of eugenics, was geneticist H. J. Muller (1890–1967). In 1932, at the Third International Congress of Eugenics in New York, Muller lambasted eugenicists for putting the cart before the horse and not recognizing that until social and economic environments are equalized for all people it is impossible to distinguish between genetic and environmental causes of social behaviors. Needless to say, the assembled eugenicists were not thrilled with Muller's view and subsequently blocked publication of his paper in the Congress proceedings (it was, however published separately). Ironically, Muller was not opposed to eugenics in principle—indeed, he was a strong proponent of selective breeding and later in his life put forward his own eugenical scheme known as "germinal choice"—but only to the simplistic, racially and ethnically biased version that had become so prominent by the 1930s. Despite some open attacks, however, the really critical questions never seemed to reach a significant sector of the reading public, leaving the impression that geneticists overwhelmingly supported eugenical claims. Eugenics gained its scientific credence as much by default of its critics as by the power of its own research claims.

The situation is somewhat better today at least in one respect. Biologists, psychologists, historians of science, and others in recent years have launched increasing attacks on claims for genetic determinism, with a level of critical analysis of the technical and social arguments and a degree of persistence unknown in the earlier period (Lewontin, Rose, and Kamin 1984). Beginning with the critiques of Arthur Jensen's study of a genetic basis for racial difference in IQ in 1969, through E. O. Wilson's sociobiological arguments about the evolution of male-female sex role differences in 1975, to recent claims about alcoholism, criminality, and schizophrenia (1985 and onward), numerous researchers from a variety of fields have openly exposed to nontechnical readers the research and methodological flaws inherent in determinist claims. We may have learned at least one lesson in the past half-century: ignoring the problems of bad research won't make them go away. Many biologists have come to realize that they have a responsibility to attack such theories, especially when inconclusive and tentative research results are reported in the public press as if they had the certainty of rigorous, experimental research.

The reason for the longevity of eugenical work, and its relative success in the United States as a political movement, must lie elsewhere than in the quality of the research work on which it was based. To understand the movement's success we turn next to an examination of its economic and political base: Who funded eugenics, and for what reasons?

ANALYSIS: EUGENICS AND AMERICAN SOCIAL HISTORY, 1890–1930

Eugenics developed during a period of considerable social and economic upheaval in the United States. It was an era that saw the rapid growth of industrial capitalism, which brought with it extensive urbanization and consequently an increase in crime, alcoholism, and prostitution. Capitalism also meant great fluctuations in prices and wages, high unemployment, increasingly militant labor union organizing, and increasing immigration, as dispossessed workers from Europe in the 1910s and 1920s sought to make their fortunes in the United States. Increasing social and economic problems brought the financial and political leaders of the United States to abandon slowly the laissez-faire economic and social policies of earlier generations and to adopt the ideas of rational planning—for both the economy and the society at large. As outlined in James Weinstein's *The Corporate Ideal in the Liberal State, 1900–1918* (1968) and Robert Wiebe's *The Search for Order, 1877–1920* (1967), modern social historians have shown that social and economic planning, particularly by a corps of trained "scientific experts," became part of the new ideology of the so-called progressive movement (roughly 1880–1930). While the idea of managed (planned, or controlled) capitalism was introduced in industry in the last quarter of the nineteenth century, it extended eventually to all aspects of society: interstate commerce, food and drug regulation, labor legislation, and education. In this era of Taylorism and the reign of the efficiency experts "scientific" management came to be held in high esteem.

It was into this environment that eugenics emerged after 1900 and in it found such a comfortable home. Because it encompassed the idea of planning human evolution, or what was called "management of the human germ plasm," eugenics was the counterpart in biology of rational control and planning in industry and society. Indeed, one of the chief arguments made by eugenicists such as Davenport and Raymond Pearl (1879–1940) was that the new science extended the concept of efficiency and control from business and technology into one of humanity's most important arenas: reproduction. The new scientific planners were to be the eugenicists; armed with Mendel's laws and pedigree charts, they were to march forth and save society from the defective classes, who were the cause of unemployment, strikes, resistance to authority, and a host of other threats to the established industrial order. Portraying themselves as scientifically trained efficiency experts, eugenicists argued that it was far more effective to prevent the dregs of

humanity from being born than to have to take care of them at the tax-
payers' expense once they became a social menace.

Particularly objectionable to eugenicists and industrial and financial leaders were the immigrants who after the 1880s came from
southern and central Europe and the Balkans. These immigrants, described as radicals and socialists, were said to be the major cause of
labor unrest and union organizing in the period from 1880 to 1930.
These were precisely the immigrant groups that Laughlin and other
eugenicists targeted for the restrictive immigration policy set by the
Johnson Act in 1924 (Allen 1983, 1987).

To support my claim that eugenics was fostered by the wealthy
and political elites as a means of instituting efficiency and control in
the social sphere, it is instructive to examine the funding basis of the
movement. Elsewhere I have documented the financial support given
to eugenics, particularly to the Eugenics Record Office at Cold Spring
Harbor (Allen 1986), so here I will present only a brief summary. The
Cold Spring Harbor operation under Davenport and Laughlin was
funded from three major sources, in the amounts indicated in table 1.
But the ERO was not the only eugenics organization in the United
States at the time. The Race Betterment Foundation in Battle Creek
Michigan was funded by J. H. Kellogg, the cereal magnate, while the
Pioneer Fund was financed by Colonel William H. Draper, a textile
millionaire, with Laughlin and Madison Grant as advisors. (By the
way, the Pioneer Fund still exists and in the late 1960s funded the
work of both Arthur Jensen and William Shockley, and more recently
that of Thomas J. Bouchard of the Minnesota twin studies and
J. Philippe Rushton of the University of Western Ontario.) Large-scale
private contributors to one or another eugenical organization included
Walter J. Salmon, a horse breeder from Kentucky, and C. M. Goethe,
a real estate entrepreneur from Sacramento, California. In addition,
the Rockefeller Foundation sponsored several eugenically oriented
projects of its own in addition to those it funded through the ERO: for
example, establishment of the Bureau of Social Hygiene and its affil-
iate, the Criminalistic Institute, to study the increase in crime in New
York City (Mehler 1987).

Just focusing on the ERO itself, table 1 indicates that between
1910 and 1940 over 1.4 million dollars was pumped into eugenics by
the wealthiest philanthropies of the day. This was a large amount of
money for a time when the dollar was worth five or six times its present value and before government funding of science had been put into
place. For comparison, the following figures indicate the scale of
other scientifically related projects or institutions being funded at the
same time: in 1906 Princeton University received a bequest of

TABLE 1   TOTAL FUNDING FOR THE EUGENICS RECORD OFFICE AT COLD SPRING HARBOR 1910–1940

Source of Funds	Amount
Harriman Family (1910–1917)	$ 641,680
Carnegie Institution of Washington (1917–1940)	474,014
John D. Rockefeller Jr. (1910–1917)	21,650
Walter J. Salmon (Lexington, Kentucky, horse breeder)	75,726
Individual Gifts of over $1,000 (1920–1930)	4,237
Total	$ 1,217,307

Source: Harry H. Laughlin, "Notes on the History of the Eugenics Record Office, Cold Spring Harbor, Long Island, New York." Mimeographed report compiled from official records of the ERO, December 1939, 5; from Laughlin Papers, Northeast Missouri State University at Kirskville; additional figures from Laughlin's correspondence in Kirksville, and from the C. B. Davenport Papers, American Philosophical Society, Philadelphia; see also Allen 1986, 260–64.

$200,000 to equip a physical science research laboratory; a decade later the operating budget for the entire physics department was only $1,600 annually. In 1915 the Carnegie Institution of Washington began funding Thomas Hunt Morgan's *Drosophila* research (studies of the chromosomal basis of Mendelian genetics using the small fruit fly *Drosophila melanogaster*) with an annual budget of $15,000 (including salaries of three full-time workers plus several postdoctoral students). In 1916 the annual budget for the entire Ogden School of Science at the University of Chicago was just over $14,000. Between 1920 and 1940 the Carnegie Institution of Washington funded the Station for Experimental Evolution at Cold Spring Harbor (Davenport's other institution) with an average annual budget of between $125,000 and $140,000. The ERO's annual budget in the same period (also from Carnegie) averaged between $22,000 and $30,000, or about 15 percent of the total Carnegie input into Cold Spring Harbor. As a single research area, therefore, eugenics appears to have received a fair share of funds during the 1910s through 1930s.

The scenario I suggest is that those with financial or political power—the elites at the top of an economic, social, and political order that was experiencing considerable instability—were searching for ways to manage and control the system without fundamentally changing it. Their search became increasingly energetic at the time of economic and social crisis, particularly just before and after World War I. One means of trying to maintain social control was to promote the view that unemployment, alcoholism, insubordination, and criminality have an inborn, or genetic, rather than a social or economic cause. This ideas was brought to the attention of the wealthy elites by eugenicists such as Davenport, who were seeking funds to carry out their research programs. The media and other means of cultural influence, which themselves, as large businesses, are under the control of the wealthy elites, became one effective means of promotion. In the non-specialist periodical literature, for example, pro-eugenics articles increased in frequency from only one per year in the period 1900–1905 to twenty per year from 1910 to 1915 to thirty per year from 1925 to 1930. To boot, Scribner's publishing house, with old-boy ties to Princeton and to the American Museum of Natural History's president, Henry Fairfield Osborn, published a number of the best-selling eugenics books, including Madison Grant's *The Passing of the Great Race* (1916) and Lothrop Stoddard's *The Rising Tide of Colour against White World Supremacy* (1922). At the same time there is virtually nothing in the standard popular press before 1925 which is strongly critical of eugenics.

When an economic system undergoes a period of crisis one of the most convenient "explanations" for the crisis and opposition to it is bad heredity: inborn defects in the victims of the system itself. Buttressed by quantitative data and the aura of established science, biological determinist arguments served to explain away defects in the economic and social system. Moreover, biological determinist arguments suggest social remedies—in the case of eugenics, legislation resulting in immigration restriction and compulsory sterilization. Research and social policy conjoined to promote a "genetic fix."

SCIENTIFIC AND SOCIAL LESSONS TO BE LEARNED

What lessons can we learn from this brief excursion into the history of eugenics? One set of lessons relates to the methodological problems inherent in what is often called the "nature-nurture" question: How much of our behavior and personality is genetically determined? Another set of lessons relates to the interrelationship between science and its social environment—that is, to the underlying political, social, and economic environment in which certain types of scientific research are promoted over others and the form that promotion takes. The second lesson asks us not to look at science primarily as an abstract search for truth but, rather, as one component of class ideology serving political and social ends.

While there are numerous methodological problems inherent in theories of biological or genetic determinism (e.g., the sloppy use of data mentioned), I will discuss only two very general ones that underlie both past and present research on this issue. One is the problem of defining the phenotype, while the other is the problem of twin research—that is, the technique of studying monozygotic twins raised apart as a means of separating genetic from environmental influences. We will examine each of the problems briefly. To carry out genetic studies it is necessary to define clearly, and objectively, the phenotype whose supposed inheritance is being followed through successive generations. Brown hair, blue eyes, or the presence (or absence) of a given enzyme, for example, are phenotypes that can be relatively easily identified in given animals or humans and therefore followed through parent-offspring lines. Complex behavioral phenotypes such as "criminality" or "alcoholism," however, are not so easily defined. What is a criminal, and what is criminal behavior? Criminal acts are totally defined by cultures and subcultures; they have no independent existence outside of a given social framework. Killing a British soldier in Boston in 1775 was regarded as a criminal act by the British and as a heroic act by colonial patriots.

The same problem exists in defining alcoholism. There has never existed a rigorous and unambiguous definition of alcoholism in either the legal or medical worlds. Current studies of alcoholism by Cloninger and his colleagues, for example, are based on data taken from Sweden (the Swedish adoption studies), in which alcoholism is defined in a legalistic way as three or more citations for public drunkenness by the police Inebriation Board. Such a definition, however, while it may or may not serve the social aims of curbing alcohol abuse, can hardly be considered as an independent scientific definition of behavior—especially if the conclusions to be drawn, as Cloninger and others claim, can be extended to human populations in general. Identification and description of behavior are always culturally dependent, something anthropologists have known for years but which geneticists (behavioral and otherwise) seem slow to learn. What, then, does it mean to propose studying the genetics of alcoholism? To be able to investigate the genetics of any trait it is first necessary to be able to identify that trait clearly, so that different researchers at different times and places can recognize the trait when it appears. If there is doubt or disagreement by different investigators about whether individuals do or do not show a given phenotype, then there can be no way to carry out a linear, genetic study between generations. All genetic studies ultimately hinge on being able to identify phenotypes in a clear and consistent way.

A second methodological problem with theories of genetic determinism is the fact that there is no way, short of controlled breeding experiments, in which environmental factors can be held constant in order to separate the effects of heredity from those of environment or human behavior. Vertebrates in general, but humans in particular, have evolved a nervous system that depends for its normal development on inputs from its environment. From a biological point of view it can be just as soundly argued that we, as a species, are genetically programmed to have flexible behavior—that is, to be able to learn—as it can be said that we inherit any rigid, stereotyped behavior. Given what we know about the enormous importance of input from the environment molding the development of the nervous system itself, the integration of genetic and environmental elements in forming any adult behavior would preclude any clear separation of the two by genetic analysis. Pedigree charts certainly do not make any such separation nor do heritability studies that purport to partition variance in a population into genetic and environmental components. Heritability estimates suggest how the partitioning might be made in particular cases but are based on the assumption of a uniform environment within the population being analyzed. Most important, though the terms *heritable* and *inherited* are continually used synonymously in the popular literature, *heritability* does not mean *inherited.* For example, since heritability relies on analysis of variance, a population of all brown-eyed guinea pigs would have a heritability of zero because there was no phenotypic variance, even though eye color might be a truly inherited trait by any geneticist's standards.

The closest researchers can get to separating the effects of heredity and environment are studies of monozygotic twins raised apart, but even these, and their corollary, adoption studies, are fraught with methodological problems that have been thoroughly analyzed by Kamin (1974) and Lewontin, Rose, and Kamin (1984). One of the major difficulties with such studies is the assumption that similar homes produce similar environments or, conversely, that different homes produce different environments, so far as the development of specific human personality and behavior traits are concerned. Psychologists admit that because we know so little about the many environmental nuances that may affect a child's behavior, to say much of anything about how similar or dissimilar two environments are over a number of years amounts to almost total speculation. Short of breeding large numbers of couples and raising their children in highly controlled environments, which for moral and ethical reasons I hope we never contemplate, to try and separate hereditary from environmental components of human social behavior seems largely futile.

A more serious drawback still to the use of twin studies is that ultimately the method relies for its analysis on the concept of heritability. Devised originally in the 1930s as a means of estimating the relative contribution of heredity and environment in determining any given trait, heritability is based on the analysis of variance within a population of organisms known to inhabit a uniform (i.e., nondifferentiated) environment. Heritability estimates (and they always remain estimates as long as there are no direct genetic studies of the trait[s] in question) require two forms of empirical knowledge to be valid: (1) accurate measurements of the phenotype in question and the presence of measurable phenotypic differences within the population; and (2) knowledge that the environment for the population is uniform throughout so that different segments of the population are not being exposed to different conditions. Lack of firm knowledge of either of these conditions renders any heritability estimate meaningless. Thus, the lack of variation for a trait in any population means that the heritability estimate will be zero, even though the trait may be largely genetic. In a population of human beings or guinea pigs with all brown eyes, the heritability of eye color would be zero. In contrast, there may be a great deal of variability in a trait, none of which is genetic— this could be due to different microenvironments (nutritional differences among members of a litter or of subpopulations within a larger population) playing on the same genetic makeup. Unless details of the entire environmental range are known, it is not a safe assumption that all members of a population, especially a population of human beings, are experiencing anything like the same environment. Investigators who assume, without empirical verification, that blacks and whites, for example, are subjected to the same general environment (as Jensen did in his original studies) or that two monozygotic twins were raised apart in significantly different environments are violating one of the basic requirements for heritability studies. What the promoters of heritability studies do not bother to mention—and this has been true from Jensen, Shockley, and Herrnstein in the early 1970s through Bouchard and Rushton today—is that heritability has nothing necessarily to say about genetics. Genetic determinists play on the similarity of the terms *heritability* and *inherited,* relying upon their readers' lack of familiarity with the statistical techniques to make their point sound more legitimate than it actually is. While this is not the place to go into a detailed discussion of all the problems with heritability, it is important to point out that the term *heritable,* in the statistical sense, is not synonymous with *inherited,* in the biological sense.

*   *   *

Among the social lessons to be learned from an examination of theories of genetic determinism are those that bear on the social, political, and economic influences that affect how science is constructed. There are three such lessons in this category which I would like to mention briefly.

The first is that scientists—from Charles B. Davenport in 1920 to Daniel Koshland in 1990—tend to become quite naive and gullible when they purport to provide technological fixes for social problems. Most eugenicists were undoubtedly sincere in their desire to provide rational solutions to persistent and disturbing social problems. But they had little idea regarding the larger social drama in which they served as actors. Moreover, the drama was being directed by social, political, and economic elites who had their own reasons for supporting one particular type of solution over others—reasons that may have been quite different from those of the scientists carrying out the work. In their zeal to provide a "scientific solution" to perceived social problems eugenicists often misunderstood the social context in which their science was being used. While many sympathized with elites' apprehension about burgeoning class warfare and social disorder, others more naively thought they were truly helping all people, even the poor and members of minority ethnic groups who were to be sterilized or deported because of so-called scientific discoveries.

A second social lesson from the eugenics case study is that biological determinists are rarely able to back up their claims with evidence that meets the usual standards of rigor customary in other areas of science. It is exceedingly important for all geneticists who wish to know what can really be said about the inheritance of human behaviors to study closely the original research reports and data on which any particular determinist claims are based. For example, with regard to Sir Cyril Burt's twin data, on which Jensen and others based their arguments about inheritance of racial differences in IQ, Kamin (1974) showed that much of the original data was collected under quite variant conditions, using different tests and methods of administration, making any aggregate analysis highly unreliable. Later investigators showed that some of Burt's data and also that of his coworkers were fabricated (Gould 1981).

Unfortunately, as mentioned, recent studies on the inheritance of criminality, alcoholism, or racial difference in family structure appear to be substantiated by no more rigorous or conclusive data than earlier claims by eugenicists or by Burt, Jensen, Shockley, and Herrnstein. Furthermore, some of the supposedly most exciting discoveries in this regard—genetic markers for both manic depression and alcoholism—were first put forward with great acclaim and then quietly retracted, both in the past two years. Thus, Daniela Gerhardt's correlation between manic depression and a marker on chromosome 11 has not been observed in a wider range of test cases, and the National Institute of Alcoholism and Alcohol Abuse has admitted that alcoholism per se is not an easily definable trait (they continue to promote a genetic hypothesis, however, by expanding the behavioral phenotype from alcoholism to obsessive-compulsive behavior). Given the sad history of research on the genetics of human social traits, it is imperative that no a priori assumptions be made about the quality of any current claims. Indeed, given the history of such theories, I believe we are justified in approaching each new determinist claim with a great deal of skepticism.

The third and final social lesson to be learned from the eugenics case is that a genetic fix, like any sort of technological fix, reflects an attitude, an approach to human problems which is at one and the same time both mechanical and irrational. The "fix" mentality shifts concern from the social and human to the technological realm. Even if the technological fix is based on some concrete and demonstrable reality, which most biological determinist arguments are not, excessive faith in such solutions creates an atmosphere of callousness and inhumanity. The Nazi genetic and physiological experiments on individuals with lives "not worth living" is an extreme, but nonetheless real, example of callousness carried to the level of horror. Formation of social and ethical attitudes, even extreme ones such as those represented by fascism, does not occur overnight. Attitudes change slowly, in small, quantitative steps, but the ultimate outcome can be a qualitative change in ethics and morality of mammoth proportions. Faith in technological fixes can play a major role in fostering such attitudes, and extreme faith in scientific solutions to human problems represents the height of rationality becoming irrational. It is no accident that eugenics found its fullest development in fascist Germany.

REFERENCES

Allen, Garland E. 1983. "The Misuse of Biological Hierarchies: The American Eugenics Movement, 1900–1940." *History and Philosophy of the Life Sciences* 5, no. 2:105–28.

———. 1986. "The Eugenics Record Office at Cold Spring Harbor, 1910–1940. An Essay in Institutional History." *Osiris,* 2d ser., 2:225–64.

———. 1987. "The Role of Experts in Scientific Controversy." In *Scientific Controversies: Case Studies in the Resolution and Closure of Disputes,* ed. H. Tristram Engelhardt, Jr., and Arthur L. Caplan, 169–202 (Cambridge: Cambridge University Press, 1987).

———. 1988. "Eugenics and American Social History, 1880–1950." *Genome* 31:885–89.

Commoner, Barry. 1975. "How Poverty Breeds Overpopulation (and Not the Other Way Around). *Ramparts* (August–September): 21–25.

Davenport, Charles B. 1919. *Naval Offices, Their Heredity and Development*, Pub. no. 259 (Washington, D.C.: Carnegie Institution of Washington).

———. 1928. "Crime, Heredity, and Environment." *Journal of Heredity* 19, no. 7 (July): 307–13.

Degler, Carl N. *In Search of Human Nature* (New York: Oxford University Press, 1991).

Dusek, Val. 1987. "Bewitching Science." *Science for the People* 19, no. 6 (November–December): 19–22.

Eckert, Elke E., Thomas J. Bouchard, Joseph Bohlen, and Leonard Heston. 1986. "Homosexuality in Monozygotic Twins Reared Apart." *British Journal of Psychiatry* 148:421–25.

Etzioni, Amatai. *Genetic Fix* (New York: Macmillan, 1973).

Faulkner, Harold U. 1977. *The Decline of Laissez-faire, 1897–1917* (New York: Rinehart).

Garver, Kenneth L., and Sandra Marchese. 1986. *Genetic Counseling for Clinicians* (Chicago: Year Book Medical Publishers).

Gould, Stephan Jay. 1981. *The Mismeasure of Man* (New York: W. W. Norton).

Jennings, H.S. 1924. "Proportions of Defectives from the Northwest and from the Southeast of Europe." *Science* 59:256–57.

———. 1925. *Prometheus, or Biology and the Advancement of Man* (New York: E. P. Dutton).

Kamin, Leon J. 1974. *The Science and Politics of I.Q.* (Potomac, Md.: Lawrence Erlbaum Associates).

———. 1986. "Is Crime in the Genes?" Review. *Scientific American* 254, no. 2 (February): 22–27.

Laughlin, Harry H. "Analysis of America's Modern Melting Pot." *Hearings before the Committee on Immigration and Naturalization, House of Representatives, Sixty-seventh Congress, 3d sess., Nov. 21, 1911* (Washington, D.C.: Government Printing Office, 1923).

Lewontin, Richard, Stephen Rose, and Leon J. Kamin. 1984. *Not in Our Genes: Biology, Ideology, and Human Nature* (New York: Pantheon Books).

Mehler, Barry. 1987. *A History of the American Eugenics Society* (Ph.D. diss., University of Illinois).

Nobel, David W. 1977. *American by Design. Science, Technology, and the Rise of Corporate Capitalism* (New York: Alfred A. Knopf).

————. 1981. *The Progressive Mind, 1890–1917,* rev. ed. (Minneapolis: Burgess Publishing Company).

Weinstein, James. 1968. *The Corporate Ideal in the Liberal State, 1900–1918* (Boston: Beacon Press).

Weissman, Steve. 1970. "Why the Population Bomb Is a Rockefeller Baby." *Ramparts* (May): 43–47.

Wiebe, Robert H. 1967. *The Search for Order, 1877–1920* (New York: Hill and Wang).

Wilson, James Q., and Richard Herrnstein. 1985. *Crime and Human Nature* (New York: Simon and Schuster).

◆ GISELA KAPLAN ◆

Irreducible "Human Nature": Nazi Views on Jews and Women

INTRODUCTION

This essay deals with two aspects of the Nazi period (1933–45)—namely, Nazi attitudes to Jews and to women. On both topics a vast separate literature now exists, although there is comparatively little on the twin-headed problem of sexism and racism (cf. Bock 1984; Gordon 1984). Not only do sexism and racism have tremendously wide-ranging implications in the Nazi regime, but there are also immediate and substantial definitional problems concerning the terms themselves. Both are problematic in the context of the "Third Reich."

RACISM AND ANTI-SEMITISM IN NAZI GERMANY

The term *racism* is more problematic than *sexism,* especially in the Nazi context. Nazi ideology was fanatically anti-Semitic. *Anti-Semitism* itself is a rather untidy term. In practice it denotes irrational hatred, fear, or dislike of one specific ethnic group, the Jews. The term *anti-Semite* was first used toward the end of the eighteenth century and was based on the myth expounded in Moses that all people stemmed from the three sons of Noah, born after the Flood: Sem, Ham, and Japheth. The descendants of Sem, called Semites, are likely to have referred to the group of peoples and tribes who, around 3000 B.C., migrated from the Arabic peninsula to Mesopotamia, Syria, and Palestine and, later, around 700 B.C., when some groups went from southern Arabia to Abyssinia on the African continent. These groups were not a "race" but, rather, a concoction of peoples including Indo-Germanic groups. Even ethnically there were vast differences, and cultural mixes between groups occurred early (around 2350 B.C.), when Sumerian and Semitic cultures were intermingled by conquest.

In European usage the term *anti-Semitism* never referred to the people on the Arabic peninsula but only to the one group from the Middle East, the Jews, who had lost their own nation and lived in the diaspora in European countries and on other continents. As a people, Jews had also intermingled with host cultures, even though they retained an identifiable culture through their religion and, in many countries, through their ghettoization.

By contrast, *racism,* as we use the term today, refers generally to the mistaken belief that: (a) different ethnic groups by way of their physical appearance and/or their culture form distinct races and (b) that some races are inherently superior to others. Racism orders the world into a hierarchy of superior and inferior ethnic groups and their cultural and social traits. It is not just the hatred of or contempt for one group but an entire worldview about the organic, anthropological, historical evolution of peoples, requiring in essence at least some form of historical consciousness. Mosse (1978, 35) rightly argued that the development of racism went hand in hand with the rediscovery of a historical consciousness in the eighteenth century.

In other words, racism and anti-Semitism may signify different things, both in terms of the historical period under consideration as well as in the overall ideological framework in the twentieth century. One needs absolutely no historical consciousness in order to hate Jews. Qualitatively, the attitude to Jews in the Europe of the late nineteenth and first quarter of the twentieth century was very different than to the peoples whose countries European nations had simply colonized, such as those living in the African nations. Imperialists indeed saw the peoples of different color and different civilizations as inferior to their own (see Kaplan and Rogers in this vol.). This was decidedly not the position adopted toward Jews.

Rather, there was fear that Jews would be *stronger* than the "host" nation and eventually take over. In Germany the myth of the Jewish "takeover" was largely based on a miniscule section of the labor force, as in a few very specific professions and economic activities in which Jews had indeed become a visible influence. In the Germany of the late 1920s 10.9 percent of all doctors and 16.3 percent of all lawyers were Jewish. If Jews "dominated" any fields, these were the German meat trade, which was to 50 percent run by Jewish traders, and the garment industry, in which 62 percent of all clothes were sold through Jewish shops and factories (Barkai 1988, 14). These job clusters had, of course, identifiable sociohistorical reasons. Suffice it to say here that, *as* clusters, they were not representative of the entire job market. But Nazi propaganda made it appear as if the Jewish "infiltration" had reached alarming proportions in *all* walks of life. The fear of domination and corruption by Jews took on paranoiac dimensions of persecution in Hitler, even though in 1933 the Jewish population of about half a million accounted for only 0.76 percent of Germany's inhabitants (Oppenheimer 1971, 162).

Hitler basically divided the world into three groups: the Aryans, the "spiritual" Jews, and the "racial" Jews. A racial Jew was a person who had three Jewish grandparents and a spiritual Jew, or the spirit of a Jew, was ephemeral but indeed something all-encompassing and dangerous which had infiltrated the European world. The "judaization" of Europe, its increasing cosmopolitanism, and the emergence of international finance were all seen as a corruption of the true inhabitants of Europe, the Aryans. There was supposedly an international conspiracy at work, fueled by "proven" plots, as shown in the forged documents of *The Elders of Zion,* which threatened to subjugate Aryans and eventually to take over Europe and even the world. This kind of "almost metaphysical force" (Gordon 1984, 92) gave every anti-Semitic debate in Nazi Germany an air of urgency and a sense that Germans were on the very brink of annihilation. Jews were seen as conspirators who, despite their insignificant numbers, would be capable of taking over and dominating the host country. At the same time we know that Nazis regarded the German "race" as superior. The two things do not go easily together, and, of course, ideologically, a few somersaults were needed to argue both at the same time.

An explanation by Yehuda Bauer is useful for our purposes. He argued: "Antisemitism was therefore not a result of Nazi racism, but the obverse was true: racism was a rationalization of Jew-hatred" (cited in Gordon 1984, 103). In this essay I will speak exclusively about Nazi attitudes to Jews, and, if this be seen as a contribution to the racism debate, then I would like it to be understood in terms of Bauer's qualification of the relationship between anti-Semitism and racism.

IMAGES OF JEWS

Many aspects of the new Nazi anti-Semitism were foregrounded in the nineteenth century and became increasingly more respectable (see Kaplan and Rogers in this vol.). Some earlier sources of important sociopolitical ideas of Nazi ideology are identified here, as far as they reflect genetic determinism.

Jews as a Foreign Race

One of these concerned the claim of a Jewish takeover of Germany and fear of an international "conspiracy," for which the forged document of *The Elders of Zion* from Czarist Russia was the only "evidence." Ironically, these fears were especially expressed within the first decades of the foundation of the German Empire. Indeed, in 1871 Germany became a unified nation for the first time in its complicated history and had every reason to celebrate its good political fortunes. But the emancipation of Jews which had taken place at a different rate and speed and in different ways in the various German principalities before had also shown that Jews had not stopped being Jews through the acts and laws of emancipation (Rürup 1975). They had become German citizens, however, and had begun to live normal lives outside ghettos and outside the previously wide-ranging occupational restrictions. While citizenship was granted to Jews formally, many writers now felt that that had been a mistake. The well-known historian H. v. Treitschke, for instance, wrote in an article entitled "Herr Graetz und sein Judentum" (Mr. Graetz and His Jewishness/Judaism) that he, Mr. Graetz, could barely be expected to be accepted as a German. Germany had been merely his "accidental place of birth." He was and remained an "oriental who will never and will never want to understand our people" (December 15, 1879, in Beohlich 1879, 43).[1] Beta went even further to argue that Jews, as a Semitic race, cannot be interbred with the Indo-Germanic race, just as two different animal species cannot interbreed and that, therefore, all attempts to absorb and "amalgamate" Jews would be in vain (Beta 1875, 19).

The new Jewish question only became a national question once a nation was in place. But these views had widespread support. In 1882 the first international anti-Jewish Congress published a *Manifest,* in which it was argued that the emancipation of Jews, especially if this had led to an acceptance of Christian religions, was even more dangerous than if they stayed within their own. For by adopting the host nation's value system, they were even more capable of ruling and destroying the cultural foundations of nations (*Manifest* 1882, thesis 4,

13). In the name of nationalism, then, anti-Semitic writers such as Stöcker proudly announced in 1888 that "we German antisemites will continue to work and struggle for the realization of our ideal, the liberation of the fatherland from the yoke of Jews" (AC, no 21, January 1888, 2). In the 1880s and 1890s concrete suggestions were made, by writers such as Fritsch and Wahrmund, to stop the progressive "judaization" of Germany and Europe. Both writers advocated mass internment and the immediate cessation of the emancipation and of the German citizenship for Jews, who, they believed, should instead be placed under alien guard and governed by Jewish laws.

The Jew as a Parasite

One of the reasons given for this attitude was that "true Semites" were allegedly a nomadic people who do not know the concept of "fatherland" and who take from their environment what they need and then move on. As Fritsch and many others wrote in the 1890s, Semites do not like to and cannot work; they will only exploit and plunder and take what they can get from their hosts (Cobet 1973, 220). Since they had acquired a position of freedom and political influence over their host nation as never before (*Sächsische Landeszeitung,* September 19, 1888), the danger was all the greater and action was more urgently needed.

The image of the parasite was readily superimposed on the concept of the nomad. For if nomads only took what they wanted and then moved on, the idea of parasitism may have appeared less farfetched, irrespective of the fact that no European Jewry had even the slightest resemblance with nomads in the Middle East. One notes, too, that the notion of a true Semite (whatever that means) as nomadic treated an economically and geopolitically very specific situation of nomadic existence as if it were an inherited, i.e., a *genetic* trait that would persist even if the environment (economic, social, or political) had changed dramatically. Only via this assumption of an unalterable, biologically immutable "racial character" was it possible to maintain a host of assumptions and to perpetrate the myth that Jews were a significant danger to German society, indeed to the European world.

The Jewish parasite was represented as an insect, gnawing away at the nation, its wealth and values, in order to destroy it (see, e.g., O. Bey 1875, 57; Ahlwardt 1890, 249). Later the image of the parasite as insect was changed to that of a vampire. Robert Ley, for instance, talked of a kind of Jew who will literally drink the blood of gentiles and their children "not for religious purposes" but, instead, "because their own chaotic blood is threatened with decay and because only

through drinking the blood of other people can they remain alive."
Writers such as Förster suggested that compromise solutions with
Jews were out of the question. Because of the destructive "nature" of
Jews as parasites, he advocated the annihilation of Jews in his article
"The Case of Ahlwardt." "Between Germans and Jews," he writes, it
was "a fight of destruction: to be or not to be! They or us" (Förster
1892, 22). In 1941, when Germany had declared war on the Eastern
front against the USSR, the *Stürmer* presented a picture and poem entitled "The Grave-Digger," explaining that the Jews had caused the demise of the USSR.[2] Stalin lies dead on the ground, the landscape is
bleak, the ruins of houses can be seen in the background, and the flag
with hammer and sickle is torn. Towering above Stalin is a grotesque
caricature of an orthodox Jew, grinning at his victim in front of him.
The poem roughly translates as:

> Make a pact with the Jew
> And the devil's work will kill you.
> The land will be covered in corpses,
> Into dirt and dust crumbles everything once standing,
> Only Ahasver with hollow eyes stares ghostlike
> Into the realms of death.
> As long as he himself survives
> He diggs the mass-grave of the world.

> (*Stürmer,* August 1941, cover page)

Presumably, the message was that the USSR had allowed Jews enough
space to bring about its own downfall, suggesting again that the fight
against Jews was a total war and that, if a nation chose to ignore the
warning, it would sign its own death sentence. Therefore, in Nazi
logic, obviously, it was a duty of Germans to kill Jews first as a measure of "self-defense," so as to avoid the fate of the Russians.

The Jew as Poison and Contagious Disease

While some of the arguments of Jewish parasitism were arrived at by
citing social, political, and economic examples, increasingly parasitism itself stood for a biological event or a medical problem that had
to be dealt with. Elsewhere we argued (Kaplan and Rogers in this vol.)
that Haeckel had devised a theoretical position that justified racial engineering, including the eradication of weak, sick, genetically undesirable, or harmful elements, so that the healthy majority may benefit. In
some early pre-Nazi examples the Jewish question appears as a "juda-
istic slime," covering all (Christian) values. In others Jews appear as

a poison that needs to be extracted so that the healthy and natural soil can be reclaimed (Wahrmund 1887, 8).

Another variant, exploited in the final phase of the "final solution," was to point out that Jews were genetically a poor race altogether. In 1942 the *Stürmer* showed faces of mentally retarded or mentally ill Jewish people, contorted faces, followed by the caption: "And they claim to be the chosen people! According to official records, Jews have the highest percentage of mentally ill of all people on this globe" (1942, no. 8, 7). This, of course, was one of the reasons given why Jews had to drink the blood of Christians to "invigorate" their own race.

Criminal tendencies in an individual were also regarded as inherited, genetic features. For this reason undesirable social "elements," amongst them prostitutes, could legally be forced into sterilization so that "the bad seed" would not spread. Since the Jews were parasites, poison, and world conspirators intent on destroying all Germans, they were of course also regarded as criminals. One of the Nazis, Johann von Leers, a German university professor at Jena, in 1942 published a book entitled *Die Verbrechernatur der Juden* (The Criminal Nature of Jews). In it he justified and defended the murder of Jews on purely biological/genetic grounds: "If the hereditary criminal nature of Jewry can be demonstrated, then not only is each people morally justified in exterminating the hereditary criminals—but any people that still keeps and protects Jews is just as guilty of an offence against public safety as someone who cultivates cholera-germs without observing the proper precautions" (cited in Cohn 1981, 207). Jewishness per se had become a contagious disease that could be caught by merely mixing with Jews. The English author Houston Stewart Chamberlain had foregrounded all this rather well as early as 1899. He said then in his influential book entitled *The Foundations of the Nineteenth Century:* "One does not need to have the authentic Hettite nose in order to be a Jew. Rather, this word describes first and foremost a special way of feeling and thinking; a person can very quickly become a Jew without being an Israelite. Some only need to busily socialise with Jews, read Jewish newspapers and get used to a Jewish attitude to life, literature and art" (Chamberlain 1899, 457).

Most of these images are well known, and while they "inspired" social and natural scientists, historians, and anthropologists alike, none of the early grossly anti-Semitic views led directly to the Holocaust. Thirty to fifty years separated the early anti-Semitic writings from Hitler's racial laws and the final solution. The "Vernichtungs-Antisemitismus" (extermination anti-Semitism) of the Hitler period was qualitatively very different from these earlier statements. A baseline was set, however, for arguing about Jews as a biological, racial entity which could neither be diluted, upgraded, reformed, modified, or converted in any way. Unalterably, then, Jews were fixed in an identity from which, as it seemed, there was no escape.

The Holocaust showed that the definition of *race* as Jewish was nonnegotiably a death sentence. The game playing with permit cards, yellow work cards that promised survival—in my opinion, and some historians would not agree with this—only gave the appearance that life and death were negotiable, and typically this tended to happen in the first phase of the Holocaust, the "rounding-up" period. In the latter part, sometimes referred to as the "internment period," of which the death camps were a specific and growing subplot (Crouch 1990), such negotiations became increasingly limited, and, if existing at all, they prolonged life for a specified period rather than sparing anyone from certain death. Jews were ultimately not persecuted because of their religion, or their economic, political, or social roles, or indeed their nationality. There was no way to save one's life by changing to Christian belief, by giving away one's personal belongings, by abdicating a social or political role, or by returning whatever nationality one held. There were no "exception Jews," no redeemable features for survival. Being a Jew, whether knowingly or not, was itself the reason for the certainty of death.

Genetic determinism was one of the main buttresses of Nazi ideology. It is one of the grim ironies that the utter devaluation of social roles and of human life itself were made possible, and more plausible, by calling upon biology, i.e., "nature," as their chief witness. Sexism and racism have at least one common denominator: genetic determinism. Biology played an important role in ideological justifications of Nazi policies and thinking. The publication *When Biology Became Destiny* captures well the treatment of women in the Nazi period (Bridenthal et al. 1984). We also know that Nazi ideology had declared Jews an alien and dangerously destructive race *(Menschenunwert),* so dangerous indeed that extermination seemed the logical and only answer. To justify a final solution, arguments tended to be couched in biological or medical language, as if the disappearance of Jews were like the cutting out of a cancer from an otherwise noble and healthy gene pool.

ATTITUDES TO WOMEN IN NAZI GERMANY

Sexism is a modern term, first used in the late 1960s by the women's liberation movement in the United States. The issue here is whether the term *sexism* is the right one to apply to Nazi views on women. The women's question under the Nazis cannot be understood without first saying that the Nazis never had a policy, let alone a consistent policy, specifically on women (cf. Winkler 1977, 28). What they had, instead, was a *racial* policy, and women, as childbearers, were fitted into that scheme. The overall plan for the destiny of the German people was the "survival of the Aryan race," and the foremost *racial* goal was to insure an "invigoration" of the "German race" and a cleansing of all undesirable elements that interfered with the gene pool. Racial hygiene quickly acquired a central position in planning and in legislation. We need only to think of the laws for the protection of German blood and of the laws pertaining to birth deformities and congenital diseases, all passed within two years of the Nazi *Machtergreifung*.

The Nazis undertook one important step of recategorizing and subdividing society. Hitler and the party despised the "unnatural" divisions that Marxists and Socialists had apparently invented, such as the discovery of class-based allegiances and competitions. Instead, the Nazis were going to abolish these class divisions and unite the German people as never before. To do so they invented racial categories. After the various phases of *Gleichschaltung* (coordination) there were to be no more socially dividing categories; only those of biology counted. Biological hierarchies were determined by health (mental and physical) and race. The mentally and physically retarded as well as Jews were biologically undesirable. But those who were Germans were indivisibly one biological and historical family. The only division that had to be made within the people itself was a gender division. Women were women, and men were men. The family was the most important, smallest unit within the state, and therefore this unit had to function harmoniously. The "invigoration" of the German race depended entirely on the strength of the bond between the sexes. In 1876 Wilmann made a statement that was to retain validity in the Nazi ideology: "The more feminine a woman, the more masculine a man, the more intimate family life becomes, and the healthier society and the state will be" (Willmann 1876, 54). Indeed, Nazi women themselves called for more masculine men and more feminine women (Koonz 1984, 213). Of course, the Nazi regime, as any totalitarian regime, only publically, but not in reality, celebrated the family. No totalitarian regime can afford a secluded, happy family unit. It could easily become a cell of resistance and of opposition. Instead, it was important that families were constantly split up and taught that their allegiance was entirely to the führer. Regular, if not excessive, meetings for children, young people, and women and separate men's meetings, activities, educational programs, outings, and gatherings insured that most of the family was constantly apart and individually tackled by Nazi ideologues. The woman's role as a wonderful homemaker—when hardly anyone who took the Nazi calls to duty for the higher good of the people seriously was ever at home—was another pretext for women having to fulfill only one role: that of reproducers of "Germanic" children.

One of the main voices for Hitler, Alfred Rosenberg, argued as early as 1930 in his book *Der Mythos des 20. Jahrhunderts* that for women national socialism represented an emancipation from the women's emancipation. Women "belonged into the total life of its people" and should be given every opportunity to find new roles and fulfillment. He argued, however: "The endeavour for a renewal of our people, after the democratic-Marxist 'sponger' system has been broken, will lead towards creating a social order in which young women are no longer forced, as is the case today, to spend their most important womanly strength in the labour force. Women must be given every opportunity to develop their strengths; but in one thing we have to be clear: the man must be and must remain judge, soldier and politician" (Rosenberg 1930, 512).

Hitler said similar things at Nazi women's congresses and meetings in the following years. Thus, he argued in 1935: "The so-called 'emancipation' of women that the Marxists had demanded, in reality was no emancipation at all but a deprivation of women's rights, for it would draw women into areas in which they would inevitably be inferior, and because this would put a woman in situations, which would do nothing to cement her position vis-à-vis the man or society, but only weaken it." He further noted that, "with every child she bears for the nation, she fights her fight for the nation. May the man stand up for his people, as a woman stands up for her family" (*Völkischer Beobachter,* September 15, 1935). A year later Hitler announced:

> An immeasurable field of work opportunities are available to women. For us, women have at all times been the most loyal work and life-companions of men. One often tells me: you want to push each woman out of her job. No, I only want to give her in the widest sense of opportunity, to co-found her own family and have her own children, because then she can be most useful to our people!
>
> If a female lawyer today achieves however much, and next door

there lives a mother with five, six, seven children, who are all healthy and well brought up, then I want to say: From the point of view of the eternal value of our people, the woman who has had children and has brought them up and who by doing so has given our people life in the future as a gift, has done more, has achieved more! *(Völkischer Beobachter,* September 13, 1936)

A woman's identity, Nazi psychologists claimed, could be achieved by rediscovering and reinforcing *"her sense of her own sex and race"* (Zuhlke 1934, cited in Koonz 1984, 232; emphasis added).

For those who did not fit the strict racial parameters of the strong new German superrace envisaged by the Nazi elite, there were provisions for eugenic sterilizations and abortions. In 1940 state health authorities were given permission to perform such eugenic sterilizing and aborting functions on women who were of inferior makeup, be this because they were prostitutes, showed a "low character" (which could include anyone from the category of small thievery to a political dissident), and those of alien race (cited in Bock 1984, 287).

Those, however, who did not have to fear being placed into any of these categories, especially if they had married German men and borne children, often saw the exalted speeches for the "new" German woman as a positive and rewarding thing. Indeed, so idolized were women in the new role of homemakers and mothers that many Nazi women believed they were given a new dignity and identity for the first time.

The question must arise at this point why so many women would have bought such a simplistic rebiologized identity, particularly since the Weimar Republic had spawned some exceptionally progressive ideas on women. We must bear in mind that the new identity, indeed, steadily removed women from the work force and from careers, although not as completely as the Nazis might have wanted to. It is worth noting here that in the early years, between 1928 and 1932, consistently fewer women voted for Hitler than men (Klinsiek 1982, 114).

Nazi ideology had at least one different source of inspiration than might have been supposed (Kaplan and Adams 1990). Again, the issue was less a social one (jobs, rights equality, and the like) than one based on one's sexual life. Writers who chose to write and preach on sexuality, particularly those in the Weimar Republic, had opened a veritable Pandora's box of evils. What many thought were new freedoms actually brought new restrictions for women. To exemplify this briefly here (for greater detail, see Kaplan and Adams 1990), in the pre–World War I era one of the most liberatory and possibly unintended side effects of a new teaching on women's sexuality was achieved by arguing that women's sexuality was linked to perceived instincts of caring and nurturing. It was regarded as a diffuse sexuality that could be sublimated into other human activities, and it was morally superior to the allegedly more primitive, and rapacious, sexual drive of men. If women's sexuality was not entirely bound to the sexual act, then women could attain the status of full adults and would not be necessarily morally suspect, even if not married. They could take up careers, albeit more readily in professions and vocations in line with their alleged innate caring nature. Social motherhood was, indeed, an identity without hidden agenda.

The sexual reform movement of the Weimar Republic, as radical as it was, initially did more harm than good because social norms had not entirely kept pace with these new discoveries. One of the new discoveries was the assertion that women have, indeed, their own sexuality and are just as driven by sexual "lust" as men. They, therefore, had a right to have this desire fulfilled. At the same time, however, a prescriptive element entered into the debate. Men had to become the teachers in sexual matters, with the goal that orgasm had to be achieved. Indeed, orgasm for women became the new yardstick for measuring successful intercourse. Women who were not married were put into an embarrassing situation. The hidden question was: What did the single/unmarried woman do about her sexual drive? The answers in turn tended to be morally disapproved: perhaps she was a lesbian or frigid or she engaged in "loose" illicit relationships. Married women, too, were put under pressure, because their femininity was tied up with the ability to display sexual pleasure and to achieve orgasm. With the reinvention of women's sex drive came the loss of social motherhood and, therefore, the loss of any justification for careers. If the diffuse sexuality was gone, then women could not find fulfillment in professions and "womanly" professions but, ultimately, only in the arms of a husband and in motherhood.

The publications by women who were early Nazi supporters are clearly concerned with defying a feminist "new woman" image promulgated in the Weimar Republic. Guida Diehl was one of the early Nazi supporters who rallied against Weimar Republican feminists as a betrayal of womanhood. She was not alone in the claim that the new teachings of feminists had allegedly instigated promiscuity of women and had led to a devaluation of motherhood. This was partly the consequence of advocating contraceptives, of pleading for the abolition of the abortion paragraph (sec. 218 of The Penal Code) and the importance of one's own sexuality, as well as a consequence of the bad habit of leaving the home to pursue a career. Effectively, this meant for her that debates and behaviors had created a shameful and artificial separation between reproduction and the sexual act. That separation was "tearing apart women's souls" and made them lose the innermost values of the "folk soul." Sexual pleasure, or as she preferred to call it, sexual lust, made women lose their motherly instinct and saw them slide into promiscuity. German women did not enter the wrong path entirely of their own accord. They were goaded and misled by "shameless" literature (usually promulgated by Jews) and by racial mixing (with Jews), which were at fault for "stimulating the female sex drive" and for "enticing women into lust" (Diehl 1932, 58–60, 97).

Behind the critique of liberal and left-wing views of the new Weimar woman was also the wish to find an image of womanhood. P. Sophie Rogge-Börner and many others found such an image in the Germanic women of legends. One was the legend of Hedwiga, who fought at the side of her husband, Odoaker, in the Battle of Ravenna in the fifth century. Here, indeed, seemed the seed for an "emancipation from the 'emancipation,' " as Rosenberg had argued, a true liberatory model for women which they alleged to have found in their own forebears. Germanic women of legend were strong, freer than their twentieth-century "descendants," and true companions of their husbands. They apparently had yet another quality. Allegedly, in sexual love Germanic tribes were "as cool as perhaps of no other people." As a result of this coolness, so she claimed, marriages of these heroes were extremely strong, long-lasting, and produced healthy babies (Rogge-Börner 1928, chap. 2; cf. Kaplan and Adams 1990, 195–97). In other words, a cool sexuality, whatever that might be, also produced eugenically fit babies, strengthened bonds, and thus made the social fabric "thrive." The alternative was to be slave to a wild, untempered sexual drive, which made those involved incapable of producing "high-quality" children. Slavery to an untempered sexual drive was linked with darkness, disorderliness, dissolution, and eugenically weak children.

Hence, without appearing frigid, the rational, cool, and strong Germanic woman would be able to ward off claims of wanting and needing sexual pleasure. Furthermore, such behavior was eugenically beneficial for all, and her sexuality was transformed into a desensualized necessity for motherhood. Motherhood, on the other hand, was firmly linked to providing a service for the people and the nation. The new image was also an abdication of the middle-class "Gretchen" model of the nineteenth century: "It is not the Gretchen type . . . who is the ideal of today's German man, but rather a woman who is also intellectually able to stand at her husband's side, comprehending his interests and his life's struggle. This is a woman who is above all also capable of being a mother" *(Völkischer Beobachter,* May 27, 1939).

Womanhood was thus advocated to be possible in (allegedly) new, rewarding ways. It was, no doubt, expressed that the identity of such womanhood was firmly based on sex and race. The ideology of race provided the model from which womanhood derived her own importance: if she belonged to the superior, exalted Aryan race, exemplified by a glorious past of the Germanic people, then she had a new moral obligation as a woman to help uplift and reinvigorate her race through childbearing and motherhood.

Nazi ideologues argued that women ought to / would want to occupy entirely different spaces than men but that she was also totally equal to men. Indeed, those who belonged to the German community by virtue of nationality and "racial" origin should consider themselves totally equal. A major Nazi publication of 1933 was entitled *The Equality of Women in National Socialist Germany,* and one of its key lines read: "Without the equality of women no German people can exist" (Beyer 1933, 21). We may reject the Nazi brand of "equality" today, but there have been feminists in the 1980s whose views on equality of women come strangely close to the Nazi views. Both argue that women are equal but different, because they have special qualities and (biological) abilities, such as for childbearing, giving birth, and nurturing; these special abilities should be recognized and valued in their difference. The Nazis did precisely that. They valued women as a differently abled and highly important component of society but only and exclusively in that difference.

The different spaces women were to occupy from the very dawn of the new Nazi reich were totally depoliticized spaces, spaces that earned no income and were most readily identified with home and hearth (Stephenson 1975, chap. 1). There were just three terms by which a new German woman could describe her identity best: as a mother, as a wife, and as an Aryan woman. In all of these functions, however, she was assured of lofty praise and possibly also of an Iron Cross should she bear many children for the German "fatherland." Her reproductive capacity became her own battleground for the nation, insuring the survival of the race and even more: a bright future for the German people, who, only through her sacrifice, would be able to withstand the onslaughts of parasites and the undermining immorality that was set to destroy the German soul.

THE LINK BETWEEN SEXUALITY AND ANTI-SEMITISM

One of the very early steps the Nazis undertook was to move the anti-Semitic debate into an imagery much more personal and intimate, and ultimately more powerful, than all the writers had done before. The key element of this portrayal of the Jewish "decomposing" influence was sexual, an observation that Andrea Dworkin would share. In her view it was the Nazi portrayal of sexuality of the Jews which provoked the German anti-Semitic response (Dworkin 1981, 147). As early as 1920, an election campaign poster of the Nazis (initialed A. H.) showed the profile of a Germanic woman and behind her the ugly profile of a caricatured, thick-lipped, older male, clearly meant to represent a Jew. The woman's tied blond hair, small lips, elongated neck, and drooping shoulder were likely to represent a beautiful, yet innocent and upright, German woman. The man's smile, and the expression of his eyes, looking at her from the corner of his eyes, signified the Jew's lecherous nature and his assurance that he will get his victim.

The point of it is not that Jews are a hated and despised minority in Germany (as they were at the time by significant subsections of German society) but, rather, that *Jews are shown as oppressors* and that the *victims* of their foul doings are good, innocent, young German *women.* The sexual connotation is all too clear, and there is no doubt left in the drawing about the Jew's ability to eventually overpower the young German woman. The sexual/reproductive connection between Jews and Germans so preoccupied Hitler that one of the early revisions of German law was the "Law for the Protection of German Blood and German Honor" of September 15, 1935, which introduced stiff penalties for so-called race defilement *(Rassenschande),* committed through sexual and/or marital connection between Germans and Jews, even though the Jews *were* Germans and often no longer associated with Judaism. "Aryans" and Jews were considered incompatible for "interbreeding," and the association could ultimately only be harmful to Germans.

By 1939 the number of court cases for race defilement went into the thousands, and the Nazi newspapers reported regularly on these events, usually making some far-reaching claims. The "case Sichel," for instance, concerned a successful businessman who had an Aryan girlfriend. The article is headed, "There are no decent Jews," and it claimed that underneath the accomplished facade of every Jew there was a criminal and a devil. When, in the same year, a merchant from Breslau was tried for racial defilement, the court judgment of three

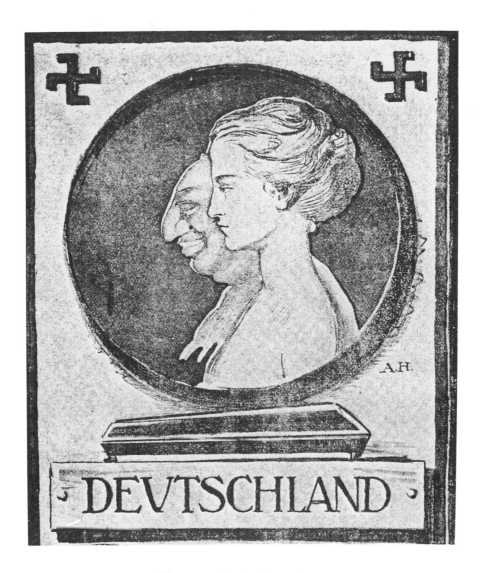

Fig. 1 1920 election poster

years of high-security prison was announced with the following words:

> There are no apparent mitigating circumstances in this case of racial defilement. Every Jew by now has to realize that he is merely tolerated as a guest in Germany and has to submit absolutely to the laws of the host country. If he nevertheless dares to lay hands on a German woman, thereby infringing the honour of the German people in its totality, he must be severely punished. *(Stürmer, 1939, no. 3; my trans.)*

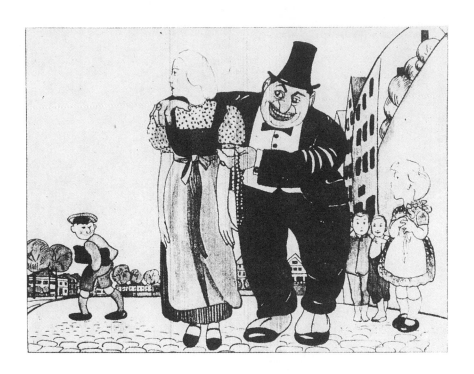

Fig. 2 Illustration in Nazi children's book

Early Nazi writing, be this for the general public or for children's books, by women and men alike, portrayed Jewish sexuality, particularly male sexuality, as lustful, lecherous, immodest, sensual, dark, sinister, dirty, passionate, evil, and disarming (cf. Kaplan and Adams 1990). Returning to the 1920 election campaign poster, we can now add another definition to the sexual plot: a Jewish male is not only an oppressor, exploiter, racial defiler, rapist, and abuser of women, but the sexual act with an Aryan woman is seen as a rape of the German people in toto. The woman is thus not just a victim as an individual; she is the embodiment of Germany and Germany's honor itself, which is being ravished and victimized by the Jewish seducer. Finally, the blond, fragile young woman is also used as a symbol of truth which "the" Jew tries to destroy.

It is noteworthy that quite often overt racism is coupled with the belief that the condemned race, such as Jews and particularly its men, are so much better lovers than the "superior" race and that, for this reason alone, they represent a danger. Underlying all these specific Nazi characterizations is the implication that a German woman would be unable to resist the advances of a Jewish man and, therefore, be forced into some kind of bondage. One wonders then, how the cool sexuality of strong Nazi Germanic women could even be at risk. To overcome this inconsistency and image problem it was fashionable to present older Jewish men with young German women. Age had explanatory function. The other was to argue that the woman did not know she was being courted by a Jew and that she only found out later or not at all. Again, innocence is the pleading mechanism why German women, despite their identity and knowledge of self-worth, could "fall" for a Jew.

A sexual relationship with a Jew carried more dangers than merely lawless passion. It has already been said that Jews were somehow contagious, both in social and in biological ways. This was expressed legally in the Nuremberg Laws and in literature. There were countless third-rate novels that instilled fear about any sexual encounter with a Jewish male, such as Artur Dinter's (1876–1948) novel *Sins against the Blood* (1918). The diseases Jews brought with them could be passed on. Thus, it was considered possible that a woman could bear a "Jewish" child even well after she could possibly have conceived a child by a Jew. This was part of the "contamination." The "Jewishness" of the child was identified by curly dark hair, and in one instance even by an "ape"-like face, because, as one pseudoscientist had claimed, Jews and apes were related, just as apes and blacks were, and a throwback into atavism was allegedly possible.

In the early phases of Nazi newspaper anti-Semitic campaigns Jewish women are rarely, if ever, mentioned. More or less every page shows Jewish men or grotesque caricatures of Jewish men; Jewish women are entirely omitted from this kind of sexual hate image making. The typical representation shows the rape of a German maiden by a Jewish man. Only in the early 1940s Jewish women began to appear in the *Stürmer,* and only then sexual relationships between German men and Jewish women began to be mentioned. In this configuration the contamination was taken literally. A 1941 edition, as part of its anti-Russian propaganda, presents Jewish women as the "wives of Satan," so the heading promises. And the subheading states: "Among the purchasable women in the Soviet Union there are thousands of sick Jewesses" (*Stürmer,* 1941, no. 32, 4). Jewish women are either ugly or riddled by sexual disease, and any self-respecting man would, therefore, keep far away from Jewish women.

Rape and prostitution were another issue. Both occurred frequently in extermination camps and were an added humiliation for women before death (Heinemann 1986, 17). But in these cases the well-instilled contempt of Jews as a race did not have to be rejected. On the contrary, Hitler had already argued in his manifesto *Mein Kampf* that prostitution was a corrupt sexuality and was comparable to the outbreak of syphilis. And it is in these situations that the general misogynist tenor of Nazi ideology could find its fiercest expression: abuse and then kill. Indeed, no special propaganda machinery had to be employed to instill contempt for Jewish women. Jewishness had been paraded as evil for long enough, and women, as a biological category, were already low on the rungs of male estimates.

Marlene E. Heinemann has noted that Hitler rarely referred to Jewish women separately (1986, 18). The exclusive portrayal of Jewish men as targets for ridicule may even be unique to the Nazi regime. I have looked at other anti-Semitic media literature and have found that anti-Semitic drawings and cartoons usually included women. (My examples come mainly from the Australian media, which had its fair share of public anti-Semitic statements.) The "long-nosed Sarah" is typically included in the "joke," and, typically, such jokes were not of a sexual nature. In these examples the specific brand of Nazi image making is illustrated even more clearly. Here were cases of intertwining racism and sexism that fitted well together because one informed the other, and each could be exploited for political purposes. Without the image of a new ideal German woman, the evil lecherous counterpart of the dark, honor-defiling Jew may not have worked. One image needed the other, both to exalt the German woman and to "reveal" the sordid nature of the Jew. The "threat" of German annihilation by Jews was effectively encapsulated by the threat of Jewish penetration into and corruption of German innocence.

Nazi ideology had not been afraid to proclaim publicly new standards for "good" and "evil." More perversely, Nazi morality was tied to a new "science," a firm belief in genetic determinism. If "human nature" was irreducibly based on one's race and gender, as Nazi propaganda relentlessly argued, then it was a matter of implementing appropriate policies. In that respect Nazi ideology was entirely and chillingly consistent.

EPILOGUE

Discussions of human nature are likely to continue in the future, and throughout the 1980s and early 1990s arguments have been put forward in some quarters of general science, and even in feminist literature, proposing deterministic explanations not too far removed from Nazi views but obviously unaware of their existence. We need to insure that the knowledge of Nazi views *and their consequences* retain the status of a reminder that ideas can be dangerous because they may have highly undesirable consequences in real life.

In addition, Nazi writing, like writing in most eras, was undertaken mainly by the educated and mostly by those who went by the name of intellectual or academic. The business of academics is to pursue knowledge scientifically, to reveal facts that can be verified, to provide measures that can be repeated and insights that can stand up to intellectual scrutiny. In the Nazi era a large number of German academics actively supported Nazi views and thereby abdicated their role as academics, shifting as they did from scholarly to propagandist writing. Facts were exchanged for opinions, and, instead of theory construction based on facts, myths were created and defended by the most spurious "evidence." Pseudoscience flourished as never before. That pseudoscience had immediate application, be this for promotion purposes for the writer, for feeling part of the general community, and/or for a sense of greater power and self-importance. A self-proclaimed political naïveté, rather than pseudoscience, was just as dangerous and despicable, not excusing men of the stature of Martin Heidegger or Konrad Lorenz. (These are complex issues, discussed at length elsewhere [Baum 1981; Bauman 1991].)

In other words, the political agenda of the day very often a priori determined the "findings." Nazi scholars also usually vindicated ethical standards, in the mildest cases simply changing some vocabulary in their writing to signal approval for Nazi ideology (and safeguarding their jobs), in the worst, as in some cases of doctors, using the opportunity of removed ethical standards to engage in human experimentation, when such human life had been declared "unworthy of life" by Nazi authorities (Lifton 1986; Müller-Hill 1988; Procter 1988). These extreme examples of academic behavior in a specific political climate in very recent times may inculcate a good measure of mistrust toward academics. For the academicians of today they reinforce the idea that none of our intellectual pursuits are value free and that we need to assess continually what we are doing.

NOTES

1. Please note that all references to nineteenth-century text have not been listed separately in the bibliography. A full bibliography on German anti-Semitic publications in the late nineteenth century can be found in Cobet 1973 and Baum 1981.

2. Throughout this article reference is made to the *Stürmer* and *Völkischer Beobachter*, the two most notorious newspapers of the Nazi propaganda machinery. The *Stürmer* was a particularly vile Nazi paper, published by Julius Streicher in Nuremberg. By the time of the *Machtergreifung* it al-

ready had a circulation of nearly half a million and was even by then one of the biggest in Germany. Moreover, the *Stürmer* was posted in display boxes in towns and villages, and "most sinister of all, it was used in schools" (Cohn 1981, 201). The *Völkischer Beobachter* was an obscure little weekly anti-Semitic paper that had existed well before World War I. In 1919 Alfred Rosenberg was its only editor. In 1920 Hitler met Rosenberg, bought the paper as a Nazi party paper, and elevated Rosenberg to one of his early prophets of national socialism.

REFERENCES

AC, no. 21, January 1888. Cf. Cobet, 1973, biblio.

Adorno, Theodor W. 1973. *Negative Dialektik.* Frankfurt am Main: Suhrkamp.

Ahlwardt. 1890. Cf. Cobet, 1973, biblio.

Arendt, Hannah. 1958. *The Origins of Totalitarianism.* Cleveland: Meridian/World.

Barkai, Avraham. 1988. *Vom Boykott zur "Entjudung": Der wirtschaftliche Existenzkampf der Juden im Dritten Reich, 1933–1943* (From Boycott to "Dejudaization": The Economic Struggle of Jews in the Third Reich). Frankfurt am Main: Fischer Taschenbuch Verlag.

Baum, Rainer C. 1981. *The Holocaust and the German Elite: Genocide and National Suicide in Germany, 1871–1945.* London: Croom and Helm.

Bauman, Zygmunt. 1991. *Modernity and the Holocaust.* Cambridge and Oxford: Blackwell/Polity Press.

Bey, O. 1875. Cf. Cobet, 1973, biblio.

Beyer, Karl. 1933. *Die Ebenbürtigkeit der Frau im nationalsozialistischen Deutschland.* Leipzig.

Bock, Gisela. 1984. "Racism and Sexism in Nazi Germany: Motherhood, Compulsory Sterilization, and the State." In *When Biology Became Destiny: Women in Weimar and Nazi Germany,* ed. R. Bridenthal et al., 271–96. New York: Monthly Review Press.

Bridenthal, Renate, Atina Grossmann, and Marion Kaplan. 1984. *When Biology Became Destiny: Women in Weimar and Nazi Germany.* New York: Monthly Review Press.

Cobet, Christoph. 1973. *Der Wortschatz des Antisemitismus in der Bismarckzeit* (The Vocabulary of Anti-Semitism in the Bismarck Period). Munich: Wilhelm Fink Verlag.

Cohn, Norman. 1981. *Warrant for Genocide: The Myth of the Jewish World-Conspiracy and the Protocols of the Elders of Zion.* Chico, Calif.: Scholars Press.

Crouch, Mira. 1990. "The Oppressors and the Oppressed in Interaction: A

Shared Dimension of Everyday Life." In *The Attractions of Fascism,* ed. J. Milfull, 21–31. New York, Oxford, and Munich: Berg Publishers.

Diehl, Guida. 1932. *Die deutsche Frau und der Nationalsozialismus* (The German Woman and National Socialism). Eisenach: Neuland-Verlag.

Dworkin, Andrea. 1981. *Pornography: Men Possessing Women.* New York: Perigee Books.

Förster. 1892. Cf. Cobet, 1973, biblio.

Gordon, Sarah. 1984. *Hitler, Germans and the "Jewish Question."* Princeton, N.J.: Princeton University Press.

Heinemann, Marlene E. 1986. *Gender and Destiny: Women Writers and the Holocaust.* New York, Westport, Conn., and London: Greenwood Press.

Kaplan, Gisela. 1992. *Contemporary Western European Feminism.* Sydney: Allen and Unwin, London: University College of London Press, New York: New York University Press.

Kaplan, Gisela, and Carole E. Adams. 1990. "Early Women Supporters of National Socialism." In *The Attractions of Fascism: Social Psychology and Aesthetics of the "Triumph of the Right."* ed. J. Milfull, 186–203. New York, Oxford, and Munich: Berg Publishers.

Klinksiek, Dorothee. 1982. *Die Frau im NS-Staat* (Women in the Nazi State). Stuttgart: Deutsche Verlags-Anstalt.

Koonz, Claudia. 1984. "The Competition for a Woman's *Lebensraum,* 1928–1934." In *When Biology Became Destiny: Women in Weimar and Nazi Germany,* ed. R. Bridenthal, et al., 199–236. New York: Monthly Review Press.

Lifton, Robert Jay. 1986. *The Nazi Doctors: A Study in the Psychology of Evil.* London: Macmillan.

Mosse, George L. 1978. *Rassismus: Ein Krankheitssymptom in der europäischen Geschichte des 19. und 20. Jahrhunderts.* Königstein/Ts.: Athenäum Verlag. *Toward the Final Solution: A History of European Racism.* New York. Howard Fertig.

Müller-Hill, Benno. 1988. *Murderous Science: Elimination by Scientific Selection of Jews, Gypsies and Others, Germany, 1933–45.* Trans. G. R. Fraser. New York and Oxford: Oxford University Press.

Oppenheimer, John F. 1971. *Lexikon des Judentums* (The Dictionary of Judaism). Published in collaboration with E. Bin Gorion, Tel Aviv, E. G. Lowenthal, London and Berlin, and H. G. Reissner, New York; Gütersloh, Munich, Berlin, Vienna: Bertelsmann Lexikon Verl.

Proctor, Robert N. 1988. *Racial Hygiene: Medicine under the Nazis.* Boston: Harvard University Press.

Rogge-Börner, P. Sophie. N.d. (approx. 1928). *An Geweihtem Brunnen: Die deutsche Frauenbewegung im Lichte des Rassegedankens.*

Rosenberg, Alfred. 1930. *Der Mythos des 20. Jahrhunderts.* Munich.

Rürup, Reinhard. 1975. *Emanzipation und Antisemitismus*. Göttingen: Vandenhoeck and Ruprecht.

Siber, Paula. 1933. *Die Frauenfrage und ihre Lösung durch den Nationalsozialismus* (The Women's Question and Its Solution by National Socialism). Wolfenbüttel and Berlin: Georg Kallmeyer Verlag.

Stephenson, Jill. 1975. *Women in Nazi Society.* London.

Der Stürmer. Melbourne University Archives, Melbourne-Parkville, Australia.

Völkischer Beobachter. Monash University Archive, Melbourne-Clayton, Australia.

Willman. 1876. Cf. Cobet, 1973, biblio.

Winkler, Dörte. 1977. *Frauenarbeit im "Dritten Reich"* (Women's Work in the "Third Reich"). Hamburg: Hoffmann und Campe.

◆ GERALD HORNE ◆

When Race and Gender Collide: The Martinsville Seven Case as a Case Study of the "Rape-Lynch" Controversy

Between 1882 and 1950, according to statistics kept by Tuskegee Institute, 3,436 Afro-Americans and 1,293 Euro-Americans were lynched. Next to homicide rape was cited as the main reason (1,937 cases of homicide vs. 910 cases of rape); overwhelmingly, most of those lynched for rape were Afro-American. In Mississippi, between 1930 and 1948, 108 people were executed, which included 90 Afro-Americans; 6 were executed by the state for rape, all Afro-Americans.

By 1892 rape had become a capital crime in the state of Louisiana. The Black Codes specified the death penalty for slaves as punishment for rape. No Louisiana-born Euro-American man was ever executed for rape, but forty-one Afro-Americans were, including twenty-nine by hanging and twelve by the electric chair, from 1900 to the early 1950s. No one at all had ever been executed for raping an Afro-American woman, and a number of the executed Afro-American men had been slain not for rape but for the "intent to commit rape." Many were found guilty of rape for hiring prostitutes; one man was charged with attempted rape for touching a Euro-American woman's arm. Another Afro-American man was convicted on a Euro-American woman's claim that he "smelled" like a Negro. In many instances Afro-American men were arrested for engaging in consensual sex. "To arresting officers, however, it is inconceivable that any white woman would voluntarily engage in an affair with a Negro."[1]

The preeminent organization fighting this trend during the twentieth century was the Civil Rights Congress (CRC); certainly, the National Association for the Advancement of Colored People (NAACP), the Association of Southern Women for the Prevention of Lynching, and other organizations were involved in this struggle.[2] But what distinguished the CRC was that it sought to show that lynching was part of an overall process of stigmatizing Afro-Americans so that they could be forced to work for less money (and be tied to the land in an inequitable fashion as sharecroppers); lynching, according to the CRC, was also part of the process of forging Dixiecrat and racist rule in the Deep South. False charges of rape followed by a lynching of Afro-American men was an essential element in forging "white unity" and glossing over class and gender contradictions in the Euro-American community. False charges of rape followed by lynching of Afro-American men was part of a process of disrupting ties between what could have been natural allies—that is, the movement for democratic rights for blacks and the movement for equality for women led by nonminority women.[3]

The CRC was itself stigmatized as a "Communist front"; that is, it was suggested that the organization had little concern for the defendants in the cases it took on but merely was seeking to advance a not too hidden agenda involving the Communist party. Strikingly, the defendants in these cases rejected these allegations. Nevertheless, the NAACP and other centrist organizations took these charges quite seriously during the cold war. By 1956 the CRC was defunct as a result of severe pressure from the U.S. government and the nation's economic elites. But by this time, partially as a result of the cold war, U.S. authorities had determined that the more egregious aspects of Jim Crow—for example, lynching because of false rape allegations—had to be curbed; this determination was motivated by the fact that the United States found it difficult to charge Moscow with human rights violations while lynchings of Afro-Americans stained these shores.

Examining the case of the Martinsville Seven, a group of Afro-American men who were executed for the alleged rape of a Euro-American woman, is revelatory, as it demonstrates, inter alia, the toxic effect of disunity between the NAACP and the CRC. Yet it is even more revealing insofar as it shows that it was not only the objective impact of the cold war which helped to extinguish the phenomenon of lynching. The drive to exterminate lynching involved tireless organizing and mobilizing—a lesson that should not be lost in the 1990s. Still, the Martinsville case demonstrated that, even if lynching—or execution without due process of law—were curbed, the fact remained that the murder of Afro-American men for false charges of rape could continue. The responsibility for these deaths was simply shifted from the private to the public sector.

The Virginia backwater town of Martinsville was the site for a turning point in the history of Afro-American/Euro-American, man-woman relations. In 1950 this community, already a hotbed of racism, received international notoriety because of a case involving seven of its black citizens. In 1949 Martinsville, near the North Carolina border, was a town of about eighteen thousand people; it was best known as the home of Bassett Furniture (controlled by the Du Ponts) and the American Furniture Company. It became the scene of another of the CRC's harbingers of the 1960s: like Mississippi and Atlanta before it, Martinsville experienced a "freedom ride" before the term became popular. And like Atlanta, Trenton, and too many other sites of CRC cases, Martinsville also was the backdrop of another conflict with the NAACP. The *Morgan* case, which had taken place in Virginia a few years earlier, had not convinced the association that legal wizardry without mass action was tantamount to the sound of one hand clapping.

The Martinsville case was an interracial rape case, and it was hardly accidental that it arose in Virginia. Prior to 1865 the state required different penalties for Euro-Americans and Afro-Americans convicted of raping nonminority women—ten to twenty years for Euro-American men, five years to death for Afro-American men. The Fourteenth Amendment forced the alteration of this legislation, but the practice continued. Between 1908 and 1951 eight hundred Euro-Americans were convicted for rape, but not one received the death penalty. From 1885 through 1951 there were Euro-American men convicted of raping a ten-year-old child (ten-year sentence), a wife's married cousin (three years), a four-and-a-half-year-old girl (three years), an eighty-three-year-old grandmother (five years), a thirty-two-year-old Afro-American woman (seven years), and so forth. In contrast, in *Woodson v. Commonwealth* the judge spoke of the "black peril" and the need to kill Afro-American rapists to prevent mob violence. Similarly, all sixteen of the state's death row inmates in 1950 were Afro-American, along with a disproportionate percentage of the prison population itself.[4] As is well known, it remains true that in 1994 Afro-American men continue to be represented disproportionately on death row.

The Martinsville case involved seven Afro-American men: Francis De Sales Grayson, thirty-seven, the father of five; John C. Taylor, twenty; James Luther Hairston, twenty; Howard Lee Hairston, nineteen; Frank Hairston, Jr., nineteen; Booker T. Millner, nineteen; Joe Henry Hampton, twenty. All were from the working class in this third-largest furniture-producing center in the nation, in which Bassett alone employed 2,500 workers, but only 150 Afro-Americans, in an area in which minority unemployment was a whopping 20 percent. The fates of these men were joined on 8 January 1949 when Ruby Floyd, a Euro-American former mental patient, went to collect a business debt. She alleged that a "squad" of Afro-American men attacked her and raped her. The seven men were arrested. The grand jury that returned an indictment was composed of four Euro-Americans and three Afro-Americans, but most of the jurors were on the Board of Directors of the American Furniture Company. The judge, Kennon C. Whittle, was a director of six of the town's leading businesses. The prosecutor, W. R. Broaddus, was one of Martinsville's richest men and also a Bassett director. The defendants were saddled with attorneys from the city's power structure, and they conducted the trial before the all-Euro-American jury with a decided lack of zeal. There were other legal curiosities. During the trial the defendants repudiated their extorted confessions, but that cut no ice. Despite the inflamed local atmosphere, the judge refused a change of venue. Two Afro-Americans were stricken from the panel during jury selection because they did not believe in the death penalty for minorities in such cases.

Ascertaining the exact relationship between the defendants and Mrs. Floyd is problematic. If one examines the issues from the vantage point of the 1990s, it would appear that the CRC sought to debase the alleged victim of the rape in order to exonerate the defendants. For example, the attorneys underscored that Mrs. Floyd, who disappeared immediately after the conviction, sold *Watchtower* magazine, a publication of the Jehovah's Witnesses, and was viewed locally as somewhat eccentric; they noted that she was rumored to be a prostitute. One researcher alleged that she "had dated one of the accused men." "The boys said she invited the relationship and did not resist." No one except the prosecutors and the police, however, had an opportunity to speak to Mrs. Floyd except during the trial. It could be argued that whatever the CRC gained in the battle for racial equality was undermined by such tactics. These issues were complicated further by the horrific racist tenor of the times and the long history of false rape charges being used for the purpose of racist executions. All of this serves to illustrate that linking the battles for racial and gender equality was not as simple as merely chanting a slogan.

At any rate, the case raised a smorgasbord of legal questions on appeal, such as the denied change of venue, forced confessions, police misconduct, inadequate cross-examinations, lack of positive identification, and the exclusion of Afro-Americans from the jury. Most of these were perennial issues for the CRC, and when the Supreme Court years later finally reversed field on many of these issues the CRC's constant prodding over the years was partly responsible. Here they highlighted constantly and incessantly the fact that, although one-third of Virginia's population was Afro-American, there were no Afro-American judges and all forty-four men executed for rape since 1908 had been Afro-American. The Martinsville case was laborious. Twice the Virginia courts denied their appeals. Twice the U.S. Supreme Court refused the case. In July 1950, forty-eight hours from death, the men got a temporary reprieve. In November 1950, after a delegation from twenty-two states descended on the state capital in Richmond, the men received a sixty-day stay of execution.[5]

The NAACP objected to the presence of the CRC in this headline case.[6] Robert Harris, who investigated the case years later, put it bluntly, and aptly. His summation could have applied to any of the groups' innumerable conflicts:

> The CRC and the NAACP approached the case from two different points of view. The NAACP felt that the state and federal laws and legal procedures were basically just. Therefore, it relied on legal appeals on the hope that somewhere along the line the miscarriage of justice would be rectified. The CRC felt that the fundamental basis of the courts and laws . . . was to preserve an unjust system of Negro oppression—a system with which the federal courts would not interfere. Thus, its approach was political, to bring the maximum public pressure to bear.

Harris went on to say that "twice during June 1950, after the first appeal to the U.S. Supreme Court had been turned down, the CRC appealed to the NAACP for a joint campaign." They were refused. But as in other cases, a de facto alliance ensued: "Even so, of course, the efforts of the two groups were to a large degree complementary." The CRC led the mass political campaign, while the NAACP did most of the legal appeals, initially with the help of CRC lawyers.[7]

As early as mid-1949, CRC leader William Patterson was complaining about a meeting with Thurgood Marshall and other NAACP attorneys. The CRC leader was "calling for cooperation . . . [but the NAACP attorneys] said that they would not work with us on any basis and if we developed a mass campaign they would publicly declare that it was detrimental to the struggle for these men's lives." Patterson's ire caused him to strike out at one of the least anti-Communist NAACP lawyers, Charles Houston: "[he] will waver until such time as he sees a significant broad mass movement as will afford him a protective cloak." Days earlier Patterson had met with local NAACP lawyer M. A. Martin and an NAACP branch leader in Richmond. They had spoken in "glowing terms of . . . joint action" with the CRC, yet the next day they repudiated their words. Indicative of the hamstringing effect of the U.S. attorney general's act in stigmatizing the CRC as a so-called Communist front was the fact that Martin, vice chair of the NAACP's powerful legal committee, said that the subversive listing barred their working with the CRC—this apparently after having received the word from on high. Patterson smoldered indignantly about this rebuff: "I repeat, CRC withdrew from this case upon your insistence that unless our organization did so, you would not proceed. . . . Yours has been a hush-hush policy without regard to the overwhelming strength which derives from the support of the people."

This blowup occurred at a time when Patterson, identified in the local press as the "Scottsboro case lawyer," was in town to file an appeal for Grayson. The case of the Scottsboro Nine involved young Afro-American men in 1930s Alabama who were charged with the rape of a Euro-American woman. Ominously, the press reported about a "mixed white and Negro meeting" with Communists, Congress for Industrial Organizations (CIO) union members, and NAACP rank and file present at a local funeral home. In any case, the high court of the state refused the NAACP's claim, rejecting the grounds of change of venue and inflammatory newspaper publicity; the court objected to their point about the trial court judge asking potential jurors if they were anti–death penalty and rejecting them if the answer was yes; it brushed aside questions of the exclusion of Afro-Americans from the jury and the tainted confession; it spurned the notion that only Afro-Americans getting the death penalty for rape was actionable. Similarly, the court did not seem to be impressed with the NAACP's sudden rush for ideological purity in disdaining the CRC.[8]

Just as the NAACP had taken their scorning of the CRC to the public, the CRC openly called for a reconciliation. While pricking NAACP leaders Roy Wilkins and Walter White about their failure to do mass mobilizing and for having forced out the CRC, Patterson extended the olive branch of cooperation. He warned forebodingly that "failure of the NAACP to organize mass action immediately" will doom the seven. He released to the press a telegram to White which called for cooperation between the two organizations beyond Virginia.[9]

As in past conflicts, the antagonism toward the CRC was expressed more acrimoniously by White, Marshall, and other top NAACP leaders, who were under the most scrutiny and pressure, than by the base of the organization. In late 1950, after the NAACP had made its hostility toward the CRC well known, Martin, the law partner of Oliver Hill and future federal judge Spottswood Robinson, was still in touch with the CRC's Ralph Powe about Martinsville and was still trying to assist the CRC in its cases.[10]

Inevitably, in a case of this character—Afro/Euro, man/woman, Communist/anti-Communist—the press flocked like moths to the light. Most of their reportage was, unfortunately, trash. Occasionally, there was a illuminating insight, as when the *Nation* noted a principal difference between the CRC and NAACP efforts: the former insisted that the men were innocent, while the latter conveniently ducked this question and simply focused on such issues as a "fair trial." Typically, *Time* called the pathbreaking Richmond vigil "517 of the faithful, masterminded by the Communist front Congress of Civil Rights." Both the *New Republic* and *Christian Century* assumed somehow that the defendants were guilty and slanted their articles in that direction.[11]

When the U.S. Supreme Court in *Coker v. Georgia* decided, finally, in 1977 that capital punishment was an improper penalty for rape, in a sense the altruistic labor of the CRC had been vindicated.[12] Raising this question during the doldrums of the transition from presidents Truman to Eisenhower was, however, an uphill climb. Nevertheless the CRC persevered. In early 1951 Patterson launched a petition campaign to save the Martinsville Seven by contacting his numerous allies in the religious community; the goal was to get fifty thousand signatures in twenty-five days. Soon petitions were flooding the CRC's office from New Jersey, Florida, Georgia, and elsewhere.

The campaign that gripped Detroit reflected its role as a leading CRC chapter, but at the same time it was not atypical. The CRC began "hitting the plant gates" with petitions that "paved the way for [its] appearances before Executive Boards and membership meetings in the shops." Chapter leader Anne Shore, a longtime progressive, who had played a role earlier in building the influential Los Angeles CRC chapter, was taken aback: "You never saw anything to equal the movement under way here. . . . [We] got money from Cadillac Local UAW. . . . [The Baptist] Ministers' Conference [is] really moving, with a special petition for circulation in all their churches. . . . [W]e have official delegates from Fur and Leather, three from Dodge 3 (the second biggest in the UAW [United Automobile Workers union]), Cadillac was sending a minimum of one [to the Virginia freedom ride]." She described the entire organization experience as "wonderful." The "steady stream of little leaflets into the auto plants here" led to the formation of a "newly formed trade union committee" of the CRC. As happened so often with CRC mass organizing for defendants, a boom in membership resulted: "We've a couple of chapters started . . . . [We are] recruiting members at mass meetings." This had an impact on the local NAACP secretary, who "said he couldn't move without New York. . . . [T]he NAACP has had a hard time of it."[13]

A major element in generating mass support was a visit to Detroit by Mrs. Josephine Grayson, family member of one of the Martinsville Seven. During her sojourn there in the fall of 1950 she had an interview with the Pittsburgh *Courier,* and spoke at the Baptist Ministers' Conference. The following Sunday fifteen churches were visited by various speakers from the CRC:

> We called the churches cold. . . . We were turned down by only one minister, who later relented. . . . The results were magnificent with several hundred dollars being collected. The white speakers were more effective than the Negro, pointing out clearly to us that we must really move the white community actively. . . . Our big weakness in working with the church groups was not to make an effort to break through to the white churches. This indicates the opportunism about which Pat spoke in Chicago.

Triggering this outpouring of activism was not only the usual energy of the chapter but also the special energy of Mrs. Grayson: "Our most significant job was done in relation to the trade unions. . . . [W]e were able to break through several [right-wing unions]. [With more time] we would have been able to break through into almost every union in the city." The Left-led Ford Local 600, the largest in the UAW, with over sixty-five thousand members, gave $358.85. Also contributing were Packard Local 190 and Local 208. All this was not greeted with catatonic passivity in the union. The *Beacon,* a local UAW paper, in a hard-hitting editorial, accused "the Communist Party and its legal arm—the Civil Rights Congress"—of being responsible for the plight of the defendants. Beneath this article was another by Walter White in which Walter Reuther called on Virginia's governor to grant a stay of execution and not be a "sucker for a left hook."[14]

This outburst of activity was replicated not only across the country but also across the globe. In Harlem there was a massive parade in the fall of 1950 on behalf of the seven accused men. There was also a production of *The Martinsville Chant,* a play directed by Ossie Davis and featuring, among others, William Marshall and Vinnie Burrows. The CRC drew connections between the Martinsville defendants and others similarly situated which had a dynamic effect on their organizing, and it was the protest from abroad during the cold war battle which was most acutely embarrassing to the United States for hearts and minds in an increasingly influential colored world. In South Africa during the same time five African men had been sentenced to death on charges of rape of a white woman. As in the United States, no white man in the Transvaal had ever received the death sentence for rape. The response from abroad was heartening. In London there were Hyde Park rallies and protests from the dean of Canterbury, the Caribbean Labour Congress, and many concerned individuals. According to Patterson, Europeans were "alarmed at the state of democratic procedure" in the United States. A familiar ally in Paris, the Mouvement Contre le Racisme, L'Antisemitisme, et pour la Paix, was in the forefront, cobbling together committees of "leading cultural, union, church and governmental figures" for both Willie McGee, another Afro-American man accused falsely of rape, and the Martinsville Seven. Eastern European groups, such as the Association of Polish Jurists, chimed in. The West Africa Students Union of Charles University in Prague and individuals from Angola and Lagos were attracted to the CRC's cause, as were a number of Latin Americans.[15]

The freedom rides to Virginia were highly publicized. The first was contemplated for the fall of 1950, as the hangman's noose awaited. The writers Howard Fast, Dashiell Hammett, and Earl Conrad were to lead this mass delegation. Patterson had traveled to Europe to rally support, and the news trickled back that 1,024 resolutions on the case had been adopted by trade unions, city councils, and organizations in Europe. Apparently, this was an effective display of strength, because the governor granted a stay of execution, and in response the CRC called off its jaunt to the South.[16]

But the stay was merely a temporary palliative, and another execution date was set for early 1951. The CRC quickly got to work. Mass open-air rallies were held in Harlem, and tables cluttered the streets there and across the country as petitions were gathered. The CRC was fighting not only this battle, but at the same time it was straining its meager resources to save the life of Willie McGee and to keep both Communists and CRC leaders out of jail. Moreover, as they were struggling to raise funds for the $15 round-trip fare to Virginia and on-site expenses, rumors had begun to percolate about the organization's having swindled money from the McGee defense; such allegations were not without effects. Undaunted, the CRC moved on with its meticulous planning for this landmark event. The "Proposed Rules for the Delegation" were mapped out carefully. It was a broad delegation going beyond the Left, so the CRC stressed that differences between people on the delegation should not divide them. Representatives of the delegation were to be selected in a democratic way. It was to be expected that intimidation would be directed at those assembled, so security was a critical concern: "During the stay in Richmond proceed in groups, not as individuals. Be dignified, orderly and disciplined. Do not give in to any provocation. Avoid arguments with anyone. . . . Put all cars in public garages at all times." Even bomb threats had to be considered.[17]

The execution dates were set for 2 and 5 February, and the delegation was set to go days before to have maximum impact. Each chapter was given a quota, and overall 250 to 500 people were expected to descend on the state. This was primarily the work of CRC leaders William Patterson and Aubrey Grossman; both were Communists and attorneys. The latter was Euro-American, the former Afro-American; both were meticulous organizers. Painstakingly, Grossman requested reports twice a week from the chapters on how their organizing was proceeding and telegraphic reports in the last ten days; he suggested reading a report on what the Detroit chapter was doing in order to get an idea of how to organize. Detroit's selection as a model was no accident. The plight of the Martinsville Seven had struck a responsive chord in that city of proletarians, its number of black residents increasing steadily and bitten by a recurrent plague of police misconduct aimed precisely at Afro-American citizens. About 20 percent of the five hundred–plus delegation was from this city, and its unions were heavily represented. This was done in the face of an NAACP denunciation of the crusade on the eve of its departure. But it was the view of many that, if the association did not want to engage in mass action, that was its lamentable right but that unity should have precluded its leaders from discouraging others from seeking to save the defendants' lives. The NAACP's maneuver did not destroy the delegation. In fact the Ford Local voted the CRC chapter a commendation for its fine work. Representatives of over 160,000 autoworkers demanded clemency and freedom for the Martinsville Seven, not to mention the steelworkers, furniture workers, and others who joined in.[18]

As the delegates were reaching Richmond, the voice of protest was becoming more insistent. The head of the Bataka party of Uganda, sixty-six members of the French Chamber of Deputies, the Zionist Democratic Federation of Israel, seventy thousand Polish youths, and the Union of Working Youth of Romania were among the protesters. The Baptist Morning Minsters' Conference of Philadelphia and the president of the National Baptist Convention joined in. But these U.S. voices were seemingly drowned out by those of Finnish parliamentarians and other groups from West Germany, Tunisia, East Africa, and elsewhere. They confronted the embattled governor, John Battle, with a five-day vigil at the Richmond capital, accompanied by an all-night vigil at the White House. The thousands of wires and phone calls to the governor from all over the world apparently swayed him to meet with the delegation. In solidarity the Afro-Americans of Richmond were sporting black armbands. Also in solidarity many taxi drivers wouldn't charge them fares, and many restaurants supplied them with free coffee. Others gave them the free use of telephones. One local Afro-American echoed the view of many and was all too accurate when he commented, "Nothing like this has happened since Grant took Richmond in 1865."[19]

The delegates from New York had traveled in Greyhound buses and had to endure Jim Crow waiting rooms and seating in the South. The others from around the nation who came to bear witness at Thomas Jefferson's state house had similar experiences. William Mandel has supplied a graphic depiction of the latter-day "vigilantes." There was a sharecropper's daughter, Fern Winston, descended from President Franklin Pierce, who had seen a similar interracial rape incident in her home state of Oklahoma; later she married Henry Winston, a Communist leader. There was an Afro-American former navy man, a young Euro-American mother from Colorado, two local Euro-American medical students, and "a Creole woman from Louisiana whose immensely wealthy tobacco-grower grandfather finally violated the family's deepest secret by telling them they were Blacks when a lynching [burning on tar-soaked ties] took place on their property." There was the CRC's principal agent in Richmond, Senora Lawson, who had just barely missed election to the City Council in 1950. Naturally, there was an FBI plant, whose wages turned out to be a down payment on college tuition.[20]

As the eleventh hour approached, Supreme Court justice Fred Vinson turned down a last-minute appeal. A spokesman for President Truman told a group led by Mary Church Terrell that he was "very familiar" with the matter but that "he was not seeing anybody about the case." In Harlem two thousand five hundred people gathered at 126th Street and Seventh Avenue to protest; the meeting was followed by a huge demonstration at City Hall. All the while a "Death Watch" bore down on the White House. Richmond was hit by a buzz saw of protest not seen since Reconstruction, as Mandel ably reported:

> Motion picture theatre owners put on the lights after each showing to urge all in the audience to phone or write the Governor. The white manager of the city-owned segregated dance hall, the Mosque, yielded to the Committee's request to make the same announcement every half hour during the evening. Men grabbed fistfuls of handbills from distributors on the streets to distribute in bars, restaurants and hotel lobbies. Taxi drivers ran out to get five dollar bills changed into nickels for phone

campaigners they had never met before. . . . Men stood by to read off numbers into telephone directories. People lined up in mass in front of the telephone booths.

As the execution approached, a mass rally that brought together hundreds was called on four-hours' notice in a city not known for its quick responses to organizers' calls. Nine hundred people showed up at a church rally then marched to Capitol Square. A hopeful sign was the fact that 10 percent of the marchers were Euro-Americans: "One of the most encouraging aspects of the whole campaign was the presence [of Euro-Americans]." Although the demonstrators did not possess a parade permit, a police force not known for its sensitivity to civil liberties did not interfere. Fueled by the overwhelming response, Mandel offered to cut the power lines into the prison in order to forestall the execution.[21]

This was the first time that Afro-American and Euro-American residents of Richmond had joined in such a public protest of Jim Crow justice. It is often assumed that the post-1955 civil rights movement led by Dr. Martin Luther King, Jr., emerged from out of the blue. In fact, the atrocity that was Jim Crow meant, in effect, that the Afro-American community had been conceded by the powers that be to the Left. The exigencies of the cold war meant that Jim Crow had to go, but this had to be done while ousting the Left from positions of influence within minority communities. Hence, CRC also had to go.

Local power brokers were not pleased and were particularly distraught with the presence of "outside agitators," many of whom were stomp-down, bona fide Communists; their reaction to this helped to set the tone for future invasions by freedom riders and the like during the tumultuous 1960s. Yet these marches, protests, and letters did not prevent all seven defendants from being marched to the gallows, strapped down in electric chairs, and juiced mercilessly until the breath passed from their bodies.

But the protests continued. In San Pedro, California, eighty Afro-American workers at the Western Cotton Compressor Company mill conducted a work stoppage. The death vigil at the White House mushroomed to five hundred people, despite "heckling and harassing" by the police. The protesters' placards reflected a recurrent theme: "Nazis Freed—Negroes Lynched" expressed their disquiet with the speedy rehabilitation of Hitler's henchmen by the United States while this nation killed its own Afro-Americans citizens.[22]

When Josephine Baker, speaking from Havana, announced, "I am absolutely horrified," she synthesized the sentiments of many about the executions. The aftermath of the tragedy saw the *Richmond News*

Leader denouncing the CRC, accompanied by a concerted campaign of intimidation against Martinsville's Afro-American community; shaken by the so-called brashness of Afro-Americans and their linkage with "whites" and "reds," local elites moved to reassert their hegemony. CRC leaders did not skip a beat in trying to use the energy generated by the crusade to save other political prisoners. Grossman thanked Frank Render of the Richmond YMCA profusely for that organization's "courtesy and friendliness" during the CRC's recent stay—yet politeness was not his only aim. He reiterated that the gesture was "particularly noted and appreciated . . . because this is a period when those who fight against jim crow are constantly being denied halls, meeting places, the right to speak, jobs and many other rights. . . . [I]t is obvious to us that pressures, small or great, must have been applied to your organizations, or you." He tried to lift his colleague's spirits and then rally him to the defense of Willie McGee. Anne Shore was pleased with the fact that the CRC had "money coming in from all over the nation . . . enough to finance all 40 people and our campaign for the whole week." But she was sad about the executions and the role of the CRC's erstwhile allies: "We decided that we could have saved the men if two things had been done . . . had NAACP really fought for the seven which they didn't and second had we really been able to move the trade union movement."

But their sweat and tears were not totally for naught. After the executions an Afro-American dentist was murdered. What ensued was singularly uncustomary, and the Martinsville episode was seen as being the determinative element. The suspects were arrested promptly, and the largest Euro-American church in town was offered for the funeral. There was a funeral of 450 Afro-Americans and 150 Euro-Americans, including the mayor, two district attorneys, and a number of police officers. The mayor went so far as to offer funds to bring Afro-American attorneys to assist the prosecution.[23]

This was part of the ultimate significance of the CRC's work in the South. In order to preempt the drawing power of the Left political elites moved to dispense concessions, principally to NAACP-led forces. This gave the impression that their no-struggle politics had produced fruits, which built them up at the same time. With this in the pocket they then moved to squash the CRC. But the organization's example of militance and mass action was not squashed, and, when others came around later in the 1960s using the same tactics, they met a community that had received a thorough education in this field. The CRC had been an able teacher.

But Martinsville provided other lessons as well. The Central Park jogger case, the St. John's rape case, and other headline-grabbing incidents in recent times remind us that when race meets gender conflict can arise. To wit, the United States is a nation in which a narrow elite rule in part because of divisions among erstwhile natural allies. Ruby Floyd, the alleged rape victim in the Martinsville case, was not a member of the elite by any means, but she was used as a symbol to subjugate the seven accused men and, by inference, the working masses of Martinsville generally. The execution of the Martinsville Seven was quite useful in forging white unity and blunting class and gender contradictions within the Euro-American community. Even today there are efforts to exacerbate conflict between the women's movement and the African-American freedom movement. Certainly, the invocation of Willie Horton, an Afro-American man displayed in ads during the 1988 presidential campaign as an example of the weakness of the prison furlough system, and the specter of darker men raping Euro-American women were helpful in electing George Bush as president. Hence, the Martinsville Seven case is instructive on a number of levels.

Fortunately, writers such as Angela Davis and Bettina Aptheker, among others, have devoted substantial attention to the contemporary manifestations of race-gender intersections. In a recent book I pointed out that, although affirmative action policies, to cite one example, primarily benefit Euro-American women, if only for the simple reason that they constitute a substantial percentage of the population, these policies are presented in the public discourse as being "black" issues exclusively benefiting Afro-Americans. The failure to underscore the true nature of affirmative action not only complicates race-gender alliances but, in a sense, represents a not unsuccessful effort by elite Euro-American men to enlist women of the same background in their regressive anti–affirmative action campaign.[24]

The case illustrates the exhaustive organizing that was required to finally put to rest the canard that Afro-American males routinely raped white women; repetition of this myth hampered relationships in the movement overall and retarded social progress. The case also illustrates that these fears and myths were overcome in practice. When large unions participated this meant that Euro-American and Afro-American men and women were joined together in a common cause. When leaflets were passed out explicating the nature of the case by Afro-Americans and Euro-Americans, men and women, this too sent a message irrespective of the content of the leaflet. When a Euro-American man by the name of Aubrey Grossman played a leading role in the global campaign to save the Martinsville Seven, this too sent a message that all Euro-American men were not content to live harmoniously with the atrocities of Jim Crow.

The international aspect of this case should not be ignored. Just as Ida B. Wells-Barnett, one of the original crusaders against lynching, had some of her biggest successes in the United States after touring Europe, the CRC recognized that capturing headlines in the international press was quite useful in penetrating the often somnolent and complacent U.S. press. Unfortunately, this is a message too often lost on political organizers today.[25]

Although the seven men were executed, they did not die in vain. While remnants of the rape-lynch syndrome continue to persist, certainly it does not rise to the level it once did. This has hampered the subordination of the Afro-American population politically and the ability to stigmatize its members economically, which has been a benefit generally for the U.S. working class. Thus, the CRC's conflict with the NAACP, its impressive level of organization, and the demonstration of interracial unity across gender lines in practice makes the Martinsville case a particularly illustrative and expressive relic of one of the more disturbing aspects of recent U.S. history.

Finally, this case is important for what it reveals about the nature of political struggle in the United States. A difficulty in saving the lives of the seven accused men was the presence of red-baiting, that is, discrediting the just cause of the seven simply because some of their prime supporters happened to be political dissidents, in this case members of the CRC. With the apparent demise of the East-West cold war it appears that the phenomenon of red-baiting may be dissipating (although the fraudulent discourse about the alleged "tyranny of the politically correct" suggests that red-baiting may be taking new forms and, in fact, broadening). Red herrings such as red-baiting hinder clear thinking and may make it more difficult to assess accurately emotionally charged questions such as the rape-lynch scenario.

The CRC perished in 1956 just as the Emmett Till case in Mississippi—a case in which an Afro-American youth was lynched for alleged improper remarks to a Euro-American woman—was helping to energize a new civil rights movement. This was a sign that the myth of the Afro-American rapist attacking Euro-American women could be given a proper burial all its own.[26]

NOTES

1. Jessie Guzman to William Patterson, 28 February 1951, reel 9, box 14, A280, CRC Papers; Memorandum from "Bella Abzug," 28 February 1951, reel 6, box 10, A201, CRC Papers.

2. For an overall view of the CRC, see Gerald Horne, *Communist Front?*

The Civil Rights Congress, 1946–56 (London: Associated University Press, 1988).

3. Oakley Johnson to William Patterson, August 1954, reel 1, box 13, A259, CRC Papers; press release, 29 January 1952, box 27, C22, CRC Papers; William Hastie to Oakley Johnson, 14 September 1951, reel 2, box 2, folder 169, Oakley Johnson Papers.

4. *Hampton et al. v. Smith,* reel 7, box 11, A230, CRC Papers; William Patterson to Bishop W. J. Walls, 1 June 1950, reel 43, box 74, N328, CRC Papers.

5. "The Case of the Martinsville Seven—Fact Sheet," reel 7, box 11, A227, CRC Papers; Robert Harris, research paper on the Martinsville Seven, 21 August 1964, box 9, folder 90, William Patterson Papers.

6. Josephine Grayson to William Patterson, 20 August 1951, reel 34, box 58, M49, CRC Papers; William Patterson to Josephine Grayson, 27 August 1951, reel 34, box 58, M49, CRC Papers; Floyd Joyner to William Patterson, 8 December 1950, reel 7, box 11, A227, CRC Papers; William Patterson to Floyd Joyner, William Patterson to Mary Kalb, 11 December 1950, reel 7, box 11, A227, CRC Papers.

7. Robert Harris, *Nation,* 3 March 1951.

8. William Patterson to Tom Buchanan, 21 June 1949, reel 46, box 80, P50, CRC Papers; William Patterson statement, 12 June 1949, reel 7, box 11, A232, CRC Papers; *Times Dispatch,* 13 June 1949, reel 7, box 11, A228, CRC Papers; undated article, *News Leader,* 14 June 1949; *Times Dispatch,* 14 June 1949, reel 7, box 11, A228, CRC Papers; *Daily Worker,* 25 June 1950; *Louisiana Weekly,* 21 May 1949; *Hampton et al. v. Commonwealth,* 190 Va. 531 (1950), 339, US 989 (1950), 340 US 914 (1950), cert. denied.

9. William Patterson to Roy Wilkins, 7 June 1950, press release, 14 March 1950, reel 7, box 11, A232, CRC Papers; William Patterson to Walter White, undated telegram, reel 6, box 10, A204, CRC Papers.

10. Martin A. Martin, 6 October 1950, reel 6, box 9, A180, CRC Papers; Anne Shore to Aubrey Grossman and William Patterson, 11 November 1950, reel 47, box 82, P92, CRC Papers.

11. *Nation,* 20 February 1951; Earl Dickerson to *Nation,* 25 July 1952, reel 34, box 57, M31, CRC Papers; *Time,* 12 February 1951; *New Republic,* 29 January 1951; *Christian Century,* 21 February 1951; William Patterson to Whitelaw Reid, 1 February 1951, reel 34, box 58, M36, CRC Papers; *Nation,* 27 January 1951; *Daily Worker,* 6 July 1949, 15 October 1950, 3 January 1951, 14 January 1951, 23 July 1950, 1 February 1951, 31 May 1949, 15 June 1950, 27 July 1950, 14 July 1950, 2 February 1951, 3 August 1950, 27 July 1950, 12 June 1950, and 17 June 1950 (naturally, the *Worker*'s coverage was most sympathetic and accurate); *Time,* 12 February 1951; *New York Times,* 14 March 1950, 11 October 1950, 6 February 1951; *Guardian,* 7 February 1951; *Sepia Record,* August 1954. William Patterson, a key member of the CRC, was

a Communist and an Afro-American leader who was catapulted into prominence during the 1930s fight to free the "Scottsboro Nine."

12. *Coker v. Georgia,* 433 U.S. 584 (1977); the most recent exhaustive examination of the death penalty concludes: "state imposed executions for rape may have become the counterpart to lynching." The success of the antilynch movement, it could be argued, forced the racists to move into "legal" channels to enforce their diktat in the face of a militant postwar upsurge by Afro-Americans. William Bowers et al., *Legal Homicide: Death as a Punishment in America, 1864–1982* (Boston: Northeastern University Press, 1984), 79; Robert Frederick Burk, "Symbolic Equality: The Eisenhower Administration and Black Civil Rights, 1953–1961 (Ph.D. diss., University of Wisconsin, 1982); Jacquelyn Dowd Hall, "The Mind That Burns in Each Body: Women, Rape, and Racial Violence," *Powers of Desire: The Politics of Sexuality,* ed. Ann Snitow et al., 328–49 (New York: Monthly Review Press, 1983). The controversial equation of black men–white women and rape had been taken up for years and is being taken up again today: petitions, ca. 1951, reel 7, box 11, A231, CRC Papers; William Patterson to pastors, 8 January 1951, reel 7, box 11, A229, CRC Papers; "Sol" to Elaine Ross, 4 January 1951, reel 7, box 11, A229, CRC Papers.

13. Anne Shore to William Patterson and Aubrey Grossman, 11 November 1950, box 62, folder M-7, 1950–51, CRC-Mich. Papers; Anne Shore to Aubrey Grossman, 17 November 1950, reel 47, box 82, P92, CRC Papers.

14. "Membership Builder Article," December 1950, reel 27, box 45, J110, CRC Papers; Arthur McPhaul to James Smith, 14 November 1950, box 62, folder M-7, 1950–51, CRC Papers; *Beacon,* February 1951, box 62, folder M-7 misc., CRC-Mich. Papers.

15. "Action Bulletin," no. 3, Harlem chapter, ca. 1950, reel 56, box 98, V128, CRC Papers; Walter Lowenfels to William Patterson, 2 October 1971, box 2, folder 57, William Patterson Papers; "Chapter Bulletin," vol. 2, 19 March 1951, reel 10, box 16, A328, CRC Papers; Billy Strachan to CRC, 1 August 1951, William Patterson to National Council of Arts, Sciences and Professions (NCASP), 22 November 1948, Aubrey Grossman to MCRAPP, 23 February 1951, Association of Polish Jurists to William Patterson, 29 September 1950, Bankole Akpata to CRC, 2 February 1951, Americo de Carvalho to CRC, 8 March 1951, Amaefuke Ikoro to CRC, 17 October 1950, reel 34, box 58, M46, CRC Papers.

16. Press release, ca. November 1950, reel 7, box 11, A227, CRC Papers.

17. "Civil Rights Action Bulletin," 1 November 1950, reel 7, box 11, A227, CRC Papers; Aubrey Grossman to Rosalee Etta Safford McGee, 6 January 1951; excerpts from interview with Rosalee McGee, including affidavit, 17 May 1951, reel 6, box 10, A207, CRC Papers; "Proposed Rules for Delegation," ca. 1951, reel 7, box 11, A233, CRC Papers.

18. Aubrey Grossman to chapter secretaries, 9 January 1951, reel 7, box

11, A229, CRC Papers; participating unions from Detroit included Plymouth Local 51, Fleetwood Local 15, De Soto Local 227, Cadillac Local 22, Bohn Aluminum Local 208, Dodge Local 3, Fur and Leather Local 38, and Packinghouse Local 69. Shore later claimed that this was an inflated estimate. Press release, 18 January 1951, Anne Shore to Aubrey Grossman, 19 January 1951, box 62, folder M-7, 1950–51, CRC-Mich. Papers; Arthur McPhaul to Mary Kalb, 17 January 1950, box 62, folder M-7, 1950–51, CRC-Mich. Papers.

19. Press release, 15 January 1951, 29 January 1951, reel 7, box 11, A233, CRC Papers; D. V. Jemison to William Patterson, 15 January 1951, reel 7, box 11, A233, CRC Papers; press release, 26 August 1950, reel 7, box 11, A233, CRC Papers; "1044 Polish organizations and groups ranging from trade unions to summer camp colonies" protested; Anne Shore report on Virginia trip, February 1951, box 62, folder M-7, 1950–51, CRC-Mich. Papers.

20. William Mandel to Gerald Horne, 20 June 1984 (in author's possession).

21. Press release, 2 February 1951, reel 7, box 11, A233, CRC Papers; William Mandel report, 10 February 1951, reel 7, box 11, A233, CRC Papers.

22. *Freedom,* February 1951; press release, undated, reel 7, box 11, A233, CRC Papers; press release, 5 February 1951, reel 7, box 11, A233, CRC Papers; *Richmond News-Leader,* 1 February 1951; press release, 13 February 1951, reel 7, box 11, A233, CRC Papers; William Patterson to pastors in Illinois, Florida, Michigan, Louisiana, etc., 29 March 1951, reel 7, box 11, A228, CRC Papers; Aubrey Grossman to Frank Render, 27 February 1951, reel 7, box 10, A220, CRC Papers; Anne Shore to Marguerite Robinson, ca. 1951, box 62, folder M-7, 1950–51, CRC-Mich. Papers.

23. *Jewish Life,* April 1951, box 9, folder 90, William Patterson Papers. Fourteen years later James Grayson, the son of one of the executed men, was himself found guilty of murder; see *Afro-American,* 21 December 1965.

24. Gerald Horne, *Reversing Discrimination: The Case for Affirmative Action* (New York: International Publishers, 1993).

25. See, for example, Alfreda Duster, ed., *Crusade for Justice: The Autobiography of Ida B. Wells* (Chicago: University of Chicago Press, 1970).

26. See also, for example, Elizabeth Pleck, "Rape and the Politics of Race, 1865–1910," *Working Paper,* no. 213, Wellesley College Center for Research on Women, 1990; Angela Davis, *Women, Race, and Class* (New York: Vintage, 1981).

· III ·

Contemporary Racism and Sexism in Different Ethnic Communities

◆ FREDERICA Y. DALY ◆

Perspectives of Native American Women on Race and Gender

Keziah*

Powhatan,
Fire Warrior
Woman.
Keziah, proud
Universal grandmother.
I want your name
On my computer.

You continue to prowl
Among my thoughts,
Even in my veins,
Fire Warrior Woman.
And I am grateful
For your genes and
For what others see in me.

They call it independence.
I know it to be survival.
These, your traits and
Now they're mine,
Have served me,
Served me very well.
As you know, grandmother,
They send a clear message.

So equipped now
With your name on

Keziah Carter, an Algonquin ancestor of the author, torched the Fairfax County, Virginia, Courthouse early in the nineteenth century. The courthouse had been built on her land without her consent.

231

My machine,
I can access you
At will.
Access you and your
Fiery, survival traits,
You, wonderful, maverick woman.

Frederica Y. Daly

INTRODUCTION

Any examination of Native Americans is made difficult because they are not an integral people, even though the United States government and Native Americans themselves often act and write as if they were. Native Americans constitute well over five hundred recognized tribes, which speak more than two hundred (mostly living) languages. Their variety and vital cultures notwithstanding, the official U.S. policy unreflectively, and simply, transforms them from Indians to "Americans" (Wilkinson 1987). Some consideration will be given to their unifying traditions, not the least of which are their common history of surviving genocide and their strong, shared commitment to their heritage.

Any discussion of Indian people requires a brief review of the history of the violent decimation of their populations as well as the massive expropriation of their land and water holdings, accomplished with rare exception with the approval of American governments at every level. To ignore these experiences prevents us from understanding the basis for their radical and profound desire for self-determination, a condition they enjoyed fully before the European incursions began.

The five-hundredth anniversary of the so-called discovery of America was met by protests from large groups of indigenous North and South Americans. Vine Deloria, in *We Talk, You Listen* (1990), writes that some Indians had wanted to celebrate 11 October as "Indians discover Leif Ericson and Christopher Columbus Day" (111). He goes on to pinpoint the critical dilemmas depending on whose eyes determine the history that is written. The discovery by Columbus, from the Native American point of view, involved the invasion of their land and its continuing occupation. In the brief historical account that follows I have drawn mainly from Charles Wilkinson's *American Indians, Time, and The Law* (1987), Vine Deloria and Clifford M. Lytle's *American Indians, American Justice* (1983), and Francis P. Prucha's *The Indians in American Society* (1985).

HISTORICAL OVERVIEW

Indian history, since the European invasion in the early sixteenth century, is replete with incidents of exploitation, land swindle, enslavement, and murder by the European settlers. The narration includes well-documented, government-initiated, biological warfare, which included giving Indians clothing infected with smallpox, diphtheria, and other diseases to which Indians were vulnerable. Starvation strategies were employed, with forced removal from their lands and the consequent loss of access to basic natural resources, for example, the Cherokee and Choctaw experiences in the famous "trail of tears."

Wilkinson as well as Deloria and Lytle assert that Indian history is best understood when presented within a historical framework established by four major, somewhat overlapping, periods. The events dominate federal policy about Indians, subsequent Indian law, and many of the formational forces described in Indian sociology, anthropology, and culture.

Period 1: 1532–1828

This period is described by Europeans as one of "discovery" and is characterized by the conquest of Indians and the making of treaties. The early settlers did not have laws or policies governing their relationships with the indigenous tribes until the sixteenth-century theologian Francisco de Vitorio advised the king of Spain in 1532 that the tribes should be recognized "as legitimate entities capable of dealing with the European nations by treaty." As a result, writes Deloria, treaty making became a "feasible method of gaining a foothold on the continent without alarming the natives" (1970, 3). Deloria explains further that inherent in this decision was the fact that it encouraged respect for the tribes as societies of people and, thus, became the workable tool for defining intergroup relationships. By 1778 the U.S. government entered into its first treaty, with the Delaware Indians, at which point the tribe became, and remains, the basic unit in federal Indian law.

The early decision by Vitorio to recognize the legal entity of the tribe no doubt was instrumental in the rejection of one of the early attempts at "scientific" racism. During the decade just before the end of the nineteenth century, the American Bureau of Ethnology, in Washington, D.C., "proposed as an official policy the theory of polygenesis—the multiple creation of the races—and argued that the separate creation of the non-white races accounted for innate inferiority of Blacks and Indians" (Prucha 1985, 6). Prucha writes that

Thomas McKinney of the Bureau of Indian Affairs (BIA) rejected poly-genesis and held firmly to monogenesis. While the polygenesist the-ory was rejected by those government officials acting in the interest of Indians, the non-Indian mainstream continued to view Indians and their cultures as inferior. Prucha asserts, "They contrasted the pre-literate Indian societies with the accomplishments of their own soci-ety and judged the Indian languages generally worthless even though of scientific interest" (8).

By this time, however, an official paternalism characterized both the language and the actions of the government in its dealings with Indians. Prucha reports that three tribes were told: "The Great White Spirit has ordained that your Great Father and Congress should be to the Red Man, as Guardian and Fathers. . . . Soon you shall be at a per-manent home from which there will be no danger of your moving again, you will receive their full benefit" (1985, 17). Furthermore, Chief Justice Marshall had also defined the Indian Nations as "domes-tic dependent nations." But even if paternalism and their legal status somewhat shielded them from the academized racism of the Ameri-can Bureau of Ethnology, Indians had already long since learned that the "Great White Father" and the Congress, racist or otherwise, had a devastating deceitfulness all their own.

Period 2: 1828–87

The second period, beginning little more than a few decades before the Civil War, witnessed massive removal of Indians from their ances-tral lands and subsequent relocation, primarily because of their resis-tance to mainstream assimilation and the "missionary efforts" of the various Christian sects.

Early in his presidency Andrew Jackson proposed voluntary re-moval of the Indians. When none of the tribes responded the Indian Removal Act of 1830 was passed. The act resulted in the removal of the tribes from the Ohio and Mississippi valleys to the plains of the West. "Nearly sixteen thousand Cherokees walked from Georgia to Eastern Oklahoma . . . the Choctaws surrendered more than ten mil-lion acres and moved west" (Deloria and Lytle 1983, 7). Soldiers, teachers, and missionaries were sent to reservations for policing and proselytizing purposes, activities by no means mutually exclusive and which represented the full benefit of the act as far as the tribes were concerned. Meanwhile, discovery of gold (especially "strikes" on or near Indian land) in the West, coupled with the extension of the railroad, once again raised the "Indian Problem." But at this point, with nowhere else to be moved, Indian tribes were even more in jeopardy, setting the basis for the third significant period.

Period 3: 1887–1928

During the final years of the nineteenth century offering land allotments seemed to provide a workable technique for assimilating Indian families into the mainstream. The Dawes Act of 1887 proposed the formula for allotment. "A period of twenty-five years was established during which the Indian owner [of a specified, allotted piece of reservation property] was expected to learn proper methods of self-sufficiency, e.g., business or farming. At the end of that period, the land, free of restrictions against sale, was to be delivered to the allottee" (Deloria and Lytle 1983, 9). At the same time the Indian received title to the land and citizenship in the state.

The Dawes Act and its aftermath constitute one of the most sordid narratives in American history involving tribal peoples. Through assimilation, swindling, and other forms of exploitation, more than ninety million acres of allotted land were transferred to non-Indian owners. Furthermore, much of the original land that remained for the Indians was in the "Great American Desert," unsuitable for farming and unattractive for any other kind of development. During this same period, off-reservation boarding schools began to be instituted, some in former army barracks, to assist in the overall program of assimilation, and the Dawes Act also made parcels of reservation land available to whites for settlement. The plan to assimilate the Indian and thereby eradicate the internal tribal nations caused immense misery and enormous economic loss. But as we know, it failed. Phyllis Old Dog Cross, a nurse of the North Dakota Mandan Tribe, mordantly puts it, "We are not vanishing" (1987, 29).

Period 4: 1928–Present

The fourth period is identified by Wilkinson especially as beginning just before the Depression in 1928. It is characterized by reestablishment of tribes as separate "sovereignties" involving moves toward formalized self-government and self-determination, and cessation, during World War II, of federal assistance to the tribes.

Prucha reminds us that, with the increased belief in the sciences in the 1920s and the accompanying belief that the sciences could solve human problems, attitudes toward Indians hardened. At this point the professional anthropologist began to be sent and be seen on the reservations to study and live with the people, alongside the missionaries. The changing attitudes continued into the 1930s with the Roosevelt administration. It was during this period that John Collier became commissioner of Indian Affairs, and the reforms of the Indian Reorganization Act of 1934 invalidated the land allotment policies of the Dawes Act, effectively halting the transfer of Indian land to non-Indians. As Deloria indicates, the Reorganization Act provided immense benefits,. including the establishment and reorganization of tribal councils and tribal courts.

After about a decade of progress the budgetary demands of World War II resulted in deep reductions in domestic programs, including assistance to the tribes. John Collier resigned in 1945 under attack from critics and amid growing demands in Washington to cancel federal support for Indians. The writer Simon Ortiz describes the period as a time when the intent of U.S. public policy was that "Indians were no longer to be Indians" (quoted in Swann and Krupat 1987, 191).

Deloria writes that Senator Watkins of Utah was "firmly convinced that if the Indians were freed from federal restrictions, they would soon prosper by learning in the school of life those lessons that a cynical federal bureaucracy had not been able to instill in them" (1970, 18). He was able to implement his convictions during the Eisenhower administration into the infamous Termination Act of 1953, in consequence of which several tribes in at least five states were eliminated. In effect, as far as the government was concerned, the tribes no longer existed and could make no claims on the government. Contrary to its original intent as a means of releasing the tribes from their status as federal wards under BIA control, the Termination Act did just the opposite, causing more loss of land, further erosion of tribal power, and literally terrorizing most of the tribes with intimidation, uncertainty, and, worst of all, fear of the loss of tribal standing.

Deloria quotes HR Doc. 363 in which, in 1970, President Nixon asserted, "Because termination is morally and legally unacceptable, because it produces bad practical results, and because the mere threat of termination tends to discourage greater self-sufficiency among Indian groups, I am asking the Congress to pass a new concurrent resolution which would expressly renounce, repudiate, and repeal the termination policy" (1970, 20). This firm repudiation by Nixon of the termination policy earned him the esteem of many Indian people, in much the same way that presidents Kennedy and Johnson are esteemed by many African Americans for establishing programs designed to improve their socioeconomic conditions.

From the Nixon administration through the Carter administration tribal affairs were marked by strong federal support and a variety of programs aimed at encouraging tribal self-determination. The Indian Child Welfare Act of 1978, which gave preference to Indians in adoptions involving Indian children and authorized establishment of social services on and near reservations, was one of the major accomplishments of this period.

Prucha believes that the tribes' continued need for federal programs is an obstacle to their sovereignty. He asserts that dependency persists but that no one knows how to eliminate it (1985, 97). Deloria insists that Indians are citizens and residents of the United States and of the individual states in which they live and, as such, "are entitled to the full benefits and privileges that are offered to all citizens" (246).

As a country, we have failed to acknowledge our despicable treatment of the Indians. This failure continues to exist in the world of science and remains a source of grave concern to Indians. An Indian leader, on the occasion of a reburial ceremony of bones at a sacred site, prayed for the time when science would stop viewing Indians as "specimens." It is hoped that the Indian quest for self-determination and proper respect will be realized, and with it will come our healing as a nation as well. There exists a tremendous need to help the U.S. public begin to understand the real significance of Indian history. The recent elaborate celebrations of the half-millennium anniversary of the arrival of Columbus in America failed wretchedly to respond to this need.

CONTEMPORARY NATIVE AMERICAN WOMEN AND SEXISM

I have just presented a very abbreviated statement of the general, post–European influx historical experience of Indians in America, drawing from the research and insights of lawyers and social scientists. Without this introduction it would be difficult to understand Native American women and their contemporary experiences of sexism and racism.

Although many tribes were matrilineal, Indian women were seldom mentioned prominently in the personal journals or formal records of the early settlers or in the narratives of the westward movement. They were excluded from treaty-making sessions with federal government agents, and later ethnologists and anthropologists who reported on Indian women frequently presented distorted accounts of their lives, usually based on interviews with Christianized women, who said what they believed would be compatible with the European worldview. Helen Carr, in her essay in Brodzki and Schenck's *Life/Lines: Theorizing Women's Autobiography,* offers some caveats about the authenticity of contemporary autobiographies of Indian women, when they are written in the Euro-American autobiographical tradition. She cautions that, in reading the autobiographies collected by early anthropologists, we need to be "aware that they have been structured, consciously or unconsciously, to serve particular 'white' purposes and to give credence to particular white views" (1988, 132).

Ruby Leavitt, writing in Gornick and Moran's *Woman in Sexist Society,* states: "Certainly the status of women is higher in the matrilineal than the patrilineal societies. Where women own property and pass it on to their daughters or sisters, they are far more influential and secure. Where their economic role is important and well defined . . . they are not nearly so subject to male domination, and they have much more freedom of movement and action" (1972, 397).

We do not learn from social scientists observing Indian communities that women also were the traders in many tribes. With this history of matrilinealism and economic responsibilities it is not surprising that some Indian women deny the existence of an oppressed, nonparticipatory tribal female role. Yet just as other North American women, they are concerned with child care needs, access to abortion, violence against women, and the effects of alcoholism on the family, all symptomatic of sexism experiences. They are also aware of these symptoms as prevalent throughout our society in the United States; they do not view them as specifically Indian related.

Bea Medicine, Lakota activist, anthropologist, and poet as quoted in the preface of *American Indian Women—Telling Their Lives,* states, "Indian women do not need liberation, they have always been liberated within their tribal structure" (1984, viii). Her view is the more common one I have encountered in my readings and in conversations with Native American women. In the middle 1970s Native American women who were in New York City to protest a U.S. treaty violation, in a meeting to which they had invited non-Indian women, were adamant that they did not need the "luxury of feminism." Their focus, along with that of Indian men, concerned the more primary needs of survival.

The poet, Carol Sanchez, writes in *A Gathering of the Spirits,* "We still have Women's societies, and there are at least thirty active woman-centered Mother rite cultures existing and practicing their everyday life in that manner on this continent" (1984, 164). These groups are characterized by their "keeping of the culture" activities.

Medicine and Sanchez concur about the deemphasis of the importance of gender roles in some tribes as reflected in the "Gia" concept. *Gia* is the word in the Pueblo Tewa language which signifies the earth. It is also used to connote nurturance and biological motherhood. The tribal core welfare role, which can be assumed by a male or a female, is defined by the tribe in this Gia context. To be a nurturing male is to be the object of much respect and esteem, although one does not act nurturing to gain group approval. Swentzell and Naranjo, educational consultant and sociologist, respectively, and coauthors, write, "The male in the gia role is a person who guides, advises, cares, and universally loves and encompasses all." The authors describe the role, saying, "The core gia was a strong, stable individual who served as the central focus for a large number of the pueblo's members . . . [for example], 'she' co-ordinated large group activities such as marriages, feast days, gathering and preparing of food products, even house building and plastering" (1986, 37). With increasing tribal governmental concerns the role of core group Gia has lessened, "so that children are no longer raised by the core group members" (39). Interestingly, the Gia concept is being used currently by social ecologists. For them it parallels the notion of Mother Earth and corresponds with the increasingly widespread understanding of the earth as a living organism.

Charles Lange, in *Cochiti—A New Mexico Pueblo, Past and Present,* says: "Among the Cochiti, the woman is boss; the high offices are held by men, but in the households and in the councils of the clans, woman is supreme. . . . She has been arbiter of destinies of the tribe for centuries" (1959, 367). The important role performed by the "Women's Society," Lange continues, includes "the ceremonial grinding of corn to make prayer meal" (283). Compatible with women's having spiritual role assignments is the fact that in some tribes the gods are women—for example, in the matrifocal Cherokee and Pueblo nations Corn Mother is a sacred figure.

A Cheyenne saying reflects the tribe's profound regard for women: "A nation is not conquered until the hearts of its women are on the ground. Then it is done, no matter how brave its warriors, nor how strong its weapons" (Kutz 1988, 143–58). Historically, in some tribes women were warriors and participated in raiding parties. The Apache medicine woman and warrior Lozen lived such a role and was the last of the women warriors (Kutz 1988, 143–58). Paula Gunn Allen, in *The Sacred Hoop* (1986), notes that "traditional tribal life-styles are more often gynocratic . . . women are not merely doomed victims of Western progress; they are also the carriers of the dream. . . . Since the first attempts at colonization . . . the invaders have exerted every effort to remove Indian women from every position of authority, to obliterate all records pertaining to gynocratic social systems and to ensure that no Americans . . . would remember that gynocracy was the primary social order of Indian America" (2–3). Later she alludes to the regeneration of these earlier roles: "Women migrating to the cities are regaining self-sufficiency and positions of influence they had held in earlier centuries" (31). "Women's traditions," she says, "are about continuity and men's are about change, life maintenance/risk, death and transformation" (82).

When Indian women deny having experienced sexism they seem mainly to be referring to their continuing historical roles within their tribes, in which they are seen as *the keepers of the culture*. There exists a general consensus that the powerful role of tribal women, both traditionally and contemporarily, is not paralleled in the non-Indian society. Additionally, they allude to the women serving in various tribes as council members, and they point to such prominent, well-known leaders as Wilma Mankiller, chief of the Oklahoma Cherokee Nation; Verna Williamson, former governor of Isleta Pueblo; and Virginia Klinekole, former president of the Mescalero Apache Tribal Council.

CONTEMPORARY NATIVE AMERICAN WOMEN AND RACISM

The relentless system of racism, in both its overt and covert manifestations, impacts the lives of Indian women; most are very clear about their experiences of it, and they recognize it for what it is. Although many are reticent about discussing these experiences, a growing number of Native American women writers are giving voice to their encounters with racism.

Elizabeth Cook-Lynn, a poet and teacher with combined Crow, Creek, and Sioux heritage, writes about an editor who questioned her about why Native American poetry is so incredibly sad. Cook-Lynn describes her reaction in her essay "You May Consider Speaking about Your Art," published in the anthology *I tell You Now:* "Now I recognize it as a tactless question asked out of astonishing ignorance. It reflects the general American attitude that American Indians should have been happy to have been robbed of their land and murdered" (1987, 60–61).

In the same anthology Linda Hogan, from the Chickasaw Tribe in Oklahoma, writes with concern about the absence of information about Native American people throughout the curricula in our educational systems: "The closest I came to learning what I needed was a course in Labor Literature, and the lesson there was in knowing there were writers who lived similar lives to ours. . . . This is one of the ways that higher education perpetuates racism and classism. By ignoring our lives and work, by creating standards for only their own work" (1987, 243). Earlier she had written that "the significance of intermarriage between Indian and white or between Indian and black [has not] been explored . . . but the fact remains that great numbers of apparently white or black Americans carry notable degrees of Indian blood" (216). And in Brant's *Gathering of the Spirit* Carol Sanchez says "To be Indian is to be considered 'colorful,' spiritual, connected to the earth, simplistic, and disappointing if not dressed in buckskin and feathers" (1984, 163).

These Indian women talk openly about symptoms of these social pathologies, for example, experiencing academic elitism or the demeaning attitudes of employees in federal and private, nonprofit Indian agencies. Or they tell of being accepted in U.S. society in proportion to the lightness of skin color. The few who deny having had experiences with racism mention the equality bestowed upon them through the tribal sovereignty of the Indian nations. In reality the tribes are not sovereign. They are controlled nearly completely by the U.S. Department of Interior, the federal agency that, ironically, also oversees animal life on public lands.

Rayna Green, a member of the Cherokee nation, in her book *That's What She Said* (1984), makes a strong, clear statement about racism and sexism: "The desperate lives of Indian women are worn by poverty, the abuse of men, the silence and blindness of whites. . . . The root of their problem appears attributable to the callousness and sexism of the Indian men and white society equally. They are tightly bound indeed in the double bind of race and gender. Wasted lives and battered women are part of the Indian turf" (10). It is not surprising to find some Indian men reflecting the attitudes of the white majority in relating to Indian women. This is the psychological phenomenon found in oppressed people, labeled as identification with the oppressor.

Mary Tallmountain, the Native Alaskan poet, writes in *I Tell You Now* (1987) that she refused to attend school in Oregon because her schoolmates mocked her "Indianness": "But, I know who I am. Marginal person, misfit, mutant; nevertheless, I am of this country, these people" (12). Linda Hogan describes the same experience, saying, "Those who are privileged would like for us to believe that we are in some way defective, that we are not smart enough, not good enough" (237). She recalls an experience with her former employer, an orthodontist, whom she says, "believed I was inferior because I worked for less than his wife's clothing budget or their liquor bill . . . and who, when I received money to attend night school and was proud, accused me of being a welfare leech and said I should be ashamed" (242). In her poem "Those Who Thunder" Linda translated the experience into verse:

> Those who are timid are sagging in the soul,
> And those poor who will inherit the earth
> already work it
> So take shelter you
> because we are thundering and beating on floors
> And this is how walls have fallen in other cities. (242)

In the United States we do not know one another, except from the stereotypes presented in the media. As a result, there is the tendency to view people of a differing group vicariously, through the eyes of media interpreters.

Louise Erdrich and Michael Dorris, both Indian and both university professors and eminent writers, reported in Bill Moyers's *World of Ideas* (1989): "We had one guy come to dinner, and we cleaned our house and made a nice dinner, and he looks and says, kind of depressed, 'Do you always eat on the table?' " (465). They used the example to demonstrate how people "imagine" (as distinguished from "know") Indians on the basis of movie portrayals, usually as figures partially dressed or dressed in the fashion of the nineteenth century and typically eating while seated on the ground. It is difficult to form accurate perceptions of the people and worldview of another group. Carol Sanchez seems to challenge us to do just that when she asks us not to dismiss Native Americans and then asks, "How many Indians do you know?" (163). How many of you in this audience know one? Ten? More than ten?

The reports in the media in May 1993 of a strange illness striking people living on reservation land in the Four Corners area bordering Arizona and New Mexico rapidly produced fear of Navajo people by many, because the illness was dubbed a "Navajo disease." The fear became blatant discrimination in some instances. Two typical cases— one in which a group of Navajo schoolchildren were "uninvited" to a program by their California host school and another in which a group of tourists visiting Gallup, New Mexico, actually put on gas masks—were reported in New Mexico's largest newspaper, the *Albuquerque Journal.* To combat these inaccuracies about the disease and its origins New Mexico TV stations initiated and continued to air public service announcements featuring Navajo children explaining the symptoms of the illness, now identified as Hantavirus, along with strong statements to the effect that it is neither caused by nor restricted to Navajo people.

The health departments of New Mexico, Arizona, Colorado, and Utah, working in concert with appropriate agencies of the federal government, have identified the disease, linking it to exposure to rodent excrement. They issued warnings and have initiated programs of rodent control. Similarly, during the early stages of the outbreak Navajo medicine men linked the illness to the year's unusually abundant piñon crop, which caused an increase in the pest population. The tourist industry continued to anticipate a negative impact on business in the Southwest because of summer visitors having associated the illness with one of the area's major tourist attractions, the Indian people.

Sanchez charges non-Indians with the wish to have Indians act like whites, so they will be more acceptable to whites, another example of accommodation, assimilation. She is describing the attitude cited by the young child care worker who said to me, "They like our food, our drum music, our jewelry, why don't they like us!?" Activist Winona La Duke, of the Ojibwa Tribe and by profession an economist, asserts in her offering in *Gathering of the Spirits:* "As far as the crises of water contamination, radiation, and death to the natural world and her children are concerned, respectable racism is as alive today as it was a century ago . . . a certain level of racism and ignorance has gained acceptance . . . in fact respectability . . . we either pick your bananas or act as a mascot for your football team . . . in this way, enlightened people are racist. They are arrogant toward all of nature, arrogant toward the children of nature, and ultimately arrogant toward all of life" (65–66). And in the same book again Kate Shanley, Assiniboine Sioux and literary scholar, wrote: "The time has come for Indian women and Indian people to be known on our own terms . . . this nuclear age demands new terms of communication for all people. Our survival depends on it" (215). There is hope that newly shared terms of communication will lead to new understanding and common insights to a more balanced history.

CONTINUING TENSIONS

That since the sixteenth century the history of Native Americans is one of racist oppression has become an integral part of contemporary historical understanding. Indian women are speaking with increasing frequency and force about their experiences of the double jeopardy of racism and sexism. I wish now to consider three factors that continue to contribute to serious tensions within the tribes and between the tribes and the so-called dominant culture. The factors are, first, the tension within the Indian community between accommodation and traditionalism; second, the erosion of tribal life which is resulting in what has become known as cultural marginality; and third, the problems that arise because of conflicts between reservation law and federal and state laws.

Tensions within the Indian Community

Indian people who wish to retain their identity and culture by continuing reservation life have constantly to struggle with choices regarding adaptation to the dominant culture. They realize that extremism in either direction will result in destruction of their ways of life. Those who resist any adaptation will be made to do so involuntarily, and those who accept "white men's ways" completely and without modification by that very fact forgo their heritage. For well over a century governmental policy favored assimilation and the concomitant dissolution of Indian tribal existence. Real estate value and greed for precious natural resources were crucial motivating factors throughout the period. Indians simply were in the way of the invaders' efforts to amass money.

To a certain degree the situation remains the same today. A California Indian cited the tensions between the Indians who live on reservations and the people who live in the surrounding communities. He reported that the dismissal and erasure of a group, even in subtle ways, is psychologically destructive. Verna Williamson, former governor of the Isleta Pueblo in New Mexico, stated that she was determined to bring an open and accountable spirit to the Isleta government, and that determination led her to run for office. Her vision of a progressive tribal government, cooperative with county, state, and federal agencies, resulted in her being attacked at times by her supporters as well as her opponents. In many ways she remained a traditionalist who presented and fostered programs to strengthen and teach traditional beliefs. But she also brought to the people new concepts such as legal advocacy training. She justified her accommodation strategies in the following statement: "The encroaching outside world cannot be ignored; its complexities affect the Pueblo's future . . . and the cultural influences from the Anglo communities . . . threaten the rich Pueblo tradition" (quoted in 1988, 5). Even though she recognized the danger to the tradition, her opponents feared that her accommodation to external community ways necessarily would erode the Pueblo way of life.

At the Flathead reservation in Montana attempts are under way to "revive the traditional Salish culture and preserve the rugged land from development" (*Utne Reader,* 1990, 54). Attempts to protect the Indian land for future generations is buttressed by the traditional, nearly universal Indian belief that we do not own the land, that we are simply caretakers of it and will pass it on to future generations. Thus, how the land is used can become an issue of deep tension between strict traditionalists and those who want to assimilate contemporary economic development thinking into tribal life and institutions. Likewise, nearly universally held precepts include the prevailing rights of the tribe over individual rights and the discouragement of aggression and competitiveness, which are seen as threats to tribal harmony and survival. Phyllis Old Dog Cross, a Sioux and a nurse, speaking at a health conference in Denver in 1987, stated: "The need not to appear aggressive and competitive within the group is still seen among contemporary Indians . . . even quite acculturated Indians tend to be very unobtrusive. . . . [If not,] they receive strong criticism . . . also anything that would seem to precipitate anger, resentment, jealousy was . . . discouraged, for it is believed that tribal group harmony is threatened" (1987, 20).

Acknowledging their need for self-sufficiency as reductions in federal funding continue, the tribes are searching intensively for economic solutions. Some have introduced organized gambling onto the reservations and the leasing of land to business corporations; others are considering storage on reservation land of toxic wastes from federal facilities. Many of these measures are resisted, especially by traditionalists within the tribes, who see them as culturally destructive.

Erosion of Tribal Life: Cultural Marginality

Cultural marginality is increasingly experienced by Indian people because of the confusion resulting from ambiguities about what defines Indian identity, individually and tribally. The questions "Who is an Indian?" and "What is a tribe?" no longer permit neat unequivocal answers.

Different tribes have different attitudes toward people of mixed heritage. In some a person with white blood may be accepted, while a person with some African-American blood may or may not be identified as Indian. Indian women, if they marry non-Indians, may or may not be identified within their tribes as Indians. To be a member of a tribe a person must meet that tribe's requirements. Many tribes require proof of a person's being one-sixteenth or one-quarter or more of Indian descent to receive tribal affiliation.

This question becomes more complicated when the issue of "Who is an 'Indian Artist'?" and it became even more confusing with the signing on 29 November 1990 of Public Law 101-644 by President George Bush. Entitled "The Indian Arts and Crafts Act," the law requires the artists to prove their "native heritage."

Halleah J. Tsinhnahjinnie, of Seminole, Creek, and Navajo heritage, writes: "I am concerned when a law regulates identity. I am reminded of the numbers tattooed on the arms of Jewish people; I am reminded of the vicious witch hunts of the McCarthy period; I am reminded of the ethnic cleansing of Bosnia" (1993, 13). This law is divisive and imposes the racist concerns of their oppressors on Native Americans, keeping current the old and useless blood quantum witch hunt.

A group or an individual may qualify as an Indian for some federal purposes but not for others. A June 1977 statement by the U.S. Department of Labor on American Indian women reads: "For their 1970 Census, the Bureau included in their questionnaire the category, 'American Indian,' persons who indicated their race as Indian. . . . In the Eastern U.S., there are certain groups with mixed white, Negro, and Indian ancestry. In U.S. censuses prior to 1950, these groups had been variously classified by the enumerators, sometimes as Negro and sometimes as Indian, regardless of the respondent's preferred racial identity." LeAnne Howe, writing in Paula Gunn Allen's *Spider Woman's Granddaughters,* says, "Half-breeds live on the edge of both races . . . you're torn between wanting to kill everyone in the room or buying them all another round of drinks" (1989, 220).

Paula Gunn Allen, of the Laguna Pueblo tribe and a professor of literature, in her essay in *I Tell You Now,* writes: "Of course I always knew I was an Indian. I was told over and over, 'Never forget that you're an Indian.' My mother said it. Nor did she say, 'Remember you're part Indian' " (1987, 144).

Conflicts between Tribal and Other Governmental Laws

The Bureau of Indian Affairs, which has specific oversight responsibilities for the reservations, has played, at best, an ambivalent role, according to its very numerous critics. There have been many rumors of mishandled funds, especially of failure of funds to reach the reservations. It is the source of endless satire by Indian humorists, who, at their kindest, refer to it as the "Boss the Indian Around" department. By federal mandate the BIA is charged with coordinating the federal programs for the reservations. Originally, it was a section of the War Department, but for the last century and a half it has operated as part of the Department of the Interior.

Continuing skirmishes occur over violations of reservation land and water rights. Consequently, the tribes continue to appeal to the Supreme Court and to the United Nations for assistance in redressing federal treaty violations. When these cases are made public they become fodder for those who continue to push for the assimilation of Indians into the dominant society as well as for the ever-present cadre of racial bigots.

Federal law and policy have too often been paternalistic, detrimental, and contrary to the best interests of the Indian people. Further, the federal dollar dominance of the tribes has a controlling interest on Indian life. Levitan and Johnston conclude that, "for Indians, far more than for any other group, socio-economic status is a federal responsibility, and the success or failure of federal programs determines the quality of Indian lives" (1975, 10).

To receive eligibility for government services requires that the person live on or near a reservation, trust, or restricted land or be a member of a tribe recognized by the federal government. To be an Indian in America can mean living under tribal laws and traditions, under state law, and under federal laws. The situation can become extremely complex and irksome, for example, when taxes are considered. The maze and snarl of legalese over such questions as whether the Navajo tribe can tax reservation mineral developments without losing its "trust status" and accompanying federal benefits would defeat, and does, the most ardent experts of jurisprudence. And the whole question of income tax for the Indian person living on a reservation and working in a nearby community requires expertise that borders on the ridiculous.

University of New Mexico law professor Fred Ragsdale, describing the relationship of reservation Indians with the federal government, compares it to playing blackjack: "Indians play with their own money. They can't get up and walk away. And the house gets to change the rules any time it wants" (1985, 1).

The outlawing of certain Indian religious practices occurred without challenge until the 1920s, when the laws and policies prohibiting dancing and ceremonies were viewed as cultural attacks. With the passage of the Indian Civil Rights Act in 1964 Indians have been able to present court challenges to discrimination based on their religious practices. Members of the North American Church use peyote, a psychoactive drug, in their ceremonies. Many consider their religion threatened by the recent Supreme Court ruling that removes First Amendment protection of traditional worship practiced by Native Americans.

The negative impact of the 1966 Bennett freeze, a federally attempted solution to the bitter Navajo-Hopi land dispute, continues to cause pain to the Hopi, who use this 1.5 million–acre land mass for grazing, and to the Navajo, many of whom have resided on this land for generations. Sue Ann Presley, a *Washington Post* reporter, describes the area as being among the poorest in the nation and notes that the people living there are prohibited by law from participating in federal antipoverty programs. She reports that 90 percent of the homes have neither electricity nor indoor plumbing, and home repairs are not permitted. She quotes Navajo chair, Peterson Zah: "There are many Navajos who want to live in what we call the traditional way. But that does not mean they want to live with inadequate sewers, unpaved roads, no running water or electricity and under the watchful eye of the Hopi Tribe" (1993, G1). The forced removal of some of the Navajos from this area to border-town housing caused a tremendous increase in the number of people who sought mental health treatment for depression and other disorders, according to the clinical observations of Tuba City, Arizona, psychologist Martin Topper.

DISCUSSION

So, what does that narrative information have to do with scientific practice? What does it have to do with scientists and educators?

Drs. Lila Wallis and Perri Klass, in *Lear's,* an upper-class "woman's magazine," in October 1989, accused the medical establishment, doctors and researchers, of practicing "MACHO MEDICINE." Their remarks were neither flip nor random, and they documented their accusations with research evidence. If their accusations that the physical health of U.S. white women is seriously underattended are true, what does that imply for minority women in general and American Indian women in particular? Wallis and Klass write that, in the area of medicine, "women have been a variant, a deviation from the concept of the human norm" (1989, 68).

Robert Hadley, a psychologist at the University of California–Los Angeles, in a letter in a 1990 issue of *American Psychologist,* condemns such gender bias in research. "Research biased by social stereotypes is faulty because it violates *general* principles of good science. Social bias is the content of the violations rather than their substance" (1990, 73).

In "Indian country" the Indian Health Service is entrusted with the care of Indians. Yet tensions created in the community by economic deprivations, sexism, racism, and federal and state interferences impact negatively on both the community health and individual health of Indian people. Historically, Native Americans have experienced medical treatment indignities and have concerns regarding the professional methods of direct inquiry, note taking, picture taking (the use of X-rays, for example), and forced separation from their families during hospital and clinic visits. For most health is a condition resulting from living in harmony with one's body, one's community, and the natural world.

Paula Gunn Allen writes: "When a community is out of balance for whatever nearest reason, its most sensitive members are most likely to suffer in their bodies and minds . . . their very sensitivity on psychic and spiritual levels makes them lightning rods, drawing the disharmony to themselves and grounding it, rendering it far less harmful to the larger community" (1991, 169). Differences in worldviews therefore result in markedly different causal factors being attributed to the same illness by Native Americans and Indian Health Service officials and other professional medical personnel. "There are powerful arguments advanced in the Indian community," Allen continues, "that many of us suffer from a variety of immune system disorders and other chronic debilitations because we are earth's children, and as she endures monstrous patriarchal abuse, we suffer as well, sharing in her pain and disease and in that way ameliorating its devastation and bringing some respite to her" (169).

The Indian Health Service supplies health data on Indian clients, and, since its transfer to the Public Health Service in 1955, improvements have occurred. Even so, according to a study published in 1987, "The health status of American Indians and Alaska Natives still lags behind that of the general population" (Stuart 1987, 95). Paul Stuart reports that accidents, alcoholism, homicide, and suicide among Native Americans are significantly above the national rate, and the death rate from diabetes has also increased.

The Navajo word for *cancer* means "sore that never heals." This sore that never heals is of great concern to Native American women living on reservations, many of whom live in areas close to uranium mining areas and the Los Alamos National Laboratories. Many have expressed suspicions because of the number of women in their immediate families diagnosed with cancer. They wonder about the proximity of the mines and the potential for contamination of their water supply. Many of these women are not monitored yearly with scheduled mammograms and pelvic examinations. As if this alone were not cause for concern, a study reported in a 1993 issue of the *New England Journal of Medicine* reports that male doctors in general are less likely to refer their female patients for these examinations.

Alcohol-related illnesses and alcoholism play significant roles in the early death of Indians; one-third of Indians die before age forty-five, according to a congressional study reported in the 18 May 1989 issue of the *Albuquerque Journal.* The Indian Health Service spends a mere 3 percent of its budget on alcohol abuse programs, according to the same study. Many of the Indians who die before age forty-five are children, whose deaths are caused by drivers under the influence of alcohol. Despite the impact of the phenomenon, the Indian Health Service does not encourage its staff to do research in this area, about which so little is known.

Alcoholism is not as prevalent in Native American women as in Native American men, yet for both the numbers affected are very high. Phillip May reports, "When behaviors which are alcohol-related are examined Indians in the United States have higher rates of death from accidents, cirrhosis of the liver, homicide, and suicide" (1989, 105). May further states that fetal alcohol syndrome was found to be the leading major birth defect among southwestern Native Americans but says this problem "is one concentrated in a small number of heavy drinking women" (106). Native American novelist and essayist Michael Dorris has written about this problem, as he encountered and attempted to live with it, in his adopted son *(The Broken Cord* [1989]). Dorris has made many educational public appearances to express his concern about the high rate of alcohol-related birth defects among Native Americans. Both the Indian Health Service and the tribes have developed programs to educate their communities about the dangers of alcohol use during pregnancy.

My own experience treating Native American clients regularly included their acknowledgment of alcoholism's multifaceted problems. Most of them were motivated to cooperate during treatment, although maintaining sobriety during weekends posed enormous difficulties for many. Of those who were successful many were members of the Native American Church and were involved in nondrinking group activities. Most of the Native Americans attributed their drinking to peer pressure, needing to "numb out," or getting away from problems by drinking to unconsciousness. None of them said they liked to drink, and environmental stress appeared to be the root cause of their problem drinking.

While many professionals have described very positive attitudes about participation in the Native American Church and recommended it to their clients, the Supreme Court recently decided that the First Amendment does not protect traditional worship by Native Americans. As a result, this indigenous adjunct to therapy is threatened by limiting the religious freedom of these people.

CONCLUSIONS

This closing decade of the twentieth century, as a promise for continuing scientific discovery and almost geometric progress, offers a special framework as a time for healing. The healing should be aligned with bias-free hope, and it should be as universally inclusive as possible. I think it a modest suggestion to say that it could well start with sharper identification and diagnosis by the scientific community of Native American women's experience of sexism and racism. Studies showing the impact of the privileged culture and dominant race on the development of Native Americans deserve continued exposure and extended development. We need medical research that investigates the health conditions and illnesses of minorities, including Native American women, whose general health status has to be among the worst in America.

Culturally significant alcoholism treatment measures need to be developed and tested along with studies on fetal alcohol syndrome. Traditional treatment approaches utilizing cooperative and nurturing values need to be investigated and formally studied under the sponsorship of the new Department of Alternative Medicine, whose first director is a Native American professional with an advanced degree in medicine. And the impending national health plan, which aims to provide basic health care to all Americans, needs to contain provisions for Native Americans in general and women in particular which answer past inadequacies and preclude continuation of practices that support or are supported by racism and sexism.

The development of new theories must include appropriate, representative definitions of the total population, free of gender bias and not derived disproportionately from the observation of middle-class white men and women. Curriculum offerings with accurate and comprehensive historical data about gender-specific Native American experiences are needed. This kind of expanded scholarship seems to me a natural and obvious priority of our scientists, who now in a special way understand themselves to be on the threshold of a new era, that of the truth seekers of the twenty-first century.

Softly Speaks My Name

Was it you, grandmother,
Who softly spoke my name?
Who paced
The length of my room,
Mumbling as you
Brought the dawn?

Could it be you,
Cousin of Pocohantas,
Grandmother of Rose,
Georgia, Marsha, Otrich
And of Grandmother too?
Was it you?

You or your beautiful
Granddaughters, strong,
Vibrant women, which
Of you, softly paces
My floor at dawn?
And what can I learn of love?

Frederica Y. Daly

REFERENCES

Allen, P. G. 1986. *The Sacred Hoop.* Boston: Beacon Press.
———. 1987. "The Autobiography of a Confluence." In *I Tell You Now*, ed. B. Swan and A. Krupat. Lincoln: University of Nebraska Press, 141–54.
———. 1989. *Spider Woman's Granddaughters.* Boston: Beacon Press.

———. 1991. *Grandmothers of the Light: A Medicine Woman's Sourcebook.* Boston: Beacon Press.

Bataille, G., and K. Sands. 1984. *American Indian Women—Telling Their Lives.* Lincoln: University of Nebraska Press.

Bergman, R. 1971. "Navajo Peyote Use: Its Apparent Safety." *American Journal of Psychiatry* 128:6.

Canby, W. C. 1981. *American Indian Law.* St. Paul, Minn.: West Publishing.

Carr, Helen. 1988. "In Other Words: Native American Women's Autobiography." In *Life-Lines: Theorizing Women's Autobiographies,* ed. Bella Brodzki and Celeste Schenck. Ithaca, N.Y.: Cornell University Press, 131–53.

Cook-Lynn, E. 1987. "You May Consider Speaking about Your Art." In *I Tell You Now,* ed. B. Swann and A. Krupat. Lincoln: University of Nebraska Press, 55–63.

Daly, F. 1980. "Relocation as a Mental Health Issue." Paper presented at the University of New Mexico, Psychiatry Department.

———. 1987. "Women and Alcohol." Paper presented at VA Medical Center, the University of New Mexico, Psychiatry Department.

Deloria, V. 1970. *We Talk, You Listen.* New York: Dell Publishing.

Deloria, V., and C. Lytle. 1983. *American Indians, American Justice.* Austin: University of Texas Press.

Dorris, M. 1989. *The Broken Cord.* New York: Harper and Row.

Erdrich, Louise, and M. Dorris. 1989. "Interview." In *Bill Moyers: A World of Ideas,* ed. B. S. Flowers. New York: Doubleday, 460–69.

Francis, D. 1990. "You, Your Doctors, and the Health Care System." *Every Woman's Health.* Garden City, N.Y.: Guild America.

Glasrud, B., and A. Smith, eds. 1982. *Race Relations in British North America, 1607–1783.* Chicago: Nelson-Hall.

Gornick, V., and B. Moran, Eds. 1972. *Women in Sexist Society.* New York: Signet.

Green, R. 1984. *That's What She Said.* Bloomington: University of Indiana Press.

Hadley, R. 1990. "Sexism in Research Is Not Only Sexism." *American Psychologist* 45:73.

Hogan, L. 1987. "The Two Lives." In *I Tell You Now,* ed. B. Swann and A. Krupat. Lincoln: University of Nebraska Press, 231–49.

Howe, L. 1989. "An American in New York." In *Spider Woman's Granddaughters,* ed. P. G. Allen. Boston: Beacon Press, 212–20.

Journal Staff. 21 July 1993. "Suspected Hantavirus Patient Now in Satisfactory Condition." *Albuquerque Journal,* 1.

Katz, W. 1986. *Black Indians: A Hidden Heritage.* New York: Atheneum.

Klass, P., and L. Wallis. October 1989, "Macho Medicine." *Lear's,* 65–68.

Kress, S. 1993. "One of the Few." *Crosswinds* 5:9.

Kutz, J. 1988. *Mysteries and Miracles of New Mexico.* Corrales, N.M.: Rhombus Publishing.

La Duke, Winona. 1988. "They Always Come Back." In *A Gathering of Spirit,* ed. B. Brant. Ithaca, N.Y.: Firebrand Books, 62–67.

Laird, C. 1975. *Encounter with an Angry God.* Banning, Calif.: Malki Museum.

Lange, C. 1959. *Cochiti—A New Mexico Pueblo, Past and Present.* Austin: University of Texas Press.

Levitan, S., and W. Johnston. 1975. *Indian Giving.* Baltimore: Johns Hopkins University Press.

Lurie, N., et. al. 1993. "Preventive Care for Women—Does Sex of Physician Matter?" *New England Journal of Medicine* 8:12.

May, P. 1989. "Alcohol Abuse and Alcoholism among Native Americans: An Overview." *Alcoholism in Minority Populations.* Springfield, Ill.: Charles C. Thomas.

Munar, D. 1988. "Verna Williamson—First Woman Governor." *Albuquerque Women in Business News* 5:3–5.

Old Dog Cross, P. 1987. "What Would You Want a Caregiver to Know about You?" *The Value of Many Voices Conference Proceedings,* 29–32.

Perrone, B., H. Stockel, and V. Kruger. 1989. *Medicine Women, Curanderas, and Women Doctors.* Norman: University of Oklahoma Press.

Presley, S. 18 July 1993. "Restrictions Force Deprivations on Navajos." *The Washington Post,* G1–G2.

Prucha, F. 1985. *The Indians in American Society.* Berkeley: University of California Press.

Ragsdale, F. 1985. Quoted in Sherry Robinson's "Indian Laws Complicate Development." *Albuquerque Journal,* 1.

Rosen, L. 1976. *American Indians and the Law.* New Brunswick, N.J.: Transaction Books.

Sanchez, Carol. 1984. "Sex, Class and Race Intersections: Visions of Women of Color." In *A Gathering of Spirits,* ed. B. Brant. Ithaca, N.Y.: Firebrand Books.

Scott, J. 1989. *Changing Woman—The Live and Art of Helen Hardin.* Flagstaff, Ariz.: Northland Publishing.

Sewell, C.M. June 1993. *Outbreak of Acute Illness—Southwestern United States.* New Mexico Department of Health memo.

Shaffer, P. January/February 1990. "A Tree Grows in Montana." *Utne Reader,* 54–63.

Stuart, P. 1987. *Nations within a Nation—Historical Statistics of American Indians.* Westport, Conn.: Greenwood Press.

Swentzell, R., and T. Naranjo. 1986. "Nurturing the Gia." *El Palacio* (Summer–Fall): 35–39.

Tallmountain, M. 1987. "You Can Go Home Again: A Sequence." In *I Tell You*

Now, ed. B. Swann and A. Krupat. Lincoln: University of Nebraska Press, 1–13.

Topper, Martin. 1979. "Mental Health Effects of Navajo Relocation in the Former Joint Use Area." Paper presented at University of New Mexico, Psychiatry Department.

Tsinhnahjinnie, H. 1993. "Proving Nothing." *Crosswinds* 5:9, 13.

U.S. Department of Labor. June 1977. *Memo on American Indian Women*. Washington, D.C.: U.S. Government Printing Office.

Wallis, L., and P. Klass. 1989. "Macho Medicine." *Lear's* (October): 65.

Wilkinson, C. 1987. *American Indians, Time, and the Law*. New Haven, Conn.: Yale University Press.

Wrone, D., and R. Nelson, eds. 1973. *Who's the Savage? A Documentary History of the Mistreatment of the Native North Americans*. Greenwich, Conn.: Fawcett.

◆ BONNIE ELLEN BLUSTEIN ◆

Educational Policy in Recent History: Reflections on Science, Ideology, and Political Action

The struggle over hereditarian theories of individual differences and social stratification has never been confined to a purely academic context. Much of this history is analyzed elsewhere in this volume. This essay takes one recent and fairly well-delimited controversy as the starting point for a more general consideration of the relations of a radical critique of hereditarianism to the practical struggle for an egalitarian society. In the first section I describe a recent debate between the educational psychologist Lloyd Dunn and his critics which revolved around the implications of genetic determinism for the education of bilingual Latino[1] children in the United States. In the second I examine the differences between liberal and radical critiques of the hereditarian position and argue that liberal approaches are dangerously flawed. Finally, I consider arguments relating to theory and practice within a radical (and specifically a Communist) egalitarian critique.

Let me say a few words at the outset about the distinction between a "liberal" and a "radical" position. Classical liberalism was developed by philosophers of the rising bourgeoisie in the eighteenth and nineteenth centuries. Its core concept is that free competition will produce the best possible social outcomes in virtually every sphere of life. In economics this has traditionally meant laissez-faire; in politics, pluralism; in ethics, individualism; and so forth. The ironies of classical liberalism soon became evident. Formal equality before the law, to the limited extent that it was implemented, together with the freedoms of the marketplace and (in the United States) the Bill of Rights, produced vast social inequalities that increased, not decreased, with time. Competitive market economies developed into tightly controlled monopolies. Racism and sexism persisted. Governments formally committed to the principles of classical liberalism proved capable of abetting and even implementing the severest repression (Knapp and Spector 1991, 43–46). In a further irony those in the twentieth century (at least in the West) who are willing to accept these consequences, maintaining their faith in classical liberalism, are now often referred to as "conservatives." Those in Eastern Europe, the Soviet Union, and China who endorse this ideology are still considered "liberals."

For those who were dissatisfied with the outcome of the policies of classical liberalism two options have existed. The first is to insist that the principles of liberalism have so far been misapplied or misunderstood; if only they were implemented consistently, in this view, society might be reformed and its problems ameliorated. The second option, radicalism, is to reject the principles of liberalism, asserting that racism and sexism, economic and political inequality, among other social ills, are implicit in the foundations (or roots) of liberal society. In particular, Marxist radicals identify the market economy—including the "labor market" or wage work—as the cornerstone of this foundation.

In the nineteenth century organized movements against sexism and against racism almost universally took the principles of classical liberalism for granted. As these have more generally become policy—for example, with the extension of the franchise and the legal abolition first of slavery and later of racial discrimination—the debates have become more complicated. In her book *Biological Politics* Janet Sayers (1983) discusses rifts between liberal and Marxist feminists, among others, over such issues as sociobiology and the "sex and brain weight" controversy (see esp. chap. 10). Elizabeth Fee (1975) provided a similar analysis of feminist approaches to women and the health care system. During the last decade, in response to the growth of the "conservative" variant of classical liberalism and of groups even further to the ideological "Right," some opponents of racism and sexism have preferred to minimize differences between liberals and radicals in the hope of building a more effective movement. I find this approach to be misguided in two respects. First, it usually means in practice that the radical analysis is suppressed for the sake of "unity," and, for reasons I shall develop in subsequent sections of this essay,

I believe that radical (not liberal) strategies will be necessary to achieve an egalitarian society. Second, while I do believe that liberals and radicals should unite in pursuit of immediate reforms, I am convinced that such unity can only be built on the basis of mutual understanding of our differences as well as of our points of agreement.

LATINO PEOPLE IN THE UNITED STATES: FALLACIES OF "RACIAL" STATISTICS

The Latino population of the United States has been growing in recent years, both in absolute numbers and relative to the total population. U.S. census data classifies individuals both by "race" and as "Hispanic" or not. Hispanics may be identified "racially" as either "white" or "black." Thus, data for whites (as distinct from "white non-Hispanics") includes some, but not all, Hispanic respondents. Differences between whites and Hispanics (e.g., in terms of income data) therefore underrepresent actual disparities between Hispanics and persons who are socially white. In addition, it should be noted that immigrants from Mexico and Central America lacking legal papers—who are undoubtedly among the most oppressed people in the country—are also the most likely to have been undercounted in census figures. This, too, contributes to an underestimate of statistical differences in social status.

Another important source of racial coding should be mentioned here, as it helps to illustrate the profoundly unscientific and ahistorical thinking on which theorizing about "inherent racial differences" rests. First of all, examination of the "racial code" guidelines issued by the National Center of Health Statistics shows that the rule of "hypodescent" is still in effect: a child of a so-called biracial mating is assigned the status of the parent with the lower racial status (except, peculiarly, in the case of Hawaiians). This rule clearly has nothing to do with inherent biological traits. In the case of Latinos the situation is still more absurd. As of 1989, parents are asked whether they are Hispanic and, if so, of what specific national identity. Dominicans are then classified as black; Central Americans and "mestizos" as "other non-white"; and Mexicans, Chicanos, Cubans, Puerto Ricans, and South Americans as white. Regardless of the response, however, they are all listed on the birth certificate as white (Byrne 1991). Presumably, this makes sense to some bureaucrat, but the logic is difficult for an outsider to discern.

In short, all so-called racial and ethnic categorizations are highly

problematic. They indicate social designations that may prove important to the lives of individuals living in a racist society, not scientific
typologies, even rough ones.

As of 1987, Latinos constituted about 8 percent of the U.S. population and nearly 11 percent of the children between the ages of five
and fourteen. Over 80 percent of these Latino grade-school-age children were Mexican or Puerto Rican in background. Their prospects in
the educational system, while better than they had been in 1970, remained discouraging. Over one in four of Latino adults in the United
States had not completed eight grades of elementary school, while
this was true of fewer than one white adult in twelve. Only about half
of the Latino adults and over three-fourths of the white adults had
completed high school. In California and Texas, the two states with by
far the largest Latino populations, both high school and college completion rates for this group were lower than the national averages for
Latino adults. These figures were not simply the results of recent immigration of large numbers of relatively unschooled adults. A 1986
survey of persons eighteen to twenty-one years of age showed that 13
percent of white youths and 31 percent of Latino youths had dropped
out of school. While the white dropout rate had declined since 1975,
the Latino rate had actually climbed (U.S. Bureau of the Census 1987,
38, 131–32, 146). In many urban high schools, Latino dropout rates
approach 70 percent.

LLOYD DUNN AND HIS CRITICS

Statistics such as these prompted the circulation early in 1987 of a
provocative monograph by Lloyd M. Dunn, entitled *Bilingual Hispanic Children on the U.S. Mainland: A Review of Research on Their
Cognitive, Linguistic, and Scholastic Development.* Dunn was professor of Special Education at Peabody College of Education in Nashville, Tennessee, from 1953 to 1969. Now in semiretirement and
affiliated with the University of Hawaii, he is best known as the author of the widely used Peabody Picture Vocabulary Test (PPVT). This
instrument takes advantage of the high correlation between scores on
vocabulary subtests on standard IQ tests and those received on the
test as a whole. It purports to assess scholastic aptitude in young children by investigating their hearing vocabulary. A series of English
words is presented orally to the subject, who is instructed to point to
the picture in a set that corresponds to that word. Among the "intelligence" tests in use in the early 1970s, noted researchers Jane Mercer

and Wayne Curtis Brown, Dunn's PPVT had the "greatest English-language and Anglo culture content" (1973, 71–72). In response to such charges and to the growing market in bilingual education, Dunn and his associates later created a Spanish-language version of the PPVT.

Dunn's monograph was likewise intended to address issues of bilingualism and in fact was meant, according to the author, to "shake up the entrenched special interest group" of bilingual educators (Dunn 1988, 304). It was printed up and copies were distributed free of charge by American Guidance Service, which publishes Dunn's testing kits, and soon found its way from educational circles to Capitol Hill. A staff member of the House Committee on Education and Labor sent a copy to James Lyons, legislative counsel to the National Association for Bilingual Education. He forwarded it to the Hispanic Research Issues Special Interest Group of the American Educational Research Association (AERA), where it evoked a storm of protest (Fernandez 1988, 179). Jim Cummins, for example, reacted with "disbelief that crude genetic explanations were again being marshalled to account for the educational failure of Hispanic students." He noted that "the reaction . . . among those who advocate for minority children and for historically brutalized communities . . . has been one of shock at the emergence of yet another apologist for discriminatory tests and school programs" (Cummins 1988, 263, 270).

Like Arthur Jensen's 1969 *Harvard Educational Review* piece—and Dunn's argument relied heavily on Jensen—the monograph was at once scientific in style and polemical in its explicit repudiation of so-called compensatory education programs, in this case bilingual education. He complained that "Hispanic pupils and their parents have also failed the schools and society, because they have not been motivated and dedicated enough to make the system work for them."

Dunn also speculated that Mexican-American and Puerto Rican children might be inherently incapable of academic success. "Most Mexican immigrants to the U.S. are brown-skinned people, a mix of American Indian and Spanish blood," he observed in rather crudely racialist terms, "while many Puerto Ricans are dark-skinned, a mix of Spanish, black, and some Indian." "Blacks and American Indians," he continued, "have repeatedly scored about 15 IQ points behind Anglos and Orientals on individual tests of intelligence." Thus, Dunn claimed, "the hypothesis must be entertained that many Hispanics on the U.S. mainland lack sufficient general intelligence, or specific linguistic aptitudes, to become proficient in either Spanish or English." Dunn's detailed proposals for schooling Latino youth included a plea for "realistic expectations" and a recommendation that instruction be in English only from first grade on (1987).

The use of IQ tests to stigmatize Latino children was scarcely a novelty. Beginning in the 1920s educational psychologists such as Garth Thomas and William H. Shelden had used group IQ test results to conclude that Mexican children (especially those with Indian ancestry) were mentally deficient. They were undeterred in this enterprise, even by their own recognition that cultural and linguistic issues called the testing process into serious question. "Differences in . . . mental attitude toward the white man's way of thinking and living are here made apparent," wrote Thomas in 1923, but he had little difficulty in conflating such differences with inferiority (cited in Padilla 1988). As early as 1932, however, E. Lee Davenport warned that IQ tests (including the nonlinguistic "Draw-a-Man") were not good predictors of school success among Mexican students. Garth and his coworkers were "startled" to find IQ differences between Mexican and Anglo children disappearing with the use of tests that were not language based. George Sanchez, a New Mexico educator, who was for decades the most influential writer on the schooling of Latino children in the United States, set the tone for the 1930s. He attributed lower test scores of Mexican children not to genetic deficiency nor even mainly to language experiences but, rather, to the unsuitability of the tests and testing conditions and the failure of the school system to provide equal education (cited in Padilla 1988).

Even Arthur Jensen acknowledged in 1961 that tests like the Stanford-Binet were "actually static measures of achievement" which "can be quite inappropriate for children who have not had much exposure to Anglo-American culture." He concluded from his study that the California tests did not successfully distinguish slow and fast learners among Mexican-American children and that "non-verbal intelligence tests probably discriminate unfairly against the Mexican-Americans almost as much as verbal tests" (Jensen 1961, 148, 156–57). Knowing the methods of Jensen's mentor, Cyril Burt, it is scarcely surprising to find that Jensen would, fewer than eight years later, cite (without further comment) this same study to support precisely the opposite conclusion: that IQ tests, despite biases, did after all "reflect genetically determined differences in potential" (Jensen 1969, 23). Over the next fifteen years Jensen would devote considerable energy to defending IQ tests from charges of bias against African Americans. Dunn, accepting these arguments uncritically and applying them to "brown-skinned" or "dark-skinned" Latinos, felt justified in concluding that "about half of the IQ difference between Puerto Rican or Mexican school children and Anglos is due to genes that influence scholastic aptitude, the other half to environment" (Dunn 1987, 7).

Members of the Hispanic Issues Research Group organized an interdisciplinary forum at the April 1988 meeting of the American Educational Research Association to rebut Dunn's monograph. The event was carefully planned to maintain academic conventions of impartiality. Dunn was invited to be present to respond to his critics. Previous commitments on his part rendered that impossible, but the papers to be presented were submitted to him in advance for comment, and his written remarks on them were read aloud at the symposium (Fernandez 1988). The revised papers and Dunn's comments on them (also revised) were published as a special issue of the *Hispanic Journal of the Behavioral Sciences* six months later. At least one of the participants was troubled by this exercise. While a "reasoned academic response" to Dunn's monograph was "appropriate and necessary" at one level, Cummins noted, it "entirely misses the point" at another, "since the very act of responding validates the academic credibility of Dunn's case." "A more appropriate response," he hinted, would be a boycott of Dunn's Peabody Picture Vocabulary Test and its publisher, American Guidance Services. In this way Latino parents and educators might "exercise at least some choices that empower both themselves and their children" (Cummins 1988, 271).

The need for direct action as well as academic argument had been an issue in the Jensen-Herrnstein-Shockley debate in the 1970s. "While part of our struggle is to expose and destroy the ideology which makes us tools of oppression," wrote Al Weinrub about the Herrnstein controversy in December 1971, "the other part is to create programs of action which follow from our political understanding" (1972, 5). An editorial collective of SESPA/Science for the People urged: "It is in workers [*sic*] interest to refuse to submit to such [IQ] tests. Destroy the tests, refuse the tests!" Teachers, they suggested, must "expose the system of tracking, of occupational channeling. . . . [D]eny the I.Q. tests and the whole battery of devices used to categorize the essential commodity of the capitalist system, human labor" (SESPA 1972, 10). The introduction to the third edition of *Racism, Intelligence, and the Working Class* notes that this pamphlet "was written when the emerging movement against campus racism had to confront the twin task [*sic*] of refuting the racists on their own terms and discrediting their pretensions to 'science.' " *"The movement against campus racism that began as an assault on the academic nazis must now extend beyond the purely ideological field,"* it emphasized, *"(without for a moment abandoning the ideological struggle) and at the same time spread far beyond the campus"* (Progressive Labor party 1974, 5).

I shall focus on the arguments of Dunn's critics rather than those of Dunn himself. This is particularly appropriate since the prompt and coordinated attack organized by the Hispanic Research Issues group so discredited the monograph that the author himself acknowledged that it had "suffered extremely heavy damage" and promised to withdraw it from circulation, pending revisions. It was therefore deprived of the mass publicity that Jensen and Herrnstein have received, and its impact on policy was muted. The fight against racist ideology is important.

LIBERALISM AND RADICALISM: CRITICIZING THE CRITICS

Critiques of theories of racial or gender inferiority have come both from liberals and from radicals. The distinction between these is crucial, not only for the sake of theoretical clarity but because it bears directly on how we go about our work. The debate over Dunn's monograph—particularly the critiques by Jane Mercer and Henry Trueba—will illustrate this point.

Mercer used many familiar arguments. She berated Dunn for his conclusion that Latinos are genotically inferior to Anglos with respect to scholastic aptitude. She identified the "major fallacy in the Jensen-Dunn argument" as the leap from "variance *within* groups to . . . *between* group differences." She pointed out that g is defined arbitrarily and that so-called IQ and achievement tests both measure learned behaviors, that heritability studies are seriously flawed, and that "IQ is highly malleable" with early intervention (Mercer 1988).

But Mercer was nonetheless fully committed to intelligence testing. She asked, "Is there any way to deal with all this conceptual and linguistic confusion short of abolishing the use of the concept of 'intelligence' in educational settings?" and answered yes. She is the author of the System of Multicultural Pluralistic Assessment (SOMPA), from which she thought that nonracist "inferences *can* be made about intelligence A/capacity *if* learning opportunities can be held constant statistically." She neither called for actual equality of learning opportunities nor questioned the class biases in testing and schooling (Mercer 1988).

Henry Trueba, in contrast, did attack the notion of a universal standard of intelligence and called the concept of race itself "obsolete and incongruent with anthropological evidence." He summarily rejected the "genetic position" as "discredited time and time again." Dunn's remarks about "realistic approaches," he warned, lead to lower expectations that "may justify social abuses by power elites." "This position," he continued, "turns the school into a brutal mechanism for the exploitation of certain human beings by others; that is, schools will perpetuate social injustice and human inequality." He sketched the long and sordid history of discrimination against immigrants in the United States, including jailings in the 1920s in many states for violations of "English-Only" laws. "The arrogance of white supremacists," he concluded, "is in itself a more serious threat to our democratic system that [sic] all the presumed academic failures of Hispanics and blacks" (Trueba 1988).

True enough. But do the schools not already "perpetuate social injustice and human inequality"? Were not school systems structured from the outset to do just this? (Katz 1968; Apple 1982). Mary K. Vaughan (1979) has described how the Mexican public school system at the turn of the century was "highly explicit in its intent to create an efficient and pliable modern labor force to meet the needs of private capital accumulation" and, in particular, how the "education of women was intended to strengthen their primary role in the home." In the United States "liberal strategies for achieving economic equality have been based on a fundamental misconception of the historical evolution of the educational system," wrote Samuel Bowles and Herbert Gintis. "Education over the years has never been a potent force for economic equality." On the contrary, they argued, it played a central role in the perpetuation of the inequalities of capitalism (Bowles and Gintis 1976, 8, 11). For that matter many high school students today already consider their schools to be unjust and oppressive, though they would not use precisely those words.

Let us hear again from Trueba. "Both Jensen and Dunn," he said, "live in a democratic society which has publicly and consistently demonstrated its commitment to the equality of all human beings with regard to social, political and economic participation in our society" (Trueba 1988, 258). What happened to that long history of discrimination? In spite of it all, Trueba shares with Dunn a basic faith in American institutions. "Minority students," he writes, "must internalize the values associated with successful schooling" (258). This comment raises three broad questions: Is there empirical evidence of the extent to which schooling itself is effective in combating the racist oppression faced by most Latinos in the United States? What values are, in fact, associated with school success, and which of them, on reflection, do we want our young people to internalize? And what attitudes and values might Latino students, for better or worse, already share with their white counterparts?

There is considerable empirical evidence that schooling will not solve the problems facing Latinos in the United States as a group, nor is it a guarantee of success for any particular individual. For example, 1970 figures showed no linear correlation between education and mean earnings among Latinos. A Latino man with one to three years of college earned an average annual salary of $9,924, considerably less than a white male high school graduate with no college ($12,377) and less even than a Latino man with only a high school diploma ($10,386). A Latina woman with eight years of schooling averaged about 12 percent greater annual income than one who had attended some high school. If she completed high school, graduation from a two-year associate degree program (frequently advocated by teachers and counselors) might have garnered her an additional pretax income of $122 per year. And at every level of educational attainment Latinas earned far less than Latino men, with their percentage of male income peaking at 56 percent for those with some college but no degree. The economic inequality between men and women among Latinos was generally less, however, than that among whites (National Center for Education Statistics 1980, table 4.16). This casts doubt on common stereotypes that hold Latino culture to be notably more "macho" than non-Latino communities.

Employment statistics reinforce these conclusions. For men and women of virtually every level of schooling Latinos were more likely to be unemployed than non-Latino whites. The official unemployment rate for Puerto Rican high school graduates (18.2 percent) was much higher than that for Puerto Rican dropouts (12.3 percent). Again, women in almost every demographic group were more likely than comparable men to be unemployed—that is, jobless but still in the labor market (National Center for Education Statistics 1980, table 4.13). It would be hard to argue from these statistics that Latinos are more accepting than whites of the notion that a woman's place is in the home, despite the utility of that notion to employers, who benefit from the maintenance of women as a reserve of inexpensive labor (Apodaca 1979; Latin American and Caribbean Women's Collective 1980; Towner 1979).

More recent figures correlating family income with the schooling of the "householder" show that this situation had not changed much by 1987. At every level of schooling the Latino family median income was lower than median white family income, although the Latino family averaged 4.10 members compared with 3.44 members in the average white family (U.S. Bureau of the Census 1989, 446). The disparity was greatest among families in which the householder had some high school education or a high school degree (Latino family income was about 80 percent of white family income) and least at lower levels of schooling (about 88 percent). At every level of educational attainment Latino families were far more likely than white families to fall below the government-defined poverty level. While the poverty rate for Latino families in which the householder had graduated from high school was substantially lower than that of others (16.3 percent for those without postsecondary work), it was still higher than the rate for white families in which the householder had only completed grade school (14.4 percent). And again the discrepancies between Latino and white families increase steadily with level of schooling (U.S. Bureau of the Census 1989, 455). Education is no panacea for the many ills created by a racist society.

The question of values is considerably more complex, and neither Dunn nor his liberal critics go much beyond platitudes, stereotypes, or vague generalities. Yet there are some research findings, as well as considerable anecdotal evidence, concerning values and attitudes that are rewarded in actual school practice. Bowles and Gintis, for example, correlated student personality traits with grade-point average in a New York high school, controlling statistically for IQ and Scholastic Aptitude Test (SAT) scores. They found that creative, aggressive, and independent students were penalized with lower grades, while traits such as consistency, punctuality, identification with the school, empathizing orders, and external motivation were rewarded with higher grades. The students in this school were from working-class families and, the researchers concluded, were being trained for working-class jobs (Bowles and Gintis 1976, 137).

A few less formal examples will illustrate this point. Well-meaning liberal teachers and community leaders often tell students that the purpose of working hard at boring tasks in school is to get better-paying jobs later on. The content of this message is: "Go for the money." But the young people see for themselves that far more money is to be made by selling drugs in the street than by working hard (as their parents do in factory and service jobs) or even by going to college to become, for example, a teacher. Unfortunately, some have already internalized all too successfully the competitive, acquisitive, individualistic values fundamental to U.S. capitalist society.

Another informal example concerns the particular pressures on Latina students. School personnel understand these very superficially, if at all. *Machismo* is often seen, incorrectly and racistly, as a cultural phenomenon peculiar to Latinos (Latin American and Caribbean Women's Collective 1980). Thus, school officials, wherever possible Latinos, are dispatched to explain to girls' fathers that their daughters will make better wives if they finish high school before marriage. Families are urged not to keep older children (usually girls) home from school to care for sick younger siblings, without recognition of the problem thereby posed when all adults in the household are working at low-paying jobs with little or no leave time, paid or unpaid. In such cases school authorities are also assuming, often incorrectly, that the adult Latina's primary role is in the home. Finally, lip service to antisexism is undercut on a daily basis by the dominant school values that reward quiet obedience and passivity, often resulting in better grades for young women who have been more successfully socialized into these traits.

Those who wish to explain differences in achievement between ethnic groups in terms of different attitudes and values ought to attempt at least to provide some evidence beyond crude or subtle stereotypes of whites as "hardworking" and Latinos as "lazy," which are scarcely acceptable substitutes for stereotypes of "smart" and "dumb." In fact, available evidence points the other way: that white and Latino young people are more alike than different. For example, a national longitudinal study of the high school class of 1972 found that Latino and non-Latino white students had very similar homework habits (National Center for Education Statistics 1980, 66). The same study asked the students what they felt was important in life. Both groups ranked as their five main concerns: success at work, steady work, marriage and family life, better opportunities for their children, and strong friendships. The sixth-ranked concern for both groups, rated considerably lower than the previous five, was a desire to correct social and economic inequalities. Well below this for both groups were the goals of making a great deal of money, becoming a community leader, and either remaining close to parents and relatives or moving to a different part of the country.

There were some differences, however, between the responses of Latino and non-Latino white students. For all but two items (friendships and change of location) Latino students rated the goals as "very important" more frequently than the others. That is, they were, overall, more strongly motivated. By far the greatest difference was that 84.5 percent of the Latino respondents and only 63.9 percent of the non-Latino whites thought it "very important" to provide their children with greater opportunities than they had had (National Center for Education Statistics 1980, 74). Over 90 percent of both groups reported positive attitudes about themselves, including feelings of self-worth and equality with others in terms of abilities (241). A follow-up study in 1976 analyzing educational attainment in terms of family socioeconomic status (SES) found that only in the top SES quartile were non-Latino white students more likely than Latinos to have attended college. In the lowest quartile Latinos were 50 percent more likely to have begun postsecondary work than their non-Latino white counterparts, although white students at all SES levels were more likely to have completed a bachelor's degree within four years. To attribute lower scholastic achievement to defective values, then, as secretary of education Lauran Cavazos did in April 1990, is as much an exercise in victim blaming as is attributing it to defective genes.

These same Latino and non-Latino white students also responded similarly when asked what factors they thought interfered "somewhat" or "a great deal" with their schoolwork. The item most frequently listed by both groups—whether out of conviction or because it seemed to be the "right" answer—was "poor study habits" (59.7 percent of the Latinos, 57.2 percent of the non-Latino whites). The rank ordering of the fourteen items was nearly the same for both groups, although again the Latino students cited almost every problem more frequently (an average of 5.3 apiece, compared with 4.4 for the non-Latino white students). They were about twice as likely (20–22 percent compared with 10–12 percent for whites) to agree that external factors limited their prospects; the other 80 percent may have been unduly optimistic. White students were slightly more likely to cite "poor teaching," but Latino students more often mentioned that "teachers don't help enough," which may have meant almost the same thing. White students also complained more about the lack of appropriate course offerings. The largest difference between the two groups was that nearly half of the Latino students (45.5 percent) and about a quarter of the non-Latino white students (27.4 percent) mentioned money problems as an obstacle to their education (National Center for Education Statistics 1980, 70, 241). In fact, 27.8 percent of Latino youth under the age of eighteen in the United States lived below the official poverty level in 1973, double the rate for whites. By 1987 nearly two out of five Latino children were officially designated as poor, compared to 15 percent of white children. Their median family income (in constant dollars) had actually shrunk (U.S. Bureau of the Census 1989, 454–55).

David Berliner suggested that Dunn's own data may be interpreted to show that "schools, as presently constituted, can be injurious to the intellectual functioning of some of our students." They have to be—to keep large numbers of minority youth in the "front rank" of the exploited and to funnel them into the front lines of the army (Bowles and Gintis 1976, 11). Perhaps the most "intelligent" young people, if we must use that word at all, are to be found among those who resist and rebel against this process rather than those who learn to conform and test well.

Dunn's critic Ricardo Fernandez warns that "the nation can ill afford the continuation of unacceptably high rates of failure of Hispanic, black, and other minority students." Dunn is also concerned with the nation's economic health, hoping that Latino youth will become, in his words, "first-rank, productive contributors to American society." But the use of the word *productive* in this context bears closer scrutiny. Has Dunn reflected on who picks the fruits and vegetables he eats, sews the clothes he wears, or cleans the building in which he labors so productively on the latest revision of the Peabody Picture Vocabulary Test? For Latinos, Dunn emphasized in response to his critics, *"lower class status is due far less to discrimination than to inadequate exertion."* Yet Latinos are overrepresented in precisely those occupations requiring the hardest work for the least rewards: farmwork (but not farm management), factory operatives (especially in the garment industry), and domestic service (U.S. Bureau of the Census 1989, 391). Dunn's call for Latino leaders to promote appropriate "middle-class" values in their communities may resonate sympathetically in the liberal ear—but it is pernicious, nonetheless.

Trueba and Dunn both portray what they call "American democracy" as an embodiment, albeit imperfect, of egalitarian values. As they put it: "It is difficult enough for a heterogeneous society to deal with its racial and ethnic inequalities in schooling and in the distribution of resources. But the very fabric of that society would be quickly destroyed if such inequalities were to be institutionalized through explicit policy."

But this is scarcely the case. Capitalism depends centrally on an unequal distribution of resources which forces a large class of the population to sell its labor power (on the "free market") to the very small class that controls the lion's share to begin with. It requires inequality within the working class—based on some combination of racism, nationalism, and religion—to prevent the cohesion of that class into a militant force for social change (Reich 1971; Progressive Labor Party 1974). In classical liberal terms the American statesman (later president) James Madison warned of the danger of a "majority faction" that could threaten the wealthy minority. Although the oppression of women clearly predated capitalist society, capitalist development in Latin America and elsewhere often intensified this oppression rather than alleviating it (Towner 1979). The fabric of U.S.

society is woven of a warp of class oppression and a woof of racism, reinforced with a durable thread of sexism. The "nation"—as defined and ruled by a powerful economic elite—could ill afford the destruction of racism, however much the majority would benefit from this.

The attack on Dunn's monograph presented at the AERA symposium, together with calls for a boycott of his test, achieved a modest victory. Does it matter, then, whether the arguments used were liberal, radical, or whatever? Yes, it does. As Bowles and Gintis remarked about the Jensen-Herrnstein IQ debate in 1976, "The liberal counterattack against the genetic position represented a significant retreat, for it did not successfully challenge the proposition that IQ differences among whites of differing social class backgrounds are rooted in differences in genetic endowments" (1976, 107). Similar observations can be made about the Dunn debate. By concentrating their fire on Dunn's genetic argument most of his liberal critics missed the main point of his "long prime example of 'blaming the victim' " (Willig 1988, 234).

The liberals left Dunn with a broad avenue on which to retreat and regroup his arguments. Thus, in his comments Dunn professed himself an agnostic on the nature-nurture question but asserted bluntly that, "in terms of intellectual prowess, as defined in Western culture, as groups, Asians, Jews, and upper class people, appear to be superior to Anglos and middle class people [sic], who tend to measure out superior to such underclasses as blacks, Hispanics and American Indians." "But then," he modified his stance slightly, "there are different aspects of intellectual function. For example, Anglos appear to be inferior to blacks in tasks involving memory, while blacks appear to be inferior to Anglos in abstract reasoning" (Dunn 1988, 315). Apart from Dunn's peculiar set of race/class/ethnic categories, this corresponds to Jensen's scheme of "Level I" and "Level II" intelligence. Then Dunn got to the heart of the issue as he saw it: "No matter what research does or doesn't say, the broader society [sic] is tired of being blamed exclusively for all the social ills of Hispanics. . . . [T]he underclassed [sic] must be taught what Asian Americans and the middle class take for granted—that their fate is mostly in their own hands" (321). Dunn does not seem to care whether he uses Jensen's racist hypotheses or Daniel Patrick Moynihan's; the impact is the same. (For that matter he does not seem to care about the empirical evidence either.) Liberal critics (and teachers) who accept the goal of fitting students into the system risk winding up on the same side of the fence as Dunn—and the opposite side from those whom they wish to help.

OBJECTIVITY, IDEOLOGY, AND THE QUEST FOR EQUALITY

Can reform within a capitalist framework—that is, liberal reform—create a truly egalitarian society with a correspondingly egalitarian educational system? If not, the liberal challenge to racist-sexist genetic determinism may inadvertently undermine our efforts by building illusions in a fundamentally intransigent set of institutions (Bowles and Gintis 1976, 8; Progressive Labor Party 1989, 41–45). Cummins made this point in urging activism as well as polemics in response to Dunn (1988). But we might also ask whether the boycott of Dunn's test was carried out in a way that left participants and observers with the notion that children should be sorted out for differential treatment in the schools based on some other test. Or did it leave them with a more profound understanding of egalitarian concepts and more confidence in their collective strength? To cite another pertinent example, the Caribbean Students Association of the University of Western Ontario, the Academic Coalition for Equality, and other Canadian groups rejected liberal notions of "freedom of speech" in their actions to suppress J. Philippe Rushton, the inheritor and proselytizer for the pseudoscience of Jensen and Shockley. On another level, however, if calls to fire Rushton were framed purely in terms of enforcing existing government policies—rather than in the context of advancing the class interests of the oppressed—then they would be buttressing a liberal analysis of the role of the state in capitalist society.

Dunn took pains to note that he thought it only a "tactical error" to introduce the genetic argument. Undoubtedly, the worst sort of racist hereditarianism will continue to flourish in well-funded nooks and crannies of the academy, as long as it can play a role in justifying the inherently discriminatory structure of capitalist society. "If the crudities of Social Darwinism are more or less discredited," wrote David Hawkins in 1977, "they still crop up again in subtler versions" (101). Thus, as Andrew Futterman and Garland E. Allen put it recently, academic refutations are not "sufficient by themselves to counter hereditarian trends in human behavioral sciences or to remove the class basis of modern education." "Indicting inequality, exposing a few technical errors, and providing better data, is simply not enough. What is also needed is an understanding and explanation of the relationships between the science of inequality and the political and economic forces that give such ideas [free play]" (Futterman and Allen 1988, 405).

We must also understand the relationship between the science of equality and its social underpinnings. An egalitarian social movement cannot grow without a serious fight against racist and sexist ideologies, and we have a responsibility to intensify this work. But if we are serious about defeating reactionary ideology, we must also make it our job to abolish its social basis, as Linda Burnham argues elsewhere in this volume. The racial doctrines of Samuel George Morton and Samuel Cartwright died on the battlefields of Gettysburg and Vicksburg, those of Alfred Rosenberg at Stalingrad. Let me propose that to create an environment in which a science of equality can flourish capitalism itself must be destroyed. Scientists and teachers must participate alongside youth, workers, and others in the struggle for communism as it was originally understood: the destruction of class society, the abandonment of the market economy and its wage system, and the creation of a global society based on the principle "from each according to ability, to each according to need" (Marx, Engels, and Lenin 1967, 461–63; Progressive Labor party 1989, 11).

Ann Willig noted in the Dunn episode that "a genetic explanation for school failure and low test scores becomes relevant only when it can be proved that the children in question are living and being schooled in optimal environmental conditions and are reaching their maximum level of potential" (1988, 227). In view of "our widespread failure to educate well," wrote Hawkins, "it is acutely inappropriate to assume that the causes of this failure lie in the 'disabilities' of children rather than in the educational disabilities of our society" (1977, 114–15). The establishment of optimal conditions is a priority, and the means for establishing them must be the subject of vigorous debate. As Richard Lewontin put it: "The real issue is what the goals of our society will be. Do we want to foster a society in which the 'race of life' is 'to get ahead of somebody' and in which 'true merit' . . . will be the criterion of men's earthly reward? Or do we want a society in which every man [sic] can aspire to the fullest measure of psychic and material fulfillment that social activity can produce?" (1973, 17). Implicit in this question is the choice between a liberal and a radical model of social criticism and social change.

LIBERALISM AND RADICALISM IN THE ERA OF GLASNOST AND PERESTROIKA

I have argued above that social change within a liberal paradigm cannot erase racism and sexism, much less class inequality, from our society. There is some evidence that many liberal middle-class social reformers of the 1960s and 1970s came to a similar conclusion during the 1980s, although perhaps for different reasons. Unfortunately, their response has generally been to retreat from the quest for social justice, either to a posture of passivity or to the conservative version of what I have called "classical liberalism" (Ehrenreich 1989, 192–94). This was to a certain extent inevitable in the absence of a compelling model for the effectiveness of radical social change. And despite Ehrenreich's plea for a renewal of faith in liberal reform as a means to an egalitarian and unalienated society, neither she nor anyone else has provided even a rudimentary analysis of why this might be a fruitful strategy.

What of radicalism? In the winter of 1990–91, as the original draft of this essay was being prepared, and again in late summer of 1991, as it was being revised, the plausibility of a radical alternative was openly challenged by events in the Soviet Union and Eastern Europe. Newscasters, editors, and headline writers loudly celebrated the death of communism (alternatively, of Marxism) and the triumph of liberalism there and, by extension, in the ideological realm.

Many opponents of racism and sexism in the West, especially those working within a liberal framework, found all this quite irrelevant to the issues at hand. After all, internal conflicts in other countries (however one might evaluate them) would not keep Latino students in the United States from dropping out of school or their parents from losing their jobs in the recession economy. I propose, however, that such a view is shortsighted. Consider, for example, the frightening upsurge of ethnic hostilities in regions supposedly benefiting from "liberalization." Does this suggest nothing about possible links between racism and an economy based on the principles of classical liberalism?

There is another consideration. The "liberalism" of Boris Yeltsin and his associates, for example, is the liberalism of a Milton Friedman rather than that of a Barbara Ehrenreich: it is the conservative version of classical liberal ideology. Thus, the celebration of "liberalization" in the East is actually *opposed* to liberal social reform (or what is often called simply liberalism) in the West. To put it another way, to the extent that the "spin doctors" of the Western media succeed in promoting anticommunism among liberal social reformers, they will make it that much more difficult to forge unity among those who, from varying points of view, wish to oppose race, class, and gender inequality. It is thus more important than ever that we make a serious attempt to understand the implications of an actual (not caricatured) Marxist radical position on relations between science and ideology, theory and practice, especially as they bear on the struggle against theories of genetic determinism.

SCIENCE AND IDEOLOGY: A CLOSER LOOK

Relationships between science and ideology, between ideology and social structure, have been the special study of the sociology of knowledge. Allan Buss took this approach to psychology in a well-researched piece that appeared in *American Psychologist* in 1975. "Psychology as practiced by professional academicians occurs within a social context," he wrote; "psychological knowledge is tied to the infrastructure of a society or socially defined groups" (988). Buss attempted to demonstrate this in the cases of five psychological specialties, including the "differential psychology" of the testers. Before doing this, however, he was careful to distinguish between the approach of Durkheim, Weber, and Mannheim (in which ideologies are viewed as "particular distortions of the social situation") and that of Marx (in which "the idea of socially determined knowledge does not necessarily impede the attainment of objective knowledge to the extent that his ideal of a classless society is realized"). He stressed that a major goal was "to emphasize the relationship between fact and value within psychology and thereby help to make psychologists more self-conscious of the implications their research has with respect to creating a specific image of man [*sic*] and society" (991).

Buss clearly intended his critical analysis as a contribution to the substantive debate over genetic determination of intelligence and social structure. Hans J. Eysenck took this as a serious challenge, particularly since his arch-rival, Leon Kamin, was hammering away with similar arguments (Eysenck versus Kamin 1981). He went to some trouble to rebut the Americans' argument in the pages of the *Bulletin of the British Psychological Society* in 1982.

First, a word on Eysenck, for many years one of the most dogged and dogmatic of the defenders of a genetic interpretation of social inequality. Many readers of this volume will doubtless recognize his name as a champion of racist and sexist ideology and as guru to the worst of the psychologists and behavior geneticists. They may be surprised to find him now claiming also to provide definitive interpretations of Marx, Lenin, and the Socialist experience. Some may be tempted to brush this off as amusing but irrelevant, perhaps citing the cliché that "politics isn't a line; it forms a circle where the far left and the far right come together." To do so, however, is to miss the significant role of anticommunism in buttressing the genetic determinist position. While it would be foolish to take Eysenck's personal opinions too seriously, it would be equally erroneous to dismiss arguments (even coming from such a mouth) which may have at least a surface plausibility even among many of his most determined opponents.

Eysenck was provoked by Buss's contention that "there are no absolute truths in the social sciences" and unimpressed by his distinction between Marx and Mannheim. For him sociology of knowledge and communism could be considered identical: both, he assumed, endorsed a thoroughly relativistic position and were thus diametrically opposed to the scientific pursuit of truth (Eysenck 1982). ("The Marxist interpretation maintains that there are no objective truths," parroted Arthur Jensen in 1984.) Eysenck determined to prove Buss wrong on his own terms: by showing that communism, both in theory and in practice, was perfectly consistent with Eysenck's own brand of genetic determinism. And as one of his respondents noted, he was "apparently seeking to communicate a message which goes beyond the formal content of his article" (Bulkely 1983, 62).

Eysenck never denied a causal link between genetic determinist arguments and social policy. He caricatured Buss's model as a causal chain beginning with economic structure and ending with psychological theories and proposed to show this to be historically inaccurate. Instead, he posited a chain beginning with innate individual biological differences, observed and described by value-free science, and accounting for social structure. "The marked difference in intelligence produced by genetic factors," he had written in 1981, "makes it very difficult to see how any society could exist which did not subdivide into social classes, and indeed, history shows that no society has ever existed which was not so divided" (Eysenck versus Kamin, 86). History shows no such thing, and anthropology shows quite the opposite, had Eysenck taken the trouble to investigate (Hawkins 1977). All things considered, perhaps he had a better chance with the sociology of knowledge.

Eysenck quoted Marxist authorities to contend that they shared his own view of hereditary differences. For example, he quoted Lenin's remark that "when socialists speak of equality, they understand thereby *social* equality, the equality of social position, but not at all the equality of physical and mental abilities of individual persons" (Eysenck 1982, 450). Eysenck, as to be expected, interpreted *abilities* to mean "genetically determined biological capacities," a translation that might have surprised the original author. The quotation was taken out of context: Lenin was explaining to "a liberal professor" that, for communism, "equality" was not a rhetorical slogan but a concrete demand: "The abolition of classes means placing *all* citizens on an *equal* footing with regard to the *means of production* belonging to society as a whole." His point was, thus, diametrically opposed to Eysenck's. Lenin elaborated this elsewhere, in a warning Eysenck might have taken to heart: "Bourgeois professors attempted to use the concept [of] equality as grounds for accusing us of wanting all men to be alike. They themselves invented this absurdity and wanted to ascribe it to the socialists" (Marx, Engels, and Lenin 1967, 471–72). As Eysenck remarked, with perhaps more than a bit of hypocrisy, "The devil can quote scripture" (1982, 450).

In fact, as David Hawkins has explained, "Equality depends on human individuality and thus also upon our *differences* from each other" (1977, 102). Marx and Engels had explored this concept in *The German Ideology* and elsewhere, to explain the necessity and not the impossibility of a classless society. Perhaps Eysenck honestly misunderstood the Marxist classics he cited, or perhaps he was using them opportunistically to make a rhetorical point. Perhaps he was unable to distinguish liberal and Marxist theories of equality; perhaps he identified communism as the necessary form of an egalitarian society; or perhaps he was merely red-baiting the liberals. In any case, his attempt to enlist Marx, Engels, and Lenin among the allies of the genetic determinists is ludicrous.

Eysenck was somewhat more successful in recruiting contemporary Eastern European social scientists to his cause. He gleefully cited recent studies of the heritability of IQ conducted in East Germany, Poland, and the Soviet Union which showed, he said, that, "in spite of the attempts of the communist government[s] to introduce complete egalitarianism into the school system, the health system, and every other aspect of the individual's life," the results (in terms of heritability of IQ) were virtually identical to those in capitalist countries (Eysenck 1982). He emphasized the results of Anna Firkowska and her coworkers, who had studied the scores on arithmetic and vocabulary tests and Raven's Progressive Matrices, administered in 1974 to 96 percent of all schoolchildren living in Warsaw who had been born in 1963. The city had been leveled during World War II and rebuilt along lines of "ecological equalization." This "egalitarian social policy executed over a generation," the researchers concluded, had "failed to override the association of social and family factors with cognitive development that is characteristic of more traditional industrial societies." What they called "mental performance" (i.e., test results) correlated positively with parental occupation and education. After examining such "extrinsic factors" as class size, training of classroom teachers, and location in the center city or on the margins, and finding no relation to test results, they felt justified in asserting the "need to turn to intrinsic factors" (i.e., innate capabilities) to explain individual difference (Firkowska et al. 1978).

Leon Kamin had commented succinctly on this reasoning when Eysenck presented it in 1981. "Perhaps Eysenck has never visited egalitarian Warsaw," he noted acerbically; "if he has, he has kept his eyes and his mind tightly shut" (Eysenck versus Kamin, 180). Even Firkowska and her associates had indicated that they had collected no data on family income and admitted that their "extrinsic measures [may be] too insensitive to detect effects" (1978, 1362).

Eysenck was at least aware of an important potential objection. "It might be argued," he said, "that perhaps Russian communism is developing into a kind of state socialism, resembling in many ways the capitalistic organization of labor" (Eysenck 1982). It might indeed. Almost every one of the eight published responses to his article offered some version of this argument. A change in ideology might well take place, wrote Richard Bulkely, a clinical psychologist, "with the dying out of the old generation of proletarian fighters and revolutionary thinkers, and the rise of a new generation of organization men" (1983, 62). Another clinical psychologist, Neil Rothwell, claimed that "the majority of Marxists, in Britain at least, would not regard any of the Warsaw Pact countries as good examples of Marxism in practice" (1983, 88). Yet another, H.L. Kavenaugh, referred to the "inequality of both income and opportunity" in "state capitalist" countries (1983, 88). The Eastern Bloc countries had not fully completed the transition to communism, explained Stephen M. Furner, but clearly maintained "elements of the capitalist mode" (1983, 179). Hugh C. Willmott and Adrian P. C. Atkinson explored this in more detail. "Advanced capitalist and state socialist economies," they suggested, were more alike than different, since "both treat most employees as atomised factors of production whose potential and performance must be tested and graded if their labor power is to be efficiently deployed and trained" (Willmott and Atkinson 1983, 254).

Eysenck had one card left to play. "None of the social factors obtaining in the U.S.S.R. have changed since Stalin's death," he declared. Since the Stalinist regime had, Eysenck said, shunned both IQ tests and genetic interpretations of human behavioral differences, and since the present regime embraces both, the science of IQ must be unconnected to social factors (Eysenck 1982, 450). Glasnost and perestroika have in the last few years, of course, made a complete hash of these sophistic remarks on the sociology of knowledge.

But the transformation of the Soviet Union from a revolutionary society committed to the eventual realization of egalitarian communism to one in the process of restoring formal capitalist property relations and beset with nationalist and anti-Semitic hostilities is a matter of real concern. A detailed case can be made that the qualitative change toward capitalism in Soviet society took place some decades ago (PLP International Committee Soviet Studies Project 1981). It emerged dialectically from policies not only of Stalin but of Lenin and even Marx which were at odds with central concepts in communist theory. Key among these policies were the retention of the wage system (and thereby social classes) in the name of socialism and the encouragement of nationalism in an uneasy compromise with class consciousness (Progressive Labor Party 1989). These are surely issues in need of further exploration, but the reversal of socialism in Eastern Europe and elsewhere scarcely resolves the contradictions of capitalism (R. D. F. 1990).

CONCLUSION

The present period poses a somewhat different challenge than that of the 1970s with respect to the ideological struggle against racist and sexist theories of genetic determinism and their application to social policy. Twenty years have made a difference. When the polemics of Jensen, Herrnstein, Shockley, and Eysenck originally surfaced, reform liberalism was still ascendant in the United States, and the nation was apparently strong economically and powerful internationally. Dunn's attack on Latino children and their families, in contrast, occurred in a period characterized not only by "Reaganism," as some would put it, but of the relative decline of the United States as a world power, the increasing weakness of the economy even during "growth" periods, and the rise of fascism domestically as well as in the foreign policy sphere. These changes have influenced antiracist responses in two contradictory ways.

Given the apparently rising tide of conservatism in the United States and the supposed triumph of "democracy" in the East, many on the Left are reluctant to pursue fully the logic of their arguments. Some impute ideology only to the other side—as it does to us—thereby discouraging examination of our own stance in the actual social struggle. Some take refuge in the rhetoric of liberalism; others retreat into increasingly nuanced ideological critiques with diminishing returns in practical terms. These responses can be seen in the Dunn debate.

Others, myself included, see the present social crisis as demanding more boldness, not less. We should be more critical in our approach to the principles of classical liberalism. Here we might take a cue from those Latino students and their parents, among other elements of the working class in the United States and in Latin America, who have already embraced basic concepts of revolutionary theory and who have begun to put them into practice. We should have more confidence in people like them and in ourselves.

An egalitarian—that is, classless—society is both possible and more necessary than ever. But it cannot be achieved through liberal reform nor even through radical theoretical critiques in isolation from efforts (however rudimentary) in the direction of revolutionary social change. As Steven Selden suggested in a rebuttal of Jensen's *Phi Delta Kappan* piece, we should strive to be *"both* academically able *and* politically committed."* The quest for objectivity, as Buss explained the Marxian position, must be actualized in the revolutionary struggle for communism. In so doing, as Selden predicted, "we will come to see objectivity and ideology as complementary rather than contradictory aspects of our work" (1984, 283).

NOTES

A shorter version of this essay was read at the February 1990 meeting of the American Association for the Advancement of Science in New Orleans. I am grateful to Walter Secada of the University of Wisconsin for supplying me with several invaluable references and to the students of Benito Juarez High School in Chicago, who helped to inspire this essay.

1. Terms designating social, racial, and ethnic categories will be used in this essay without quotation marks for the sake of convenience. Although *Hispanic* is the designation in official use, I have chosen to use *Latino,* as it is generally preferred among the people so designated.

REFERENCES

American Council on Education. 1988. *One-third of a Nation.* Washington, D.C.: American Council on Education.

Apodaca, Maria Linda. 1979. "The Chicana Woman: An Historical Materialist Perspective." In *Women in Latin America: An Anthology from Latin American Perspectives.* Riverside, Calif.: Latin American Perspectives.

Apple, Michael W. 1982. *Education and Power: Reproduction and Contradiction in Education.* Boston: Routledge and Kegan Paul.

Aubrey, Carol. 1983. "The Sociology of Psychological Knowledge." *Bulletin of the British Psychological Society* 36:218–19.

Barriers to Excellence: Our Children at Risk. 1985. Boston: National Coalition of Advocates for Children.

Berliner, David. 1988. "Meta-Comments: A Discussion of Critiques of L. M. Dunn's Monograph *Bilingual Hispanic Children on the U.S. Mainland.*" *Hispanic Journal of the Behavioral Sciences* 10:273–99.

Bowles, Samuel, and Herbert Gintis. 1976. *Schooling in Capitalist America: Educational Reform and the Contradictions of Economic Life.* New York: Basic Books.

Bulkely, Richard. 1983. "The Sociology of Psychological Knowledge." *Bulletin of the British Psychological Society* 36:62–63.

Burnham, Linda. 1994. "Racism and Sexism: The Limits of Analogy." In this volume.

Buss, Allan R. 1975. "The Emerging Field of the Sociology of Psychological Knowledge." *American Psychologist* 30: 988–1002.

———. 1976. "Reply [to Hans J. Eysenck]." *American Psychologist* 31:312.

Byrne, William G. 1991. "Birth Registration and Racial Identification." MS.

Cummins, Jim. 1988. " 'Teachers Are Not Miracle Workers': Lloyd Dunn's Call for Hispanic Activism." *Hispanic Journal of the Behavioral Sciences* 10: 263–72.

DeBlassie, Richard. 1980. *Testing Mexican American Youth: A Non-Discriminatory Approach to Assessment.* Hingham, Mass.: Teaching Resources Corporation.

Diaz, Joseph O. Prewitt. 1988. "Assessment of Puerto Rican Children in Bilingual Education Programs in the United States: A Critique of Lloyd M. Dunn's Monograph." *Hispanic Journal of the Behavioral Sciences* 10: 237–52.

Dunn, Lloyd M. 1987. *Bilingual Hispanic Children on the U.S. Mainland: A Review of Research on Their Cognitive, Linguistic, and Scholastic Development.* Honolulu: Dunn Educational Services.

———. 1988. "Has Dunn's Monograph Been Shot Down in Flames—Author Reactions to the Preceding Critiques of It." *Hispanic Journal of the Behavioral Sciences* 10: 301–23.

Ehrenreich, Barbara. 1989. *Fear of Falling: The Inner Life of the Middle Class.* New York: Pantheon.

Eysenck, Hans J. 1976. "Ideology Run Wild." *American Psychologist* 31: 311–12.

———. 1982. "The Sociology of Psychological Knowledge, the Genetic Interpretation of the I.Q., and Marxist-Leninist Ideology." *Bulletin of the British Psychological Society* 35: 449–51.

Eysenck, Hans J., versus Leon Kamin. 1981. *The Intelligence Controversy.* New York and Toronto: John Wiley and Sons.

F., R. D. 1990. "Understanding Events in Eastern Europe." *Communist* 2: 71–88.

Fee, Elizabeth. 1975. "Women and Health Care: A Comparison of Theories." *International Journal of Health Services* 5:397–415.

Fernandez, Ricardo R. 1988. "Introduction to Special Issue: Achievement Testing: Science versus Ideology." *Hispanic Journal of the Behavioral Sciences* 10:179–98.

Firkowska, Anna, et al. 1978. "Cognitive Development and Social Policy." *Science* 200:1357–62.

Furner, Stephen M. 1983. "A Contribution to Eysenck's Debate upon the Relationship between IQ and a Marxist Interpretation of Ideology." *Bulletin of the British Psychological Society* 36:179–80.

Futterman, Andrew, and Garland E. Allen. 1988. "Genetics, Race, and IQ: A Final Answer to an Old Question." Review of Michel Schiff and Richard Lewontin, *Education and Class: The Irrelevance of Genetic Studies of IQ* (Oxford: Clarendon Press, 1988). *Journal of the History of the Behavioral Sciences* 24:402–6.

Hawkins, David. 1977. *The Science and Ethics of Equality.* New York: Basic Books.

International Committee Soviet Studies Project, Progressive Labor Party. 1981. "Classes and Class Struggle in the U.S.S.R." *Progressive Labor* 14:48–69.

Jensen, Arthur R. 1961. "Learning Abilities of Mexican-American and Anglo-American Children." *California Journal of Educational Research* 12:147–59.

––––––. 1969. "Intelligence, Learning Ability and Socioeconomic Status." *Journal of Special Education* 3:23 35.

––––––. 1984a. "Objectivity and the Genetics of I.Q.: A Reply to Steven Selden." *Phi Delta Kappan* 66:284–86.

––––––. 1984b. "Political Ideologies and Educational Research." *Phi Delta Kappan* 65:460–62.

Katz, Michael B. 1968. *The Irony of Early School Reform: Educational Innovation in Mid-Nineteenth-Century Massachusetts.* Cambridge: Harvard University Press.

Kavenaugh, H. L. 1983. "The Sociology of Psychological Knowledge." *Bulletin of the British Psychological Society* 36:88.

Knapp, Peter, and Alan J. Spector. 1991. *Crisis and Change: Basic Questions of Marxist Sociology.* Chicago: Nelson-Hall.

Latin American and Caribbean Women's Collective. 1980. *Slaves of Slaves: The Challenge of Latin American Women.* Trans. Michael Pallis. London: Zed Press.

Lewontin, Richard C. 1973. "Race and Intelligence." In *The Fallacy of IQ,* ed. Carl Senna, 1–17. New York: The Third Press.

Marx, Karl, F. Engels, and V. I. Lenin. 1967. *On Scientific Communism.* Moscow: Progressive Publishers.

Mercer, Jane R. 1988. "Ethnic Differences in IQ Scores: What Do They Mean? (A Response to Lloyd Dunn)." *Hispanic Journal of the Behavioral Sciences* 10:199–218.

Mercer, Jane R., and Wayne Curtis Brown. 1973. "Racial Differences in IQ: Fact or Artifact?" In *The Fallacy of IQ*, ed. Carl Senna, 56–113. New York: The Third Press.

National Center for Education Statistics. 1980. *The Condition of Education for Hispanic Americans*. Washington, D.C.: National Center for Education Statistics.

Padilla, Amado M. 1988. "Early Psychological Assessments of Mexican-American Children." *Journal of the History of the Behavioral Sciences* 24:111–16.

Progressive Labor Party. 1974. *Racism, Intelligence, and the Working Class*, 3d ed. Brooklyn, N.Y.: Progressive Labor Party.

———. 1989. *The Road to Communist Revolution: Twelve Articles*. Brooklyn, N.Y.: Progressive Labor Party.

Reich, Michael. 1971. "Economic Theories of Racism." In *Schooling in a Corporate Society*, ed. Martin Carnoy. New York: McKay.

Rothwell, Neil. 1983. "The Sociology of Psychological Knowledge." *Bulletin of the British Psychological Society* 36:88.

Sayers, Janet. 1983. *Biological Politics*. London: Tavistock.

Selden, Steven. 1984. "Objectivity and Ideology in Educational Research." *Phi Delta Kappan* 66:281–83.

SESPA (Scientists and Engineers for Social and Political Action). 1972. "Science in the Justification of Class Structure." *Science for the People* 4: 6–12.

Towner, Margaret. 1979. "Monopoly Capitalism and Women's Work during the Porfiriato." In *Women in Latin America: An Anthology from Latin American Perspectives*. Riverside, Calif.: Latin American Perspectives.

Trueba, Henry T. 1988. "Comments on L. M. Dunn's *Bilingual Hispanic Children on the U.S. Mainland: A Review of Research on Their Cognitive, Linguistic, and Scholastic Development*." *Hispanic Journal of the Behavioral Sciences* 10:253–62.

U.S. Bureau of the Census. 1989. *Statistical Abstracts of the United States: 1989*, 109th ed. Washington, D.C.: U.S. Government Printing Office.

Vaughan, Mary K. 1979. "Women, Class, and Education in Mexico, 1880–1928." In *Women in Latin America: An Anthology from Latin American Perspectives*. Riverside, Calif.: Latin American Perspectives.

W[einrub], A[l]. 1972. "Open Letter AAAS Philadelphia '71." *Science for the People* 4:4–5.

Willig, Ann C. 1988. "A Case of Blaming the Victim: The Dunn Monograph on Bilingual Hispanic Children on the U.S. Mainland." *Hispanic Journal of the Behavioral Sciences* 10:219–36.

Willmott, Hugh C., and Adrian P. C. Atkinson. 1983. "The Sociology of Psychological Knowledge, the Genetic Interpretation of IQ, and Marxist-Leninist Ideology." *Bulletin of the British Psychological Society* 36: 253–54.

♦ CARMEN LUZ VALCARCEL ♦

Growing Up Black in Puerto Rico

There is something deeply spiritual in knowing about these women's lives; in knowing that there were Black women who named themselves so clearly that every time one of them said, "I am," the after-silence vibrated with the words that did not need to be said aloud: ". . . and, therefore, you are too."

—*Noliwe Rooks*

Recently, I was surprised to hear that the governor of Puerto Rico, the Honorable Rafael Hernandez Colon, during the Martin Luther King birthday commemoration in Puerto Rico, expressed opposition to the racism so prevalent in the United States. He did not, however, allude to the racism in his own homeland. This is an example of the denial that still persists in Puerto Rico regarding racism. Other officials express this denial as well. At a conference at the International Festival of Caribbean Culture in Cancun, Mexico, in 1988, Elias Lopez Soba, director of the Puerto Rican Cultural Institute, said, in response to a statement by Marie Ramos Rosado that there were few blacks in finance, academia, or law, that there is no racism or classism in Puerto Rico (Anonymous 1988).

Racial discrimination in Puerto Rico is often seen as isolated acts by individuals or groups of individuals. This is an expression of the complex process of understanding racism in light of the ethnic history of Puerto Rico, derived from the relationships among the aboriginal Taino, the Spanish, and the African peoples who came later. I am using the definition of *institutional racism* given by Pettigrew (1977): "that complex of institutional arrangement that restricts the life choices of Black Americans in comparison to those of white Americans." In my case, we would compare black Puerto Ricans with white Puerto Ricans, because the colonial status of Puerto Rico in relation to the United States has resulted in white supremacist views having been adopted by our culture.

In this essay I will describe and reflect on my experiences as a Boricua* woman growing up black in my homeland and how these experiences shaped my psychological makeup. In general, I incorporated a distorted, negative self-image and only through the pain of struggle could I reconstruct a positive one. I grew up in a working-class neighborhood (barrio). The racial composition of my barrio was mostly black with a few white families. The children in my community learned racist attitudes very early in their development. From these early socialization experiences I came to know how I was seen by society.

I was the daughter of a *triguena* mother. This term may be used to describe a person who is both black and Spanish and has light skin. The term has different usages and connotations (Jorge 1979; Zenon Cruz 1974), but my mother identified with the white side of her heritage. Several of my sisters from my mother's previous marriage to a white Puerto Rican were white. Yet because I looked more like my father, who was clearly black, very early in life I came to feel that I was black. Through various negative messages I learned to understand what being black meant. My hair, for some reason, was called *malo* (bad). According to my mother, it was "difficult" to comb. For my sixth-grade graduation my hair was treated with a "relaxer" to make it appear straight and, therefore, more acceptable. When I made my first communion I was given to understand that I look like a *mosca en un vaso de leche* (a fly in a glass of milk). From that day on I avoided dressing in white.

Isabelo Zenon Cruz (1974) has done extensive and valuable research on how racism is projected in our folklore. He demonstrates how popular expressions regarding black people are used in Puerto Rico to perpetuate a notion of physical and intellectual inferiority. Some of these expressions are: *El negro/a piensa solo los viernes* (Blacks think only on Fridays); *El negro/a si no lo hace a la entrade lo hace a la salida* (Blacks are always putting their feet in their mouths); *Tenia que ser un negro/a* (If a black person did something wrong, it had to be because he or she was black). Other expressions

*Borinque was the Taino name for the island now called Puerto Rico.

relate to their skin color or "nature": *El negro/a es cosa mala* (Black is bad); *Mas negro/a que un cardero* (Blacker than an iron kettle). I heard these expressions frequently in my community. When my friends fought verbally with me or my family they used to call us *negra sucia* (dirty blacks). These insults were deep blows to my self-esteem, but one of the most demeaning experiences was to be called "Africana," because of the negative association of this term with slavery.

In my experience Puerto Ricans are preoccupied with morphological characteristics, such as facial features and skin colors. When babies were born in the barrio the older women would examine their noses and lips. If the nose was "too wide," they would advise the mother to do a kind of "manual surgery" by pressing the nose between the thumb and the index finger to make it narrower. They would also look at the color of the baby's cuticles, which was considered the first predictor of the child's color. When gradations in skin color are the criterion of self-worth, these practices increase rivalry among siblings. Thus, children in the same family were sometimes treated differently according to the color of their skin, and this was true in my family as well.

In childhood games in which one chose a partner white girls were always chosen first or at least more frequently than black girls. Black girls were never considered pretty. I learned to evaluate myself psychologically with white models, as they were considered more attractive and desirable. I never thought I was ugly, but when I compared myself with other girls I always found white girls more attractive. An old sonnet by Pablo Zaez called "The Puerto Rican Woman," cited by Zenon Cruz (1975), reveals, by its idealization of "white characteristics," the racist attitude toward black Puerto Rican women:

> A light brunette with large eyes,
> Black hair, lofty forehead,
> Small, narrow nose,
> Beautiful mouth and rosy lips.

Thus, in this sonnet blacks are denied their right to be identified as Puerto Rican women.

This attitude is still present in today's Puerto Rico, where modeling agencies are requested by public relations firms to supply women with certain measurements but are asked not to send black women. This not only represents job discrimination; it also sells the image of Puerto Ricans as white. When women are chosen to represent Puerto

Rico in international beauty pageants women who look "more Nordic" are selected. As an adolescent looking for summer jobs, I always had to send a photo along with my application, particularly when the job dealt with the public to a great extent. I was never asked to come for an interview, and it was clear to me that I was "too dark," for when I went to the department stores to which I sent applications I found that all the clerks had lighter skin colors than I. My photo was a signal for discrimination, but so was my barrio address, which was required on the applications. I understood not only the racist aspect of this discrimination but the class nature as well.

In the barrio white women generally stayed home, while black women went out to work, and most of them found work only as domestics or in factories. Thus, when I needed to earn money in order to enter the university I also could find only domestic work.

In elementary school most of the teachers were white and showed a preference for the middle-class white students. Thus, I grew up completely ignorant of my African heritage and embarrassed by my African ancestry. These feelings were exacerbated at school, where the history of black slavery was taught from a white supremacist view, sympathizing with the colonizer and the slave owner. Black slave rebellions were discussed within a negative context, describing black slaves as bad, criminal, or savage people who refused to work for their owners and often escaped to the mountains. The fact that black slaves fought for their freedom from the day they came to Puerto Rico was never seen as a positive reaction to oppression. We never learned about the slave women who participated in the Maroon communities of runaway slaves in the Caribbean (Terborg-Penn 1986). It was psychologically painful to learn about black slavery from this perspective. Thus, at school, too, I came to wonder if there was something wrong with my being black and with my feelings about the injustice of slavery. I was embarrassed by the derogatory sneers of my classmates.

Feelings of ambivalence and confusion continually plagued me, since the people around me insisted upon denying racism, asserting that we were all a mixture of Indians, Africans, and Spaniards. But my daily experience constantly reminded me of my blackness and reinforced a feeling of inferiority. I was growing up in a culture in which everybody was "ethnically equal" but racially divided. As a result, I internalized racism by buying the negative notions of blackness. In fact, I came eventually to deny a prejudiced attitude from other people. I came to believe that what I was experiencing was not racism, because racism in Puerto Rico was compared with the U.S.

racist perspective, which had a history of legal restrictions against black people.

Coming of age as a black Puerto Rican woman added further psychological burdens. I was not only facing discrimination and prejudice as a black but also as a woman. Black and white Puerto Rican men have misconceptions and stereotypes about black Puerto Rican women. I was frequently subjected to *piropos* (flirtatious remarks) by men in the street, such as *negra-blanca* (this was intended as a compliment, in that I was "not so black") or *Con un negrita asi, yo si me caso* (I would consider marrying a black like you). These racist remarks imply that the more you conform to the white standards, the better. Other *piropos* imply sexual stereotypes. Expressions such as *Esa negra es caliente* (Black women are hot) and *Buena in la cama* (Good in bed) are jibes familiar to any black Puerto Rican. In my first year at the University of Puerto Rico I was sexually harassed by one of my professors, who had typical misconceptions about the sexuality of black women, yet I was too young, embarrassed, and frightened to report this to anyone.

Another expression of these racist attitudes is the fact that white men do not choose black women as possible marriage partners. Black men are socialized to believe that they can improve their stations in life by marrying a white woman. Likewise, black women are encouraged to look for a partner lighter than themselves, so that they can *mejorar la raza* (improve the race by "whitening it.").

Several years ago Marie Ramos Rosado (1987) criticized a letter, entitled "Love, but Not Biracial," which appeared in a local newspaper. In this letter a woman criticizes a published photograph of a white woman and a black man playing a love scene. She was concerned about the effect of this on children and adolescents, because of the great troubles that children of biracial marriages encounter in Puerto Rican society. She supports her position by saying that "God created three races, and people should not change what God has done" (quoted in Rosado 1987).

I grew up in a very cohesive group of black cousins and friends who did not "approve" of dating white men. Peer pressure was strong on this issue. There was a well-worn motto: *tira para tu raza* (stick to your own kind). The explanation for this may have been the fear of being rejected not only by the white man, if we showed interest in him, but also by the group. Dating a white man was not my goal, because it was clear to me that white men were not interested in black women as lifetime partners. There is a saying, *Mujer blanca, perdición del negro,* which means that a woman's black boyfriend or husband is ready to leave her at any time if he has the opportunity to get involved with a white woman. This belief further devalued the black Puerto Rican woman in comparison with the white woman. In my barrio young black women dated within the boundaries of their community. The white girls, however, had the choice of crossing the boundaries and dating the *blanquitos* (whites) from the surrounding lower-middle-class community. On the other hand, while my dating choices were limited to black men, my black male friends in the barrio could be encouraged to consider marrying a white woman from the barrio but not from the middle class. As a poor white, you still had more freedom of choice than if you were a poor black.

As a result of redistricting the school system, I spent my last year of junior high school in a school located in an upper-middle-class neighborhood. This situation taught me about race, class, and social interaction. When I attended a Christmas party organized by my class I was not asked to dance by any of the young men; this had never happened to me before. Of course, the young men were all white. I was humiliated. Needless to say, I never again attended parties at that school. In his book *Requiem por una cultura* (1972) Eduardo Seda Bonilla reports the results of research in which the following question was asked of black Puerto Ricans: If you attended a party at which the majority of the couples were white, how would you feel? Of the 110 people interviewed, 70, or 63 percent, answered that they would feel bad or uncomfortable (125).

The literature on the lives of female African slaves in the United States illustrates that this history has left its impact through racist beliefs and attitudes (Davis 1981; hooks 1981). Although there is a record of the treatment of slaves in Puerto Rico, there is no published research on the conditions of African female slaves. Since the experience of slavery was one of exploitation and oppression, I can conclude that the experience of the black slave woman in Puerto Rico was similar to that of the black slave woman in the United States. Although some Puerto Rican historians claim that the black slaves of Puerto Rico were not treated as cruelly as those in other colonies and in the U.S. South, the following quotation from the writings of Brother Inigo Abbad y Lasierra in 1796 describes the condition of the black slave on the island of Puerto Rico:

> When all is said and done, there is nothing more ignominious; a white person insults any of them with impunity and in the most contemptible terms; some masters treat them with despicable harshness, getting pleasure out of keeping the tyrant's rod always raised and thereby causing

disloyalty, desertion and suicide. (Quoted in Maldonadol-Denis 1972, trans. Elena Vialo)

In addition, Zenon Cruz (1975) reports that black slaves were brought to Puerto Rico in ships rampant with such disease that both female and male slaves died in large numbers. One of the most barbaric procedures used was that of *el carimbo,* the branding of black slaves when they landed on the island. The Spaniards had done the same to the Tainos. The use of the whip was also a common practice by the slave owner as a means of intimidation. Research on black women in U.S. slavery shows that the roots of contemporary myths and stereotypes about African-American women are in that period. Although published research on the treatment of slave women in Puerto Rico does not exist, there is no reason to think that the Spanish slave owner provided a benevolent situation for the black female slaves. As the literature regarding other slave systems has shown (Terborg-Penn 1986), slave owners exploited women in many ways: Slave women were exploited sexually through rape and impregnation by slave owners. They were also exploited as field workers, house servants, and wet nurses for the slave owners' children. The fact that black Puerto Rican and black U.S. women are stereotyped as having a strong sexual drive may be attributed to that history.

This exploitation continues to be a reality in contemporary Puerto Rican culture. Fewer black Puerto Rican women go to the university because they cannot afford the private preparatory schools, and frequently their early education is insufficient to achieve entry to the university. As a consequence, they end up in jobs that are traditional for working-class women. The black Puerto Rican woman is portrayed in a negative manner on television and in the newly developed Puerto Rican film industry. In most of these new films the black Puerto Rican woman is practically absent. In fact, when I was a child I saw the roles of black women played by white women, who painted their faces and bodies. Today many black actors play the roles of servants in the soap operas. Such subtle and overt forms of racism and sexism, reinforced by our lack of knowledge of our history, heritage, and important contributions to the Puerto Rican culture and economic development, undermine our sense of worth and identity.

Rivera Ramos (1985), in her study of life satisfaction in elderly black and white Puerto Rican women in rural and urban areas, found the color of the woman's skin correlated with income, health, husband's occupation, and whether or not their children went to the United States. Among the light-skinned women the higher income, better health, more professional husband's occupation, and having children in the United States were accompanied by self-esteem and satisfaction with one's life. These findings reflect the increasing discrimination based on being black and a woman in Puerto Rico, both of which tend to lower self-esteem and satisfaction with life.

Even in church, where equality before the eyes of God was proclaimed, there was an open practice of discrimination (Denton, Denton, and Massey 1989, 792). Segregation was practiced every Sunday. The upper-middle-class white people, some of them North Americans, who lived in fancy houses nearby, had a section in the church reserved for them. The people of the barrio were not expected to cross the boundaries of the reserved section. No explanation was given for this—it was taken for granted—yet my friends and relatives knew it as "self-explanatory." Given this situation, Reverend Hector Lopez (1989), a Baptist minister, has proposed a theology for decolonization which acknowledges racism as an oppressive race and class problem: "The theology of decolonization analyzes class domination on the basis of exploitation of Black women and men and creates a pastoral mission from which will emerge a political project of human liberation."

Class and race are intertwined in Puerto Rico. Black Puerto Ricans constitute the poor sector within the society's class structure. We need only visit my barrio, Yambele, and many other barrios in the metropolitan areas, or such towns as Loiza and Carolina, to see the large concentrations of poor black Puerto Ricans. In 1959 Bonilla found that 100 percent of the upper class identified themselves as white (10 people); among the middle class 78.3 percent identified themselves as white, 15.7 percent identified themselves as *intermedio,* and 6 percent identified themselves as black (from a sample of 213); in the category of "lower class" 68.7 percent considered themselves white, 22 percent called themselves *intermedio,* and 9.2 percent said they were black (314 people). The percentages probably reflect that, at that time, black Puerto Ricans were less likely to identify themselves as "black." As Denton, Denton, and Massey (1989) point out, black Puerto Ricans identify themselves as white whenever possible (792–93). Since 1970, however, all Puerto Ricans have been considered a "race," and skin color is not recorded by the authors. This omission may be a reflection of societal attitudes. In another study by El Centro de Investigaciones Sociales it was found that in the upper-middle-class section of Morro 94 percent of the population were white, and 6 percent were black. In Las Marias area 94 percent of the upper-middle class were white, and 6 percent were black. In Monacillo, a huge barrio, 40 percent were white, and 60 percent were black (Seda Bonilla 1972). It is important to point out that in Puerto Rico many barrios are physically separated from a middle- or upper-class neighborhood by a high cement wall. When black people walk in those neighborhoods they are viewed with suspicion. Middle-class *blanquitos* express fear about walking to the barrios.

When I enrolled in the university I had my first opportunity to develop my racial identity. It was then that I started to explore my black heritage from a positive perspective. At the same time I analyzed the false notion of physiological and psychological inferiority. I looked at the problem in the light of colonialism, and this helped me to confront the double burden of being colonized as a Puerto Rican, and as a black woman. Through solidarity with other women and my reading, I learned to develop a positive self-image. I went through a period of being born again black, of experiencing a transformation. My relaxed hair was changed to an Afro look. My mother felt scandalized, and my family and friends looked at me suspiciously. They asked me if I were an *independenista.* This was the beginning of a period in my life of feeling the rage, coming to terms with the guilt, healing the shame, and breaking the silence. And then I realized how beautiful a black woman looks when she wears white.

As a black Puertorriquena, my becoming a person was a very painful process but worth the cost. I learned to look into my own inner strength and to develop the power to fight all kinds of racism. I felt motivated to make changes, accept risks, and take challenges. I am committed to developing myself as a full human being based on my own potential and capabilities. I believe that this potential is derived from the historical experience of being part of the past generations of black female slaves who had no other choice than to survive by any means.

It is ironic that in his Martin Luther King Day speech, the governor of Puerto Rico was so concerned about racism in the United States, when in his own political party, Partido Popular Democratico, racial discrimination has been practiced since its beginning. Black representation in the cabinet does not reflect the proportion of the black population in Puerto Rico. And of course, finding a black woman in political power is like finding a needle in a haystack. Since Puerto Rican history has been written by white men, the role of the black Boricua woman in the labor force as well as in the arts has been ignored. The emancipation of the black woman has to be carried out by us. Black women must speak out; they need to discover the history of slavery and the ways in which black women rebelled, and bring the results of their discoveries to Puerto Rican society today. Marie Ramos Rosado (1990), director of the Puerto Rican Council against Racism, writes of the need to include in the new educational reform a program to eradicate racism and sexism in school textbooks. It is especially necessary in the elementary public schools, where all poor children get much of their education. During International Working Women's Week ("Que Hacer" 1992) there were meetings that affirmed the resistance of black women against oppression as well as analyses of the image of black women in Puerto Rican literature. Through such activities the black Puerto Rican woman defines feminism in her own terms, by our grassroots struggles.

REFERENCES

Anonymous. 1988. "En Puerto Rico pocos tienen acceso a la superacion; existe un racismo sutil." *Novedades de Quintana Roo.* Mexico.

Davis, Angela Y. 1981. *Women, Race, and Class.* New York: Vintage Books.

Denton, Nancy A., Douglas Denton, and S. Massey. 1989. "Racial Identity among Caribbean Hispanics: The Effect of Double Minority Status on Residential Segregation." *American Sociological Review* 54:790–808.

hooks, bell. 1981. *Ain't I a Woman: Black Women and Feminism.* Boston: South End Press.

Jorge, Angela. 1979. *"The Black Puerto Rican Woman in Contemporary Society."* New York: Praeger.

Lopez, Hector. 1989. "Racismo, colonialismo y teologia negra de la descolonizacion." *Claridad* (August 18–24): 33.

Maldonado-Denis, Manuel. 1972. *Puerto Rico: A Socio-interpretation.* Trans. Elena Vialo. New York: Vintage Books.

Pettigrew. 1977. In *Racism and Mental Health,* ed. Charles U. Willie, Bernard M. Kramer, and Bertram S. Brown. Pittsburgh: University of Pittsburgh Press.

"Que Hacer." 1992. *Claridad* 33, 40.

Rivera Ramos, Alba Nydia. 1985. *La mujer Puertorriquena: investigaciones psico-sociales.* Rio Piedras, P.R.: Centro para el Estudio y Desarrollo de la Personalidad Puertorriquena (CEDEPP).

Rooks, Noliwe. 1988. "The Women Who Said 'I am.' " *Sage,* student supp. 30.

Rosado, Marie Ramos. 1987. "Por una sociedad mas justa, no sexista y no racista." *Todo Carolina–Rio Piedras,* March 5, 27.

———. 1990. Reacciones al Proyecto de la Reforma Educativa. *Todo Carolina– Rio Piedras,* February 22.

Seda Bonilla, Eduardo. 1972. *Requiem por una cultura*. Rio Piedras, P.R.: Ediciones Bayoan.

Terborg-Penn, Rosalyn. 1986. "Women and Slavery in the African Diaspora: A Cross-Cultural Approach to Historical Analysis." *Sage* 3: 11–14.

Zenon Cruz, Isabelo. 1974. *Narciso Descubre su Tracero*. Vol. 1. Humacao, P.R.: Editorial Furidi.

———. 1975. *Narciso Descubre su Tracero*. Vol. 2. Humacao, P.R.: Editorial Furidi.

◆ CHOICHIRO YATANI ◆

School Performance of Asian-American and Asian Children: Myth and Fact

Americans first impressed by the quality of Japanese cameras then TV sets then cars and stereo equipment are now beginning to hear about another top-quality product, the school performance of Japanese children. Educators and business leaders believe that Japan's competitive economic edge can be attributed to its citizens' academic performance. This is best symbolized by the report of the education summit called by President George Bush with fifty U.S. state governors (U.S. Department of Education 1987). The last five years in particular showed the poor academic performance of young students in the United States, not only in science and mathematics but also in social sciences and humanities, including foreign languages. The results were very disappointing when compared with those of other nations.

In mathematics, for example, only the top 3 percent of United States high school students achieved the standard reached by more than half of their Japanese counterparts (International Association for the Evaluation of Educational Achievement 1988). In a 1989 study by the Educational Testing Service (ETS) similar results were obtained (Anrig and Lapointe 1989). The ETS administered a standardized test of math and science to twenty-four thousand thirteen-year-olds in six countries—Britain, Canada, Ireland, South Korea, Spain, and the United States. Koreans did the best and U.S. students the worst in average mathematics scores. In science teenagers in the United States placed near the bottom. According to a seventeen-nation study by the

U.S. Department of Education in 1986, United States high school graduates fall short in their literacy and communication skills as well as in their knowledge of sciences, mathematics, geography, world history, and foreign languages.

Examinations designed to check only the school performance of young people in the United States have not presented encouraging results, even when not compared with other countries. A 1987 study under contract with the National Endowment for the Humanities (NEH) showed that the average student received an F grade on both history and literature tests (*New York Times,* September 8, 1987). The study, entitled "What Do Our Seventeen-Year-Olds Know?" used multiple-choice items, including 141 history questions and 121 literature questions. A representative national sample of 7,812 seventeen-year-old students correctly answered 55 percent of the history and 52 percent of the literature questions, which meant an F if transferred to the usual letter grading.

A simple but serious question has been raised: Why is the school performance of United States children so poor? Moreover, facing the age of global economic competition, concerned people of other ancestries in the United States have started to question why their children do not do as well as Asian children educated here and in Asia.

SCHOOL PERFORMANCE, BRAIN SIZE, AND DILIGENCE

A recent article by Rushton (1988) appears to have given a reductionist explanation to declining educational performance and rising economic competition from abroad, especially from the Pacific Rim. He attributes these problems to the relatively larger brain size of "Mongoloids" compared to those of ""Caucasoids"" and "Negroids." Rushton provided the following grounds: "It is reasonable to hypothesize that the bigger brain evolved to increase intelligence ... and mammals with larger brains learn faster than those with smaller brains (i.e., chimp > rhesus monkey > spider monkey > squirrel monkey > marmoset > cat > gerbil > rat ≥ squirrel)" (1010). Using available data on cranial capacity provided by Coon (1982) and Molner (1983), Rushton calculated the average brain sizes of 1,448 cm³ for Mongoloids, 1,408 cm³ for Caucasoids, and 1,334 cm³ for Negroids. Rushton contends that the differences in educational attainment between students in Asia and the United States and between U.S. white and African-American students are attributable to the differences in their cranial capacity, that is, their different brain sizes. This biological determinism also conveys a strong message that environmental efforts to ameliorate the poor performance of students are of little use. Insofar as the task of education is concerned, however, Rushton's contention is probably least appreciated by Asians, if not by Americans.

Culturally and institutionally, Japanese, who are members of what Rushton calls Mongoloids and a major target population in respect to the issue of education in the United States, have hardly paid attention to the presumed association of brain size and school performance, of cranial capacity and intelligence, or even the heritability of intelligence. "In Japan, poor performance in mathematics was attributed to lack of effort; in the United States, explanations were more evenly divided among ability, effort, and training at school. Japanese mothers were less likely to blame training at school as a cause of low achievement in mathematics" (Hess 1986, 161). The strong emphasis of the Japanese on diligence is a well-known fact, as indicated in an extensive three-year study under the general sponsorship of the United States–Japan Conference on Cultural and Educational Interchange (CULCON), resulting from an agreement at the 1983 summit meeting between President Reagan and Prime Minister Nakasone (U.S. Department of Education 1987). The U.S. government acknowledged that Japanese education has succeeded in motivating students to learn and in teaching them effective study habits as well as in creating and maintaining a productive learning environment that includes effective school discipline (U.S. Department of Education 1987).

The Japanese believe that education is a powerful instrument of cultural continuity and national policy. The origins of the Japanese commitment to education lie in the country's Confucian and Buddhist heritage, in which great respect is accorded learning and educational endeavor as means to personal and social improvement. Therefore, quite different from the United States, education in Japan aims at moral education and character development as central concerns along with the acquisition of academic knowledge. Even a certain amount of difficulty and hardship is believed to strengthen student character and their resolve to do their best in learning and other important endeavors. "The amount of time and effort spent in study are believed to be more important than intelligence in determining educational outcomes" (U.S. Department of Education 1987). Consequently, the high educational achievement by most Japanese students in international comparisons provides considerable support for the beliefs and expectations that hard work, diligence, and perseverance are more important for success in education than a level of "inherited" intelligence or relative brain size.

For the Japanese the issue is not whether Rushton's (1988) argument is acceptable but, rather, that it discredits the task of education (Zuckerman and Brady 1988). In other words, the poor educational results of young U. S. students are believed to be attributable to a lack of effort, ineffective study habits, and poor learning environment, not brain size. "How do they work in school?" would thus be an appropriate question.

SCHOOLWORK VERSUS PAID EMPLOYMENT

For the past two years I have had the opportunity to ask over three hundred senior high school and junior high school students about their school lives. The students, from Middle Country School and Commack school districts on Long Island, New York, represent a mixture of middle-class and working-class family backgrounds. The majority of the students told me that they had not studied as much as or as hard as they were supposed to. Compared with the Japanese students I had taught in middle schools in New York, I can say that U.S. students in my "Gifted and Talented Programs" in New York did not study as hard or as seriously as they should have. Schoolwork was not their major concern.

Every teacher working in a school setting is in a fortunate position to observe students' work behavior at school. Having spotted inappropriate behavior, fatigue, poor grades, failing, and other "problems" of their students, faculty members of Seaford High School, a school not far from those at which I taught, conducted a survey and found that almost 90 percent of the seniors had a part-time job. Over 60 percent of the juniors, 40 percent of the sophomores, and 39 percent of the freshmen were found working for an average of twenty hours, seventeen hours, and fourteen hours per week, respectively. This 1988 survey, conducted in a typical suburban town of middle-class residents on Long Island, New York, also found that 72 percent of the freshmen who held jobs failed two or more school subjects. The same was true of 53 percent of the sophomores, 34 percent of the juniors, and 13 percent of the seniors. It has been found, however, that an expected 75 to 80 percent of Seaford graduates go to college (Seaford Senior High School 1988).

The CULCON study reported that only 12 percent of Japanese high school students worked part-time during the school term, compared with 63 percent in the United States (U.S. Department of Education 1987). Part-time jobs held by young students in the United States are not performed out of any "urgent financial need to put bread on the table, . . . but for money for going out, food, soda, gas, clothes, tickets, jewelry. . . . All across the country it's a major phenomenon" (*Newsday,* January 24, 1988, 4). Schools and parents in Japan discourage students from working on the grounds that "it distracts them from study and exposes them to dubious influences in the adult community" (Stocking 1986, 145). Consequently, even those Japanese parents who are not economically well-off tend to sacrifice to cover school costs for their children.

Bishop (1989) has reported that the typical senior high school student in the United States spent ten hours per week in a part-time job and about twenty-four hours a week watching TV. Over three-quarters of U.S. high school seniors spend less than five hours per week on homework. Thirty-five percent of their Japanese counterparts do so (*Wall Street Journal,* March 10, 1987). Considering the fact that the length of the school year is 180 days in the United States and 240 days in Japan, it is not surprising that teenagers in the United States do not give schoolwork a high priority, in view of the fact that the adults in authority devalue time spent at school.

It may be that educational outcomes are determined not only by the length of schoolyear or study hour but also by the study behavior of the students. Students in the United States have been reported not to have effective study habits or well-disciplined behavior. Based on 1,200 to 1,600 hours of observation in the first- and fifth-grade classrooms in Minneapolis (U.S.), Sendai (Japan), and Taipei (Republic of China), H. W. Stevenson (1987) and his colleagues found that children in the United States spent nearly 20 percent of their classroom time in first grade and 15 percent in fifth grade engaged in irrelevant activities (e.g., being out of their seats, talking to classmates, or otherwise behaving inappropriately). Chinese and Japanese children were less likely to be "off-task." W. C. Frederick (1979) reported that in Chicago public schools with high-achieving students averaged about 75 percent of class time in actual instruction, while in schools with low-achieving students the average was 51 percent of class time. Other studies presented similar results: average engagement rate in reading and math instruction is about 75 percent in the United States. About 46.5 percent of potential learning time was wasted in absence, lateness, and inattention (Frederick, Walberg, and Rasher 1979). It is safe to conclude that in the shorter length of the schoolyear the students are not using their class time effectively. Could we expect better educational outcomes from these students who are not engaged in schoolwork as much as they are supposed to be?

MOTIVATION IN STUDENTS

Albert Shanker (1989), president of the American Federation of Teachers, once said: "No matter how good the teaching, students will not learn unless they work at it, unless they're engaged. . . . Yet in a large number of high schools across the country students are docile, bored, passive, lacking interest" (New York Times, Op-Ed, March 5). He argued the importance of student motivation and stressed rewards for good educational outcomes—"a good job for a good grade" at the time of graduation from high school. The behavioral scientist B. F. Skinner (1986) argued that present cultural practices in the United States have eroded the contingencies of reinforcement.

In Japan perhaps the most important work for a teacher is to motivate students. The CULCON study reported: "The cultural emphasis on student effort and diligence is balanced by a recognition of the important responsibility borne by teachers, parents, and school to 'awaken the desire to try.' Japanese teachers . . . believe that the desire to learn—like character itself—is something which can be shaped by teachers and influenced through the school environment" (U.S. Department of Education 1987, 4). A major method of motivating students in Japan is the encouragement of group activities. A strong sense of shared identity, along with the opportunity for individuals to influence group goals and activities and other group-oriented behavior, including the use of school uniforms, contribute to the process of motivating students. Difficult entrance examinations at the secondary level provide special motivation for study. Students know that the results of these examinations will strongly influence the paths of their future economic lives in the highly organized society of Japan. Parental involvement in urging their children to study hard, by creating and maintaining home environments conducive to study and by financing extra lessons (e.g., juku, a private school after school), is also important (White 1987).

J. H. Bishop, after his extensive study of why high school students in the United States are not motivated, argued that, "although there are benefits to staying in school, most students realize few benefits from working hard while in school" (1989, 7). The lack of incentives for effort, he explains, is a consequence of three phenomena. First, when hiring, employers pay little attention to "reading, math, and reasoning ability," evidenced by the grades and performance on academic achievement and aptitude tests of high school graduates or of students seeking part-time jobs while they are in school. Second, peer group activity discourages students from academic effort. Third, admission to selective colleges is not based on an absolute or external standard of achievement in high school subjects. It is based on aptitude tests that do not assess the high school record on such measures as student performance, class rank, and grade point averages, which are defined relative to classmates' performance, not to an external standard.

Although most research clearly shows the strong relationship between competence in reading, mathematics, science, and other subjects and productivity on the job, the business community in the United States rarely rewards high school students' academic performance and achievement. This is quite contrary to the process in Japan as well as in such Western countries as Canada, Australia, and Germany. Obviously, the social system in the United States is not functioning to motivate U.S. students to study hard but, rather, encourages apathy toward their schoolwork.

THE POLITICS OF BRAIN SIZE

Recently S. Sue and S. Okazaki (1990) cast some doubt on cultural explanations for the better achievements of Asian Americans born and educated in the United States, giving two reasons for their view: first, culture is difficult to define and to test, although it may affect learning and performance; second, when the very characteristics associated with Asian culture (e.g., parental pressures for achievement and not embarrassing the family) were investigated, available research gives little support for cultural interpretations of the phenomenon. For example, parenting style was a weaker predictor of grades for Asians than for whites in the United States (Sue and Okazaki 1990).

As indicated, however, the difference in scholastic achievement between Asian students in their homeland and American students in the United States can be largely attributed to the differences in their actual schoolwork and learning environments. Despite these findings, Rushton's (1988) argument on brain size and behavior received wide publicity, as if it had been a substantial scientific discovery. It seems that history repeats itself in "scientific" contributions to racism.

About twenty years ago, when racial tension was at its peak in the midst of the civil rights movements in the United States, a group of studies provided so-called scientific evidence for the notion that intelligence differences between blacks and whites were genetically determined (Jensen 1969; Eysenck 1971; Herrnstein 1971). These reports implied that any environmental improvement would be no remedy for the socially underprivileged. Not only are IQ tests and their results very questionable, but these studies also distort science to achieve racist and eugenic goals (Hearnshaw 1979; Kamin 1974; Lewontin et al. 1984). B. Mehler (1983), in his look at the Pioneer Fund, a New York–based organization with racist and eugenic goals, pointed out the presence of a powerful association of scientists propounding a genetic base to racial differences. In 1988 Rushton added "Mongoloids" to the racist comparison.

For the past ten years people in the United States have been saying, "The Japanese are coming, the Japanese are coming." When the longtime obsession of Americans with "the Russians" was weakened in the middle of the 1980s, the Japanese seemed to take the Russians' place. Recent national opinion surveys such as the *New York Times/ CBS News* polls (1990) indicated that people in the United States had increased their unfavorable attitudes toward the Japanese. For those who sound such an alarm Rushton's argument might give a satisfying explanation: people in Asia are doing better than others because the average brain size of Asians is larger than that of people in the United States. By making such an argument, Rushton probably accomplishes another important goal—that is, he reinforces the old notion of the intellectual superiority of whites to blacks within the United States (i.e., Caucasoids have a larger brain size than the Negroids do).

Such studies contribute to the increasing racial and ethnic tensions within the United States (e.g., blacks vs. whites, Jews vs. blacks, Koreans vs. blacks). Although Rushton's study would seem to praise high academic achievement by Asians and Asian Americans, the "Yellow Peril" prejudice and discrimination in the United States is well documented (Yee 1992, 1). S. Sue, D. W. Sue, N. Zane, and H. Z. Wong (1985) have reported that Asian Americans perceive limitations in their career choices and chances for upward mobility, despite their high educational achievement. If they were without education, their future would surely be a dead end (Hirschman and Wong 1986; Wang 1980).

Despite their ethnic diversity, Rushton regards Asians as homogeneous. In his 1988 paper he uses the concept of "a cranial size for Mongoloids," implying an average brain size for all Asians and Asian descendants; he also speaks of high educational achievement by Japanese, Chinese, and Koreans, which gives the impression that all so-called Mongoloids (i.e., all Asians and those of Asian ancestry) are "smart." Obviously, his sample did not represent all Asians, nor did the claim of "smart Asians" represent all Asians and Asian descendants.

Mongoloids, as a category, must include not only Japanese, Chinese, and Koreans but also Vietnamese, Tibetans, Inuits, Polynesians, those of the indigenous nations of the United States, and probably hundreds of other ethnic groups in Asia and other areas of the world. Until now, however, there has not been a single study that was conducted to compare educational achievement among all these Asians and Asian descendants in countries other than their homelands. Without comparative studies of education within the category "Mongoloids" generalizations of research findings based on Rushton's three groups—Mongoloids, Caucasoids, and Negroids—is extremely misleading.

Curiously enough, North American scientists are extremely fascinated with the school performance of young children in Japan, China, and Korea, but not with that of children in other Asian countries. There are some reports, however, that indicate considerable differences in school performance among Asians. I. Scott (1989), for example, reported that the poor school performance of young students in Hong Kong has become a serious social problem. The International Association for the Evaluation of Educational Achievement found that, in tests in the area of the natural sciences, ten-year-old students and fourteen-year-old students in Hong Kong ranked thirteenth and sixteenth out of a total of seventeen countries (Holbrook 1989). The failure of the Hong Kong students was attributed to the territory's corruptive sociocultural climate and not to their brain sizes (Scott 1989; Yee 1991).

Japanese students are not necessarily "whiz kids," despite the impression given by comparative national studies of school performance and media reports. The Japanese high school teacher T. Oomura (1990), after more than ten years of teaching and professional experience, gave a different picture of his students and those of his colleagues. Particularly notable was the disparity of educational outcomes between high school students in large cities and those in small locales. Because competition is greater in large cities and *juku,* private testing centers, libraries, and a more developed educational climate are more widely available, high school graduates in large cities are much more likely than those in rural towns not only to enter prestigious colleges and universities in large cities but also colleges and universities in rural areas, although the primary objective of the latter is to educate the children of local residents. Since educational achievement is the single most powerful determinant for getting a "better" job, and thus having a "better" life, in Japan, this disparity has become a serious social problem for Japanese in areas with fewer academic advantages.

The keen competition in school performance, best symbolized by the *Juken Jigoku* (exam hell); the parental and school pressure felt by students; and the well-organized structure of the Japanese society, without much flexibility in social mobility, have caused mental health and other problems. *Ijime* (bullying behavior), physical violence, and even suicide by victims of *ijime* are some examples of such problems (Oomura 1990; Ohta 1986; Buruma 1988). Mental health problems such as anxiety, school phobia, psychosomatic disorders, and neurotic disorders have been found to be much higher among high school students in Hong Kong and Taiwan than in the United States (Cheung 1986). Similar problems caused by high educational achievement pressure were also greater for Asian-American students, as well as students in Asia, than for non-Asian students (Chen 1987; Yee 1992). These are the negative aspects behind the story of the higher success of Asian-American and Asian schoolchildren.

The wide publicity surrounding Rushton's contention about race and intelligence coincided with the increased attention being paid to economic aspects of U.S.–Pacific Rim relations, particularly the challenge to the United States posed by Japan's growing economic strength in the global market and the resulting anxiety about U.S. economic competitiveness.

In the late 1970s and early 1980s quite a number of U.S. scientists attempted to understand the worldwide success of Japanese products, the nation's high productivity, and the efficiency of its economy by "demystifying the oriental secrets." Japan, a small island nation, has almost no natural resources aside from its huge population. It suffered greatly during World War II, and, given the extent of the devastation, the country's recovery and later economic growth seem mystical indeed. That this country, which Douglas General McArthur predicted would at best be the "Switzerland of Asia," has rebounded as it has really is "miraculous." What U.S. researchers have found to explain Japan's success, to their surprise and contrary to what the general public would like to believe, are significant sociocultural factors, such as a work ethic much like the Protestant work ethic (Spence 1985), a system of "manufacturing ABC's" (Hayes 1981), group-oriented work activities (Ouchi 1981; Pascale and Athos 1981; White and Trevor 1983); quality-oriented high standards for products (Y. Tsurumi 1981), and the importation of United States management practices (Ringle 1981; R. R. Tsurumi 1982). Obviously, and interestingly, what is going on at Japanese schools is being repeated in the workplaces of Japan. As U.S. management, rather than workers, was criticized as being mainly responsible for the economic problems (Yankelovich and Immerwahr 1983; Y. Tsurumi 1981), one could see that American educational problems were derived from students' educational environment, including parenting, not their biological components including brain size.

Most comparative studies have pointed out that the problems within the United States do not stem from Japanese biological "superiority" but, rather, from sociocultural factors (Vogel 1979; Hayes 1981; Ouchi 1981; Pascale and Athos 1981; Y. Tsurumi 1981; White and Trevor 1983; Yatani 1989). Thus, Rushton's biological determination distorts the reality in the classrooms and helps to further aggravate racial and ethnic conflicts in all aspects of life in the United States today.

REFERENCES

Anrig, G. R., and A. E. Lapointe. 1989. "What We Know about What Students Don't Know." *Educational Leadership* 47:4–9.

Bishop, J. H. 1989. "Why the Apathy in the American High School?" *Educational Researcher* 18:6–10.

Buruma, I. 1988, June 5. "Obsessed With Exams Whatever the Price." *Far Eastern Economic Review:* 46–7.

Chen, S. 1987. "Suicide and Depression Identified as Serious Problems for Asian Youth." *East/West* (April 9): 6.

Cheung, F. M. C. 1986. "Psychopathology among Chinese People." In *Psychology of Chinese People,* ed. M. Bond. Hong Kong: Oxford University Press.

Coon, C. S. 1982. "Racial Adaptations." Chicago: Nelson-Hall.

Eysenck, H. J. 1971. "Race, Intelligence, and Education." London: Temple Smith.

Fortune. 1986. "America's Super Minority," November 26.

Frederick, W. C. 1977. "The Use of Classroom Time in High Schools above or below the Median Reading Score." *Urban Education* 11: 459–64.

Frederick, W. C., H. Walberg, and S. Rasher. 1979. "Time, Teacher Comments, and Achievement in Urban High Schools." *Journal of Educational Research* 73:63–65.

Hayes, R. H. 1981. "Why Japanese Factories Work." *Harvard Business Review* 60:57–66.

Hearnshaw, L. S. 1979. *Cyril Burt, Psychologist.* Ithaca, N.Y.: Cornell University Press.

Herrnstein, R. J. 1971. *IQ in the Meritocracy.* Boston: Little, Brown.

Hess, R. D., et al. 1986. "Family Influences on School Readiness and Achievement in Japan and the United States: An Overview of a Longitudinal Study." In *Child Development and Education in Japan,* ed. H. Stevenson, H. Azuma, and K. Hakuta. New York: W. H. Freeman.

Hirschman, C., and M. G. Wong. 1986. "The Extraordinary Educational

Attainment of Asian Americans: A Search for Historical Evidence and Explanations." *Social Force* 65:1–27.

Holbrook, J. 1989. *Science Education in Hong Kong: The National Report of the Hong Kong Science Study*. Vol. 1. Hong Kong: Education Department, University of Hong Kong.

International Association for the Evaluation of Educational Achievement. 1988. *Science Achievement in Seventeen Nations*. Englewood Cliffs, N.J.: Prentice-Hall.

Jensen, A. 1969. "How Much Can We Boost IQ and Scholastic Achievement?" *Harvard Educational Review* 39:1–123.

Kamin, L. J. 1974. *The Science and Politics of IQ*. Hillsdale, N.J.: Erlbaum.

Lewontin, R. C., S. Rose, and L. J. Kamin. 1984. *Not in Our Genes*. New York: Pantheon Books.

Mehler, B. 1983, May–June. "The New Eugenics." *Science for the People*, 18–23.

Molnar. S. 1983. *Human Variation: Race, Types, and Ethnic Groups*. Englewood Cliffs, N.J.: Prentice-Hall.

Newsday. 1988, January 24. "It's Work versus School Work in Seaford," 4.

———. 1989, February 1. "No U.S. Gold Medals in Math," 4 and 14.

New York Times. 1987, September 8. "School Criticized on the Humanities," A1 and B8.

———. 1990, February 6. "Poll Detects Erosion of Positive Attitudes toward Japan among Americans," B7.

Nielsen, A. C., Company. 1987. Unpublished raw data.

Ohta, T. 1986. "Problems and Perspectives in Japanese Education." *Comparative Education* 22, no. 1: 27–30.

Oomura, T. 1990. Personal communication.

Ouchi, W. 1981. *Theory Z: How American Business Can Meet the Japanese Challenge*. Reading, Mass.: Addison-Wesley.

Pascale, R. T., and A. G. Athos. *The Art of Japanese Management: Applications for American Executives*. New York: Warner Books.

Ringle, W. M. 1981. "The American Who Remade 'Made in Japan.' " *Nation's Business*, 70–76.

Rushton, J. P. 1988. "Race Differences in Behavior: A Review and Evolutionary Analysis." *Personalities and Individual Differences* 9:1009–24.

Scott, I. 1989. *Political Change and the Crisis of Legitimacy in Hong Kong*. Hong Kong: Oxford University Press.

Seaford Senior High School. 1988. *Job Survey*. Seaford, N.Y.: Seaford High School.

Shanker, A. 1989. "How Business Can Motivate Students." *New York Times*, March 5, Op-Ed.

Shields, J. J. 1989. *Japanese Schooling: Patterns of Socialization, Equality, and Political Control.* University Park, Pa.: Penn State University Press.

Skinner, B. F. 1986. "What Is Wrong With Daily Life in the Western World?" *American Psychologist* 41, no. 5: 568–74.

Spence, J. T. 1985. "Achievement American Style: The Rewards and Costs of Individualism." *American Psychologist* 40:1285–95.

Stevenson, H. W. 1987. "America's Math Problems." *Educational Leadership* (October): 4–10.

Stocking, C. 1980. "Comparing Youth Culture: Preconception in Data." In *Educational Policies in Crisis,* ed. W. K. Cummings et al. New York: Praeger.

Sue, S., D. W. Sue, N. Zane, and H. Z. Wong. 1985. "Where Are the Asian-American Leaders and Top Executives?" *Pacific/Asian American Mental Health Research Center Review* 4:13–15.

Sue, S., and S. Okazaki. 1990. "Asian-American Educational Achievements." *American Psychologist* 45, no. 8: 913–20.

Tsurumi, R. R. 1982. "American Origins of Japanese Productivity: The Hawthorne Experiment Rejected." *Pacific Basin Quarterly* 7:14–15.

Tsurumi, Y. 1981. "The U. S. Trade Deficit with Japan." *World Policy Journal* 5: 207–30.

Time. 1987, August 31. "The New Whiz Kids."

U. S. Department of Education. 1987. *Japanese Education Today.* Washington, D.C.: U.S. Government Printing Office.

U.S. News and World Report. 1988, March 14. "What Puts the Whiz in Whiz Kids?"

Vogel, E. E. 1979. *Japan as Number One: Lessons for America.* Cambridge: Harvard University Press.

Wang, L. C. 1980. "Federal Exclusionary Policy." In *Civil Rights Issues of Asian and Pacific Americans: Myths and Realities,* ed. U.S. Commission on Civil Rights, 21–24. Washington, D.C.: U.S. Government Printing Office.

White, M. I. 1987. *The Japanese Educational Challenge: A Commitment to Children.* New York: Free Press.

White, M., and M. Trevor. 1983. *Under Japanese Management: The Experience of British Workers.* London: Heinemann.

Yankelovich, D., and J. Immerwahr. 1983. *The World at Work: An International Report on Jobs, Productivity, and Human Values.* New York: Octagon Books.

Yatani, C. 1989. "American National Character and Japanese Management: Individualism and Work Ethnic." *Organization Development Journal* 7, no. 1:75–79.

Yee, A. H. 1991. Personal communication.

————. 1992. "Asians as Stereotypes and Students: Misperceptions That Persist." *Educational Psychology Review* 4, no. 1: 95–132.

Zuckerman, M., and N. Brady. 1988. "Oysters, Rabbits and People: A Critique of 'Race Differences in Behavior' by Rushton." *Personalities and Individual Differences* 9:1025–33.

◆ SIMONA SHARONI ◆

Feminist Reflections on the Interplay of Racism and Sexism in Israel

Despite the Israeli government's persistent attempts to paint to the world a picture of a democratic, pluralistic state, Israel is far from engaging in practical plans for the implementation of its public relations campaigns. Inequalities and injustices, when pointed out, are usually justified as inevitable because of Israel's intractable security problems. The special needs, historical narratives, and cultures of Oriental Jews, Palestinians, and women have been systematically excluded from Israel's national agenda, mass media, and educational system and from the history of the state and its self-image.

The term *Oriental Jews,* translated from the Hebrew word *mizrahim,* is used in this essay to refer to Jews who immigrated from Arab countries, mainly North Africa, the Mediterranean, and the Middle East. It covers various groups of immigrants with different languages, cultures, social structures, and histories. This term is being used more and more by Oriental activists who struggle for their equal rights and self-determination. The choice of this particular term highlights the common social experience that non-Ashkenazi Jews have gone through and reflects an assertion of a new collective identity that has emerged as a result of this oppressive experience (Elbaz 1980; Shohat 1989; Swirsky 1989).

The term *Palestinians* refers to Palestinians who live in the pre-1967 borders and who constitute 16 percent of Israel's population. But despite their Israeli citizenship, they are treated as second- (or third-) class citizens (Lustick 1980). The choice of the term *Palestinians* to refer to this particular group is still contested, especially in Israel, which regards them as Israeli Arabs. Research on the collective identity of Arabs in Israel, however, has yielded consistent results; the vast majority (around 90 percent) of people in this identity group regard themselves as Palestinians (Smooha 1989; Rouhana 1991).

Israel's Declaration of Independence was among the earliest constitutional documents to include sex as a group classification for the purpose of equal social and political rights. The right to equality between the sexes, however, was not recognized as "a fundamental principle" by the Israeli Supreme Court until 1987, and even then it was given a relativist interpretation (Raday 1991). The state of Israel has reinforced patriarchal legal systems that grant priority to religious values over egalitarian values. Consequently, women in Israel, whether they are Jewish, Muslim, or Christian, are excluded from full participation in the public sphere and subordinated to male authority in the private sphere (Polan 1982).

Despite the differences within and between the three groups in their experiences of discrimination, there are some measures of inequality which forge a common denominator of domination and resistance among these groupings. Yet, although Israeli society is clearly structured around ethnic, racial, and gendered differentials, attempts to critique this reality rarely focus on the linkages and relationships that exist between sexism and racism. Instead, most studies look at these phenomena as separate, dealing with incidents and policies of discrimination against women *or* Oriental Jews *or* Palestinian citizens of Israel.

In recent years feminists, especially women of color and non-Western women, have called attention to the fact that racism and sexism have been used worldwide and in specific contexts to reinforce the politics of power and privilege through mechanisms of exclusion, discrimination, and oppression (Davis 1983, 1990; hooks 1984, 1989, 1990; Mohanty, Torres, and Russo 1991). Such critiques have opened space for innovative thinking and urged feminist scholars and activists to engage in discussions that interpret "racism and sexism [as] interlocking systems of domination which uphold and sustain one another" (hooks 1990, 59). Recognizing that race and sex have always been overlapping poles of political identity and understanding the conditions that have facilitated this relationship require a careful but critical exploration of the dynamic interplay of racist and sexist ideologies in a given sociopolitical context. bell hooks also points out that, "when we talk about race and class in convergence and conjunction with gender, we really struggle for a new language" (1990, 67). To create the discursive space in which such a language could emerge we need to challenge the hegemonic discourses and ideologies of governments which have been used to reinforce gender, race, class, and other inequalities.

Feminist interpretations of the dynamic relationship between racism and sexism can become very useful in the process of developing effective strategies of struggle. Such strategies may include uncovering alternative information that will open new space for interpretations of histories from the victims' standpoints. In addition, it is important to underline the commonalities that stand out in these stories of discrimination and suffering. In the specific context of the present work this strategy might lead to further research on the social and political construction of racism and sexism in Israel and to the creation of political coalitions and alliances that will work together to dismantle institutionalized and internalized racism and sexism.

The present critique of sexism and racism in Israel critically explores the ways in which patterns and ideologies of discrimination have been constructed, maintained, reinforced, and justified. Therefore, while taking into consideration the differences in the ideologies and operations of sexism and racism, it is particularly concerned with the similarities and shared characteristics of the ideologies and structures of discrimination which have been used against three groups of Israeli citizens: Oriental Jews, Palestinians, and Israeli women. This is done through a critical interpretation of the intersections between different types of racist and sexist discourses in the Israeli context. I also intend to address the "contribution" of militarism to dynamic interplay between racism and sexism and the state's institutionalized use of military service and "national security" as excuses that are intended to maintain and reinforce gender, race, class, and other inequalities.

While referring to ideologies, patterns, and practices of discrimination, however, the scope of this work is not just to provide alternative information and challenge existing myths concerning the democratic character of the Israeli state. In articulating examples of daily humiliation, echoing silenced voices, and documenting stories that have been systematically erased from dominant representatives of Israel's history and from the Israeli-Jewish collective memory, I wish to engage in an archaeological project of uncovering human suffering, discrimination, and pain and searching and struggling for a new language to describe human experiences, resistance, and visions of social and political change.

LIFE EXPERIENCES AS CRITIQUE

A new genre in feminist critique which is particularly concerned with the politics of representation insists on experience as a location for the construction of theory (Bulkin, Bruce-Pratt, and Smith 1984; Mohanty and Martin 1986; Russo 1991). This challenging mode of thinking and writing is still struggling for its own existence and recognition, since "in academia . . . there seems to be an odd refusal to respect the ways in which the confessional can lead to the conceptual and the political" (Childers and hooks 1990, 77). The reference to self-reflexive storytelling and oral histories as strategies of political resistance and alternative theory building has been very inspiring for me. As a political activist, I find personal experiences useful for engaging skeptics in critical discussions and for exploring alternative ways of coping with complex sociopolitical contexts. Thus, in exploring and remembering my own encounters with racism and sexism in Israel, I seek to open up space for critical reflections on processes, forces, and dynamics that have shaped my identities and my critiques of the constructions of Israeli collectivity. My selective life experiences, however, placed in the complex political context of Israeli society, do not intend simply to reveal what motivates me to speak out against racism and sexism but also to highlight some aspects concerning the social and political climate in Israel which usually remain unaddressed in most academic work and media accounts.

My fractured identities—the different social and political roles I have engaged with throughout my diverse experiences in Israel, in the occupied West Bank and Gaza Strip, and in the United States—are woven together in this multilayered text. As an Israeli feminist and peace activist who is politically committed to the struggle for a Palestinian self-determination, as a former immigrant and a daughter of a Holocaust survivor, and as a psychotherapist and a conflict resolution scholar, I speak in many voices and raise questions more than I provide answers. Full of contradictions and question marks, passion and despair, hopes and fears, this text offers a glimpse of my own personal and political journey. By voicing my deep concerns, I struggle against the denial and complicity that have accompanied the deeply ingrained racism and sexism in Israel.

"NEVER AGAIN": "NATIONAL SECURITY" AS A TOP PRIORITY

While critically reflecting on my upbringing in Israel, I cannot forget the painful "absorption" process that my family and I had to go through when we immigrated from Romania to Israel in 1963. As refugees, with no knowledge of the language, my family, as most immigrants, was easy to manipulate. We became human resources, tools in a propaganda campaign, and crunched numbers supporting demographic projects and political policies we knew nothing about. We had no choice but to identify with the oppressive structures of the hegemonic Zionist establishment. In order to belong to the collective, or in many cases simply to survive, many immigrants had no other choice but to "buy the government's line" and go through the difficult and painful "transformation" process to become a "new" Jew and a "real" Israeli. To facilitate this process of cultural transformation the Zionist ideology created educational material based on a historical narrative that uses powerful cultural symbols and linguistic metaphors to elaborate on what being an Israeli Jew means. These strategies and others were implemented under the euphemism of *unity*, reinforcing a battlefield mentality of "us" versus "them": the Jewish people in "their" homeland surrounded by threatening Arab "enemies" and the new, strong, masculine Jew of the present shorn from the weak, feminine, and confused Jew of the past. As I recount my personal story, however, I am aware that the obstacles and hardship that we had to deal with as new immigrants cannot be compared to the structural discrimination, humiliation, and cultural domination faced by entire communities of Oriental Jews who came to Israel in the early 1950s and 1960s.

The rhetoric invoking memories of Holocaust suffering and victimization became enmeshed with contemporary political propaganda, reinforcing the myth of Jews as the eternal victims and of every non-Jew as a potential enemy. This rhetoric was projected onto "the Arabs" particularly, who were portrayed as just waiting for the right opportunity to destroy the state of Israel and throw its citizens into the sea. Being the victims once justified the use of all means necessary to protect the Jewish collective from the terrible memories of the past. This nationalistic-militaristic (and, of course, masculinist) discourse and line of reasoning became an integral part of Israeli collective thinking and ways of coping with criticism. The popular Hebrew song "The Entire World Is against Us" *(Holam Kulo Negdenu)*, is a typical example of this phenomenon in Israel's popular culture. The song was written and became popular in 1975 as a response to the United Nations equation of Zionism with racism. The average Israeli reaction to the international charge of racism was defensive and tautological; Jews viewed the charge of racism as racist. The official Israeli response did not deny racism but, rather, affirmed Zionism. For example, Haifa's main boulevard, UN Boulevard, was renamed Zionism Boulevard. Marcia Freedman, a Jewish feminist who lived in Israel during that period and a former member of Parliament explains: "Though they may or may not be racist, most Jews agree that with reference to Jews—the historical victims of anti-Semitism and survivors of genocide—the question cannot arise" (Freedman 1990, 180).

My father was thirteen when he witnessed his father being killed in a concentration camp in Eastern Europe. Outraged and frustrated with his powerlessness and helplessness, he made a decision never again to face a similar situation. For me the Holocaust was not something I learned about from history books; the horrors were part of my daily childhood and adolescence. Growing up with hardly any relatives on my father's side, I listened to my father's stories time and again. On one hand, I tried to empathize with his pain and memories of suffering, and, upon the other, I searched for explanations for his antisocial behavior and his protectiveness of me and my sister. Although I still cannot accept parts of his behavior, I can better understand now that his decision to become a policeman in the Jewish state was not merely a random choice of vocation, nor was his alliance with the right-wing Likud party simply a political statement.

The hegemonic Zionist ideology of the state and its establishment placed "national security" as a top priority and as a matter of survival. The dominant interpretation of *national security,* which became a core concept in the state's ideology, depended, however, on a particular historical narrative concerning the birth of Israel. That narrative has been sustained through the reinforcement of unchallenged myths that are located at the core of Israel's self-perception. Simha Flapan, an Israeli scholar and peace activist, drawing on recently declassified material from former Israeli prime minister David Ben-Gurion's war diaries and from the minutes of his secret meetings, challenged some of the dominant myths regarding the birth of Israel: that the Zionists welcomed the partition of Palestine, that the Palestinians fled Israel despite the efforts of Jewish leaders to get them to stay, and that, when after its victory in 1948 Israel extended its hand in peace, not a single Arab leader responded (Flapan 1987; Morris 1988; Segev 1986).

In the introduction to his book *The Birth of Israel* Flapan explains why it is so difficult for Israelis and Jews to challenge such myths: "Like most Israelis, I had always been under the influence of certain myths that had become accepted as historical truth. And since myths are central to the creation of structures of thinking and propaganda, these myths had been of paramount importance in shaping Israeli policy" (1987, 8). The state's dominant historical narrative regarding the creation of Israel hardened into an ideological shield, which was projected onto Israeli society and the Jewish diaspora. The "Israeli Defence Forces" were a major agent in facilitating this process. Consequently, the military became a central institution in Israeli society and a major force in shaping the identities of new generations.

The "Sabra" symbol, named after the indigenous cactus fruit, refers to native-born Israeli Jews and came into its own after the establishment of the Israeli state in 1948; it has played an important role in the construction of Israelis' national identities. The new race of Jews was portrayed as the antithesis of the weak, persecuted, and helpless Jew. Lesley Hazelton refers to the role of the Sabra image in shaping Israeli identity. She characterizes the ideal-type Sabra as exceedingly masculine, pragmatic, assertive, and emotionally tough: "Action and strength were to be [the Sabras'] bywords; passivity and weakness were to be unknown. Impassive except on questions of their nation's survival . . . the Sabras were to know their own minds and, above all, would be freed of the doubts of constant self-questioning. They were to have their softer side too. Underneath the prickly, tough exterior of the cactus fruit after which they are named" (Hazelton 1977, 92).

The establishment of the state and the Jewish reassertion of manhood that is symbolized by the Sabra image was intended to rescue the new Jewish immigrants from the impact of the Holocaust on their lives. Instead, it prepared the ground for the rise of militarism and chauvinism, for aggressiveness, chutzpah, and lack of tolerence for difference. My father's own experiences and Holocaust nightmares blended with Israel's ideological shield; like most Israelis, he accepted the state's interpretation of *national security* as the only viable alternative for survival. The militaristic discourse of "never again," which was later exploited by the theocratic racist rabbi Meir Kahane, made my father and most Israelis feel stronger and safer while exposing Palestinians in Israel, in the West Bank, along the Gaza Strip, and in Lebanon to further terror, suffering, and pain. This discourse, fixated on a manipulated conception of Israeli security and a narrow interpretation of the Holocaust, contained no room for empathetic understanding of Palestinians.

The emphasis on national security as a matter of survival has implications not just for Palestinians but also for Oriental Jews and women in Israel. In fact, any attempt to call for social and political change in Israel is either suppressed, dismissed, or marginalized under the same excuse. Therefore, Israeli feminists in Israel are not joking when they explain that feminism in Israel is perceived as a threat to national security (Freedman 1990). Israeli feminists have occasionally threatened the status quo by resisting the masculinist and militaristic discourse of national security and by destabilizing the gender identities, relations, and politics that are inscribed in this discourse (Swirsky and Safir 1991). The struggles of Oriental Jews for equal rights have been treated in a similar manner. Demonstrations calling for "bread and jobs" and more militant social movements challenging the status quo of the state's priorities and the existing disparities of power and privilege were dismissed as agitations, while the organizers were harassed by the police. These attempts to alter the inscribed ethnic politics that have been promoted under the banner of national security have been sanctioned, perceived, as they have been, as a threat to the existing status quo and power relations (Swirsky 1989).

BEHIND THE "MELTING POT":
RACISM AND THE POLITICS OF POWER OF PRIVILEGE

I was born in a small village, Tecut'i, in Romania on March 8, 1961, and immigrated to Israel with my family in 1963. Until the last few years I haven't mentioned the fact that I am not a "Sabra," suppressing unpleasant memories from my early childhood as a newcoming immigrant to Israel. In fact, I even remember lying on several occasions in elementary school, telling others that I was born in Israel. I managed to forget my mother tongue, Romanian, refusing to use the language with my parents and demanding that they not use it in the presence of my friends. I think even at that young age I understood that, in order to belong and to be accepted, I had to become a Sabra, and the sooner the better.

Indeed, despite its declared objectives, the Zionist movement appeared more than ambivalent in its relation to diaspora Jews in general and Oriental Jews in particular. Research on immigration policies and on ethnic relations in Israel point out that the segment of diaspora Jews which did emigrate in large numbers or as entire communities were Jews from Africa, Asia, and the Middle East who were perceived by the Zionist establishment as potential problems for the goal of fusion. "At worst, the immigrants were referred to as the 'generation of the desert,' likened to the Israelites who were forced to wander until a new, purified generation arose, able to enter Canaan. More optimistically, it was argued that even the adults might become

Israelis. But the definition of 'Israeli' was a decidedly European, Ashkenazi one" (Avruch 1987, 328).

The policies employed by the Israeli establishment to absorb the new immigrants, in fact, prepared the infrastructure for a comprehensive and systematic plan of internal colonization and cultural domination. These implicitly ethnocentric and racist policies also directed where people would live. European Jews, because of their professions and "culture," were placed in the developed center of the country and usually were given a chance to choose where they wanted to live. Oriental Jews, more dependent upon the state, were relegated to the "pioneer" areas, in most cases against their will. In some cases they had a choice between living in the frontier areas along Israel's borders or in a remote underdeveloped town in the south or in the north (Elbaz 1980; Swirsky 1989).

Despite their attempt to present an image of a progressive pluralistic state, the veterans of the state claimed assimilation as their goal; they designed programs that encouraged immigrants to relinquish their previous languages, cultures, and ways of coping and to adopt the "modern" ways of the state. Thus, to cover its ambivalent position toward immigration in general, and immigration of Oriental Jews in particular, the Israeli establishment launched propaganda campaigns in Israel and in the diaspora; the contradictions between the declared intent to create a plural society in Israel and its imposition of "melting pot" strategies were not addressed. Such immigration policies were portrayed as a general state policy, although in practice they clearly discriminated against Oriental Jews and laid the foundations for an ethnic division of labor and clear class divisions in Israel (Elbaz 1980). Becoming part of such a process was not a matter of free choice. Governmental policies were created to reinforce this ideology as the central ideology of the state and as an entry ticket for membership in the Israeli collective.

Oriental Jews as a group have been considered by the Ashkenazi ruling elite to be marginal citizens whose social and cultural contribution runs contrary to the European character of the state of Israel. Israeli official leaders repeatedly voiced their fears of the possible cultural influence of Oriental Jews on Israeli society. For example, in a 1950 speech to senior military officers Ben-Gurion referred to Oriental Jewish immigrants as a "semblance of people . . . without a trace of education, Jewish or human" (Brown 1983, 6). More examples of racist statements by the Labor elite and followers are by now so well documented that they hardly need repeating. What the fathers of Zionism had in mind was to establish a state based on immigration of the predominantly secularizing Jewish masses of Eastern and Central Europe, not those traditionally religious masses from Asia.

Theodore Herzl had set the tone in *The Jewish State* (1895): "The state would form part of a defensive wall for Europe in Asia, an outpost of civilization against barbarism" (quoted in Brown 1983, 6). Another Zionist leader, Zeev Jabotinsky, founder of the Revisionist party, had clear views about Oriental Jews: "Even with the real Ishmael we have nothing in common. We belong to Europe, thank God: for 2000 years we helped to build European civilization" (quoted in Brown 1983, 7). And the quotable Golda Meir not only lived in fear of Arab babies being born but also cried in relief when Russian Jews began arriving in Israel in the early 1970s: "At last real Jews are coming to Israel again . . ." (quoted in Yuval-Davis 1987, 78). By implementing melting pot strategies and speaking of "fusing" the exiles, the founding fathers' state of Israel negated differences in the name of the unity of the Jewish people. These strategies contributed to the project of masking the historical and material foundation of the dominance of both the world Zionist movement and the Israeli society by European Jews.

"CHOSEN PEOPLE," "PROMISED LAND"

Since it became clear that Palestine was not, as the Zionist cliché promised, "a land without people for a people without land," a major concern of the Zionist movement, especially the Labour Zionist movement, has been the creation of a Jewish majority in Israel. Thus, the immigration of Jews to the country *(aliya)* became the major strategy to secure a Jewish majority in the country. The Law of Return, which grants automatic citizenship to every Jew, served to reinforce the special relationship between the Israeli state and the Jewish people in the diaspora. The emphasis on Jewish identity, which links the communities together, influenced the development of policies according to which people have been included or excluded from positions of power and privilege within Israeli society but also opened a Pandora's box: a never-ending debate around the question "Who is a Jew?" Nira Yuval-Davis points out in her critical essay on Jewish collectivity that the modern ideological and legal debate on the definition of *the Jew* had already started by the time of the French Revolution, when the question of legal emancipation of the Jews came to the fore. It focused on the question of whether or not the Jews constituted a nation or merely shared a religion (Yuval-Davis 1987). In many ways this debate has not been fully resolved up to this day, and two Israeli governments have fallen as a result of disagreement on the question of who is a Jew.

Listening carefully to the rhetoric of the public relations campaigns that Israel has been launching throughout the world around the recent immigration of Soviet and Ethiopian Jews, I began to unshelve my own memories from being a new immigrant in Israel twenty-eight years ago. This summer in Israel I met them everywhere, recognizing the fears and hopes in their eyes as they struggle for survival in the "promised land." The national and international festivities around the immigration of Soviet and Ethiopian Jews seem like an updated attempt to revive the Zionist ideology of the "chosen people" who are returning to "their" land. Meanwhile, Palestinians in the West Bank and Gaza Strip, like those who hold Israeli citizenship, are reminded that they are not chosen and therefore have to pay the heavy price of this immigration, losing their jobs and land and their limited rights. Any attempt to draw linkages between the massive immigration, the lack of housing in Israel, and the likelihood of settling the immigrants in the West Bank and Gaza Strip is either silenced or dismissed as lacking humanitarian consciousness or as being anti-Semitic.

Looking back, it becomes clear and much more painful and outrageous to realize how the Law of Return and the declared immigration policies became legal justifications for cultural imperialism and multilayered discrimination justified by the ultimate sacred goal of securing a Jewish majority in Israel. To achieve this goal the Zionist establishment used Jewishness as the major criterion for granting basic rights and privileges such as automatic right for citizenship, loans and housing, and child support. Judging from these ideologies and practices, it appears that, as long as Israel does not address the contradictions in terms between a Jewish state and a democratic state, Palestinians who hold Israeli citizenship will remain second- or third-class citizens.

The Palestinians who hold Israeli citizenships and constitute 16 percent of Israel's population are perceived as "threats" to the Zionist project in more ways than one. Their presence is a continual reminder that Palestine has not been an empty country waiting for two thousand years for "its sons" to return, as the Zionist myth has it. Palestinians who managed to stay in the Jewish state that was established in 1948 lived under direct Israeli military rule until 1966. During these years they were forced to live in relative geographic isolation and had to obtain special permission from the Israeli military in order to travel outside their home zones.

Despite the fact that Israel portrays itself to the international com-

munity as a parliamentary democratic welfare state, it has been systematically using apartheid-type discrimination and exclusions in the
supply of amenities, state resources, and supplementary benefits for
its Palestinians citizens. Moreover, plans for a population expulsion
("transfer") of the Palestinians outside the Zionist state have existed
in more or less muted forms throughout the history of Zionism
(Yuval-Davis 1987). Such ideologies and plans have usually been introduced as alternative ways for resolving the political contradiction
of a Jewish state with too many non-Jews in it. But although racist
ideologies have become part of Israel's official political discourse with
the emergence of neofascist parties such as Kach and Moledet, the
majority of Israeli society still refuses to believe that population expulsion is an option that an Israeli government might not rule out.
Unfortunately, after looking at the underlying assumptions of Israel's
demographic policies, it is my opinion that such an option cannot be
dismissed.

THE "DEMOGRAPHIC WAR": EXPLICIT
MANIFESTATIONS OF RACISM AND SEXISM

Although official records of Israel's demographic policies are available now, it is important to set them in their context in order to critique their racist and sexist nature. Until the early 1960s the major
form through which the Jewish majority in Israel was secured was by
aliya, the immigration of Jews into the country. Gradually, however,
Israeli-Jewish national reproduction has come to rely more and more
on Israeli-born babies. This change has contributed to a political debate that focuses on the "ultimate threat" of the gradual demographic
growth of the Palestinian community in Israel and the erosion of the
Jewish majority. The Israeli establishment formulated two major types
of demographic polices: one aimed at directly combating the Palestinian population and the other in the form of a "demographic race" and
national campaigns to encourage national reproduction of Israeli Jews
(Yuval-Davis 1987).

The official plan to implement the former type of demographic
racism was initiated in the 1960s by Levy Eshkol, then prime minister, under the slogan "Judaization of Galilee." In 1976 a confidential
report, which became known as the "Koenig memorandum," was sent
to the Israeli Ministry of Interior by its district representative in the
northern part of the country, Yisrael Koenig. In the document Koenig
expressed his alarm that Arabs do and would continue to constitute
a majority in the Galilee and suggested various ways of combating this

tendency. Koenig went beyond demographic policies that were already in place and encouraged Jews to settle in areas densely populated by Palestinians; he offered to encourage Palestinians who hold Israeli citizenship to emigrate from the country by limiting their prospects for employment and studies, cutting their national child insurance benefits, and more (Merip Reports 1976).

Yisrael Koenig's headquarters was in Nazareth Elit (also referred to as Upper Nazareth, since it is built on the hills overlooking Nazareth, the largest Palestinian town inside Israel). Since its establishment the Israeli state has been expropriating Palestinians lands using various excuses (very common among these are security reasons). These lands have been used to expand Jewish settlement and to prevent the emergence of excessive concentrations of Palestinians within Israel. Nazareth Elit is the place where my family was sent upon our arrival in Israel; there I grew up, and my parents still live there. Nazareth Elit was established in 1956, on expropriated Palestinian land, as part of the comprehensive plan to Judaize the Galilee.

In the early 1980s a racist organization named Mena became active in Nazareth Elit under the slogan Don't Sell Your Flat to an Arab! The word Mena means "prevention" in Hebrew; it became known to the media as an anachronism for "the defenders of Nazareth Elit," and to its supporters it offered an additional interpretation: "War against the Arabs." This group did not hesitate to use violence and encouraged others to do so in order to expel Arabs from the town. To justify their blatant racism Mena offered the Israeli public a history lesson, reminding people that Ben-Gurion's government, which had founded the town, intended it to be purely Jewish (Keller 1983).

The emergence of the Mena racists in Nazareth Elit is not a unique example. Around the same period Jewish residents of a newly built building complex in Jaffa, one of the few cities in which Israelis and Palestinians have been living side by side, opposed the sale of flats to Arabs and were backed publicly by a rabbi, Ephraim Zalmanovich, who claimed that segregation is ordained by Jewish religious law. Meanwhile, in another part of Israel, at Ya'ara, a Galilee settlement in which Bedouins have been living beside Jews for over thirty years, some Jews suddenly claimed that the Bedouins have too many children and are becoming too numerous and that something must be done about it (Keller 1983). Yet in the context of these descriptions of blatant racism in Israeli society it is important to note that Palestinians have not been the only victims of this particular wave of racism. In the western part of the town of Safad, in northern Israel, a "neighborhood committee" was organized to oppose the entry of dark-skinned Ethiopian Jews, because of their "primitive culture" and "primitive mentality," and in a fashionable Tel Aviv pub the gatekeepers have been instructed not to admit anyone with an "Oriental appearance" (Keller 1983).

To understand the wave of racism and violence which was directed against Bedouins, Palestinians, and Ethiopian Jews, we must tie it into the larger political climate in Israel at that time. In the 1981 elections the hostility between Labor and Likud supporters became blatantly ethnically based. What was referred to in the media as "the war between the Jews" was partly one between Ashkenazis and Orientals, and both parties tried to use ethnic symbols of animosity and, indeed, hatred. A whole vocabulary of racial slurs referring to the Oriental Jews became commonplace. Moreover, the whole vocabulary of ethnic strife, employed by both parties and accepted by most Israelis, served the interests of the government. Mordechai Gur, a Labor candidate and former chief of staff, warned a heckling group of Oriental Jews, Likud supporters, in a development town: "We'll screw you like we screwed the Arabs in the Six Day War" (Brown 1983, 7). By using such rhetoric, Gur and other government officials have, paradoxically, highlighted the connections that exist between the treatment of Palestinian Arabs and Oriental Jews. The racist discourse that surfaced called attention to a deeper context: systemic structures of discrimination and inequalities from which both groups have been suffering.

The second official demographic policy that encourages Israeli-Jewish reproduction lies at the intersection of racist and sexist ideologies in Israel. In the early 1950s Ben-Gurion initiated a plan according to which symbolic money rewards were granted to "heroine mothers," those who had ten children or more; Ben-Gurion was known for his continuous calls for Israeli-Jewish mothers to have more children. In this spirit a government committee was set up to review the demographic situation, and in 1967 the Center for Demography was established. This center coordinated studies on demographic trends in Israel and in the Jewish diaspora and promoted various pronatal policies. These policies were carried out along with a propaganda campaign promising material incentives such as housing loans for families with more than three children, and increased child allowances. It is important to note that these benefits were granted only to Jews belonging to "families who have relatives who have served in the Israeli Army" (Yuval-Davis 1987, 80).

These demographic policies do not only embody sexism, racism, and class distinctions but have also served to legitimize and reinforce further discrimination of Israeli-Jewish women, Oriental Jews, and Palestinians. In the case of the Palestinians the Israeli establishment hardly tried to hide its intentions to block their access to a whole line of state benefits; the oppressive and discriminatory policies were usually justified by the "ultimate argument" of defending against possible threats to Israel's national security. This argument became a powerful tool that has been used extensively by the state of Israel to draw the borders of Israeli collectivity and to construct the identity of the "new" Jew in contrast to the non-Jewish population.

In the case of the Oriental Jews there was a deliberate attempt to hide the discriminatory nature of some state policies, including the demographic ones. On the surface Oriental Jews were to be rewarded, since their families were relatively larger than those of Ashkenazi Jews, but, in fact, this was a trap. The incentives offered to families with more than three children were indeed based on the size of the family but failed to take into consideration the size of the combined family income. This factor legitimized another economic gap, since the combined family incomes of Oriental Jews tend to be much lower on the average than those of Ashkenazi Jews. Another factor that was omitted from these supposedly encouraging incentives was a long-term program that would guarantee financial resources and the essential living conditions necessary for actually raising a child and not simply giving birth to another soldier.

From a feminist standpoint demographic policies can work for and against women depending on the context and on a woman's choice. Since in this particular case women did not choose to volunteer their wombs to the demographic struggle, this could serve as a clear example of women's subordination in Israel as a result of the militarization of their lives; it clearly highlights the interplay between racism, sexism, and militarism. Israeli-Jewish women have been "recruited" to join the "demographic war" by bearing more children. Their role has been defined by the hegemonic discourse of the state as a national duty to the Jewish people in general and to the state of Israel in particular. Ben-Gurion raised the issue of women's fertility to a level of a woman's national duty: "Increasing the Jewish birthrate is a vital need for the existence of Israel, and a Jewish woman who does not bring at least four children into the world is defrauding the Jewish mission" (Hazelton 1977, 63).

In the 1980s the "Efrat Committee for the Encouragement of Higher Jewish Birth Rate" became powerful enough to establish centers and branches all over Israel and incorporate into its ranks major elite figures from all professional fields, both religious and secular; it also managed to gain official status as a governmental consultative body on natal and demographic policies. This committee gained a great deal of its public power by linking the debate on encouragement of the Jewish birthrate to the public campaign against abortions. In addition to the usual reasoning of the antiabortion lobby, whose members treat abortion as murder, there came an emotive call to Jewish women to fulfill their national duty by replacing the Jewish children killed by the Nazis. An extreme (and narrowly defeated) example of how this ideology was put into practice was a suggestion by then advisor to the minister of health, Haim Sadan. He proposed to force every woman considering abortion to watch a slide show that would include, in addition to other horrors such as dead fetuses in rubbish bins, pictures of dead children in the Nazi concentration camps (Yuval-Davis 1987).

While addressing this point, I remember how my father, a Holocaust survivor and a self-proclaimed Israeli patriot, always stated that he wanted to have more children to compensate for the loss of his family. Another detail that comes to mind is his assertion that he would like to have a boy, who could carry his family name to the second generation. In this particular case the Holocaust has been used not only to justify racist and sexist state policies but also to reinforce patriarchy. And if this is not enough, the security argument can always be appropriated to silence possible voices of dissent. As Nira Yuval-Davis eloquently points out, "The development of the specific ideological construction of women as national reproducers in Israel has had a lot to do with the specificity of the development of Israeli society as a permanent war society" (1987, 86).

MILITARISM AND THE POLITICS OF EXCLUSION

Israel's written history and my recollections of my life there tell a story of wars and conquest, not simply self-defense. The Israeli military is probably the most significant social and political institution in Israeli society. The army and its practices have an impact on every single sphere of Israeli life: education, economy, culture, among others. In recent years critics of the impact of militarism on Israeli society argue that military service is so pervasive that it has become the main socializing agent in the society (Katriel 1991). The centrality of the military in Israel remains unchallenged as Israel continues to appropriate the discourse of "a nation under siege" surrounded by threatening evil enemies.

Since defense matters continue to receive first priority and only Israeli men are perceived as qualified to make decisions concerning them, Israeli women's lack of political power is perpetuated. Moreover, while excluding Palestinians and marginalizing Oriental Jews, Israel reinforces Ashkenazi male hegemony not only in the military but also in political, economic, and technological decision making. Israel has developed a large defense industry, run exclusively by retired career officers, most of whom are upper-class Ashkenazi men who retire at the age of forty to begin second careers in administrative positions in the public and private sectors. In Israel retired military men are almost invariably preferred over any other candidates for top jobs in national defense (Waintrater 1991).

In addition to its above functions as a social and political catalyst, the Israeli army, as other military forces, makes an "important contribution" to the institutionaliztion of gender (and race and class) inequalities in Israeli society. Thus, the image of Israeli men, whose identities are constituted through a discourse that emphasizes masculinity, pragmatism, protectiveness, and assertiveness, is contrasted with that of women, who should be prepared to function as primary caretakers, fertile wombs, and supporters of Israeli men. Women are socialized to contribute to national efforts by fulfilling first and foremost their traditional roles, which are confined to the private domain. Any woman with an adult Israeli male between the ages of eighteen and fifty-five in her life will see him leave for the army at regular, scheduled intervals, for reserve duty for one to three months a year, according to the circumstances. When the men in their lives are in service Israeli women must deal by themselves with the everyday problems of existence (Waintrater 1991). This caretaking role, which has been imposed on women both in the private and in the public domains, is usually taken for granted, as a "natural" contribution women should make.

Israel was, however, the first, and still is, one of the few states in which women are recruited to serve in the army through a national recruitment law (Yuval-Davis 1982). This phenomenon is one of the reasons for the existence of the myth of the equal status of women in Israel. But the overwhelming majority of military tasks in which women are engaged present a mirror image of the roles Israeli women occupy in the civilian work force: office work, technical and operational duties, and caretaking roles (Bloom 1991; Yuval-Davis 1982, 1985). There is also a similarity in status: in the military, too, women are found in positions inferior to those of men. Another aspect of the complex relationship between Israeli women and the military is suggested by the name of the Women's Corps, whose initials in Hebrew mean "charm." Indeed, Israeli women soldiers are expected to "raise the morale" of the male soldiers and to make the army "a home far away from home." Thus, during the basic training of women they are coached to emphasize their feminine characteristics and their neat appearances and they even receive cosmetic guidance to help them in this respect (Yuval-Davis 1982).

The Hebrew language highlights some of these underlying assumptions concerning gender roles in Israel. For example, it makes its contribution to the constitution of women as fertile wombs in the service of the state; the word for "motherland" in Hebrew is *moledet,* which is a feminine noun derived from the verb meaning "to give birth." The social and political construction of Israeli women vis-à-vis the state was best summed up by MP Geula Cohen, the founder of the neofascist Tehiya party and a former member of the terrorist Stern gang in the prestatehood period: "The Israeli woman is an organic part of the family of the Jewish people and the female constitutes a practical symbol of that. But she is a wife and a mother in Israel, and therefore it is her nature to be a soldier, a wife of a soldier, a sister of a soldier, a grandmother of a soldier. This is her reserve service. She is continually in military service" (quoted in Hazelton 1977). Indeed, Geula Cohen's statement could serve as a clear indication for the legitimization of the relationship between sexism and militarism and the militarization of women's lives in Israel.

Numerous social scientists, as well as journalists, have commented on the high level of violence in Israeli society. In most cases, however, the verbal and physical manifestations of violence were attributed to the stress caused by living in a constant state of siege (Waintrater 1991). This reason alone falls short in explaining why men are those who usually exercise violence. I, too, see violence as a way of coping, and I do not believe that a tendency to be violent is something men are born with. Rather, I tend to attribute the high level of violence in Israeli society to the significant role the army plays in the socialization process of Israeli men. During their military and reserve service, and maybe even before, Israeli men learn that violence is a legitimate way of dealing with problems.

The intifada (Palestinian uprising), which began in December 1987, confronted Israelis with their image as brutal occupiers who shoot Palestinian children and carry violent ways of coping home to their families and friends. Israeli men didn't like these images, but, instead of challenging the unjust structure of the occupation, they used their defense mechanisms and blamed the victims for triggering the violence in them. Israeli women, however, began to see, feel, and understand more clearly the interconnectedness of militarism and sexism. The message started to reach home: the violent patterns of behavior that were being used by the Israeli army against Palestinians in the West Bank and Gaza Strip were part of a widely spread culture of violence and oppression which terrorizes their daily lives (Sharoni 1991). The Israeli establishment does not encourage Israelis to recognize such connections, since the separation of one set of inequalities from another reduces possible threats to its unchallenged regimes of power and privilege. But even if it is risky to point them out, these connections, like those between racism and sexism, do exist.

UNLEARNING PRIVILEGES, BUILDING BRIDGES

What can be done to change the present reality of discrimination in Israel? A critical discussion of the problem, as it has evolved in its particular context, is the first step. I have tried to open some space for such a discussion while emphasizing the need to look at the intersections of the histories and present realities of the three groups of Israeli citizens. While Oriental Jews, Palestinians, and women have been discriminated against and kept in disadvantaged political positions, the Labor party, which dominated Israeli politics from 1948 to 1977, has placed most key positions in political and economic life in the hands of privileged Ashkenazi men. Their leadership and control have largely remained unchallenged, since they literally were there first and managed to stake their claims and build a party machine to maintain them. Accordingly, Oriental Jews, Palestinians, and Israeli women have been excluded and placed in disadvantaged positions, primarily because they lack power and insiders' knowledge of the political and economic systems.

Since the primary purpose of this essay was to describe the interplay of racism and sexism in Israel, I did not focus here on the struggles of Palestinians, Oriental Jews, and women to end the reality of inequality and injustice. Because Israeli public relations campaigns usually fail to address internal dynamics and conflicts within Israel, I decided to provide some background and historical information regarding the complex social and political climate in Israel. Since my goal was to highlight the shared experiences of these three subordinate groups, I have not addressed the significant differences between the groups and the multiplicity of voices and perspectives within each one.

In exposing the exclusions, discrimination, and resistance in each particular case (for Palestinians, Oriental Jews, and women) and making the linkages between them, I see a potential for coalition building and solidarity which may lead to joint struggle against racism and sexism. Learning to recognize relationships and linkages between different structures of discrimination and between different communities is an important strategy in combating racism and sexism. Another crucial strategy of struggle is the development of an insider's perspective and "way of knowing" so that disenfranchised people can engage in social and political critiques and acts of resistance that challenge myths portrayed by the state as the ultimate truth. By developing critical and counterhegemonic political perspectives, the subordinate group empowers itself to reshape its passive "victim identity" and engage in a struggle for social and political change.

The crucial question is: How can those of us who are not members of subordinate groups join their struggle? What I find very effective when I talk to people about these issues are stories, similar to the ones I have woven throughout this essay. What is even more important is to discuss the location from which the story is told. I am not a Palestinian nor an Oriental Jew, yet, as an Israeli woman, I have had to confront discrimination. The process of critically examining the construction of my identity as an Israeli woman triggered my understanding of how other identities have been constructed in Israel and how different systems of discrimination sustain and reinforce one another. I began to understand and appreciate differences while recognizing connections and linkages.

When I first met Palestinians who hold Israeli citizenship I was shocked at my ignorance regarding their life conditions and history. I had to go through a painful process of confronting my fears and mistrust and also their fear, anger, suspicion, and sometimes hatred directed at me. In many ways I had to engage in a process of unlearning my privileged upbringing as an Israeli-Jewish woman. When I listened to their stories of suffering, to their family histories, I had to let go of the learned defense mechanisms of protecting the state. I felt guilty for not knowing. Sharing the stories that I hadn't known and visiting again and again Palestinian friends who lived in villages that I used to regard as frightening have contributed to the painful process of liberating myself from the collective Israeli identity which was imposed on me. Once I realized that the exclusion of Palestinian histories from my education was part of a planned strategy, I had to engage in a process of transforming my guilt feelings into responsibility and commitment to struggle against the injustices committed in my name.

Although I have learned a great deal through my personal relationships with Palestinians and Oriental Jews, I want to stress that one cannot build bridges of solidarity through dialogue alone, especially not in situations with great disparities of power and privilege and which contain violence, as in the particular cases described here. To build coalitions power and privilege, as well as other spheres of differential access, need to be addressed. It is not enough anymore to bring people together under an agreed-upon banner to create an illusion of unity against a common "enemy." As we critically reflect upon the social and political construction of our own fractured identities, we must confront enemies within and negotiate agreements between competing identities. Engaging in a self-reflexive process is essential, in my opinion, for deciding to unlearn privileges and build alliances to struggle for change and transformation.

NOTE

This project was completed while the author held the International Fellowship from the American Association of University Women.

REFERENCES

Avruch, Kevin. 1987. "The Emergence of Ethnicity in Israel." *American Ethnologist* 14, no. 2: 328.

Bloom, R. Anne. 1991. "Women in the Defense Forces." In *Calling the Equality Bluff: Women in Israel*, ed. Barbara Swirsky and Marilyn P. Safir. New York: Routledge.

Brown, Kenneth. 1983. "Iron and a King: The Likud and Oriental Jews." *Merip Reports* (May 1983).

Bulkin, Elly, Minnie Bruce Pratt, and Barbara Smith, eds. 1984. *Yours in Struggle: Three Feminist Perspectives on Anti-Semitism and Racism.* New York: Firebrand Books.

Childers, Mary, and bell hooks. 1990. "A Conversation about Race and Class." In *Conflicts in Feminism*, ed. Marilyn Hirsch and Evelyn Fox-Keller. New York: Routledge, 77.

Davis, Angela. 1983. *Women, Race, and Class.* New York: Vintage Books.

———. 1990. *Women, Culture, Politics.* New York: Vintage.

Elbaz, Mikhael. 1980. "Oriental Jews in Israeli Society." *Merip Reports* (November–December 1980): 15–23.

Flapan, Simha. 1987. *The Birth of Israel: Myths and Realities.* New York: Pantheon Books.

Freedman, Marcia. 1990. *Exile in the Promised Land.* New York: Firebrand Books.

Hazleton, Lesley. 1977. *Israeli Women: The Reality behind the Myths.* New York: Simon and Schuster.

hooks, bell. 1984. *Feminist Theory: From Margin to Center.* Boston: South End Press.

————. 1989. *Talking Back: Thinking Feminist, Thinking Black.* Boston: South End Press.

————. 1990. *Yearning: Race, Gender, and Cultural Politics.* Boston: South End Press.

Katriel, Tamar. 1991. *Communal Webs: Communication and Culture in Contemporary Israel.* New York: State University of New York Press.

Keller, Adam. 1983. *The Other Israel* (November–December 1983): 15–16.

Lustick, Ian. 1980. *Arabs in a Jewish State: Israel's Control of a National Minority.* Austin: University of Texas Press.

Merip Reports. 1976. Excerpts from the "Koenig Memorandum." *Merip Reports,* no. 51 (October 1976): 11–14.

Mohanty, Chandra Talpade, and Biddy Martin. 1986. "Feminist Politics: What's Home Got to Do with It?" In *Feminist Studies / Critical Studies,* ed. Teresa de Lauretis. Bloomington: Indiana University Press.

Mohanty, Chandra Talpade, Ann Russo, and Lourdes Torres, eds. 1991. *Third World Women and the Politics of Feminism.* Bloomington: Indiana University Press.

Morris, Benny. 1988. *The Birth of the Palestinian Refugee Problem.* Cambridge and New York: Cambridge University Press.

Polan, Diane. 1982. "Toward a Theory of Law and Patriarchy." In *The Politics of Law,* ed. D. Kairys. New York: Pantheon Books.

Raday, Frances. 1991. "The Concept of Gender Equality in a Jewish State." In *Calling the Equality Bluff: Women in Israel,* ed. Barbara Swirsky and Marilyn P. Safir. New York: Pergamon Press.

Radford-Hill, Sheila. 1986. "Considering Feminism as a Model for Social Change." In *Feminist Studies / Critical Studies,* ed. Teresa de Lauretis. Bloomington: Indiana University Press.

Rouhana, Nadim. 1991. "Palestinization among the Arabs in Israel: The Accentuated Identity." Paper presented at the conference on "The Arab Minority in Israel: Dilemmas of Political Orientation and Social Change." Tel-Aviv University, Israel, June 1991.

Russo, Ann. 1991. "We Cannot Live without Our Lives: White Women, Antiracism and Feminism." In *Third World Women and the Politics of Feminism,* ed. Chandra Talpade Mohanty, Ann Russo, and Lourdes Torres. Bloomington: Indiana University Press.

Segev, Tom. 1986. *1949: The First Israelis.* New York: Free Press.

Sharoni, Simona. 1991. "To Be a Man in the Jewish State: The Sociopolitical Context of Violence and Oppression." *Challenge: A Magazine of the Israeli Left* 2, no. 5.

Shohat, Ella. 1989. *Israeli Cinema: East/West and the Politics of Representation.* Austin: University of Texas Press.

Smooha, Sammi. 1989. *Arabs and Jews in Israel: Conflicting and Shared Attitudes in a Divided Society.* New York: Westview Press.

Swirsky, Shlomo. 1989. *Israel: The Oriental Majority.* London and Atlantic Highlands, N.J.: Zed Books.

Waintrater, Regine. 1991. "Living in a State of Siege." In *Calling the Equality Bluff: Women in Israel,* ed. Barbara Swirsky and Marilyn P. Safir. New York: Pergamon Press.

Yuval-Davis, Nira. 1982. *Israeli Women and Men: Divisions behind the Unity.* London: Change Publications.

————. 1985. "Front and Rear: The Sexual Division of Labour in the Israeli Army." *Feminist Studies* 11, no. 3.

————. 1987. "The Jewish Collectivity." In *Women in the Middle East,* ed. Khamsin Collective. London and Atlantic Highlands, N.J.: Zed Books.

♦ GEORGINE SANDERS ♦

Millennium Foretold
the Brooklyn Botanic Garden

The warm day's harvest of this long cold spring:
Trees are barely starting but the flowers last,
golden bushes, bridal bower of magnolias.
Ducks in the lily pond, where goldfish swim again.

A dark and stately woman striding down the path,
dark children, in their Easter best, playing on the grass.
Where early tulips bloom, some tourists from Japan
are taking pictures, posing one by one.

Further down, a row Yeshiva pupils on a bench,
they laugh and push each other, waiting for their lunch.
On every path the strollers, babies fast asleep,
pass by in convoy with their families.

Someone mows the lawns today, the grass smells sweet.
The children's garden has been plowed, its dark soil waits
for little hands to tend the beds, to plant the seed.
The Garden holds and saves us all. We are at peace.

Notes on the Contributors

GARLAND E. ALLEN is Professor of Biology at Washington University in St. Louis, Missouri. His field is history of science, with a special interest in the history of biology in the post-Darwinian period (1880–1950). His current research projects include a social history of the U.S. eugenics movement, 1900–1950; a comparative study of Darwin, Marx, and Wagner; and completion of a volume for the Harvard Source Book series on Heredity, Development, and Evolution, 1880–1960. He is presently a member of the Council of the History of Science Society, and he served as a trustee of the Marine Biological Laboratory in Woods Hole, Massachusetts, from 1986 to 1993.

BONNIE ELLEN BLUSTEIN received her Ph.D. in History of Science from the University of Pennsylvania in 1979. Her publications about the history of U.S. biology and medicine include *Preserve Your Love for Science: Life of William A. Hammond, American Neurologist* and *The Preventive Perspective: A Social History of the Department of Community and Preventive Medicine at the Medical College of Pennsylvania,* as well as numerous articles. She is currently completing a book about the history of neurology in the United States between the Civil War and World War II. Since 1974 she has been an active member of the International Committee against Racism.

LINDA BURNHAM is cofounder and director of the Women of Color Resource Center. She has worked for twenty-five years on issues of racial justice and gender equity and she has published numerous articles on African-American women, African-American politics, and feminist theory. Burnham is an editor of *Crossroads* magazine. She also teaches yoga.

FREDERICA Y. DALY was born under the Rest and Cleansing Moon in Washington, D.C., on Valentine's Day in 1925. She received her formal education in public schools, and at Howard University and Cornell University. Her professional life has included teaching positions at Howard University, State University of New York College at Cortland and Empire State College, and the University of New Mexico. Most of her career has been spent doing trench work in therapy as a practicing psychologist in clinics and hospitals, and with troubled adolescents at a treatment center in upstate New York. In her retirement, she writes poetry, keeps a journal, and does genealogical research in search of her African and Indian ancestries.

BEVERLY GREENE is Associate Professor of Psychology at St. John's University and a clinical psychologist in private practice in New York City. She has served as Director of Impatient Child and Adolescent Psychology Services at Kings County Hospital in Brooklyn, New York. A fellow of the American Psychological Association, she is coeditor of the Sage series titled Psychological Perspectives on Lesbian and Gay Issues, coeditor of *Women of Color: Integrating Ethnic and Gender Identities in Psychotherapy,* and an author of *Abnormal Psychology in a Changing World.*

GERALD HORNE is Professor and former Chair of the Department of Black Studies at the University of California at Santa Barbara. He formerly served as special counsel of Local 1199 of the Hospital Workers Union in New York City. He received 305,000 votes in his race for the U.S. Senate in California in 1992. He is author of numerous books, including *Reversing Discrimination: The Case for Affirmative Action.*

RUTH HUBBARD is Professor Emerita of Biology at Harvard University, from where she retired in 1990. She has edited several collections of feminist writings about science, including (with Marian Lowe) an earlier volume in the Genes and Gender Series, *Genes and Gender II: Pitfalls in Research on Sex and Gender.* Her other books include *The Politics of Women's Biology* and, with Elijah Wald, *Exploding the Gene Myth.* She has also published scientific papers and reviews, as well as articles about the sociology of science, the politics of health care, and various health issues, especially as these relate to women.

GISELA KAPLAN is Foundation Professor of the School of Social Science at the Queensland University of Technology in Brisbane, Australia. Her publications include *Contemporary Western European Feminism* and *Hannah Arendt: Thinking, Judging, Freedom.* She is editor-in-chief of the *Australian Journal for Social Issues* and has been joint editor of the *Australian and New Zealand Journal of Sociology.* Her chief research interests lie in the areas of ethnicity and gender, political sociology, and comparative psychology.

PAMELA TROTMAN REID is Acting Associate Provost and Dean for Academic Affairs at the Graduate School and University Center of the City University of New York, where she also has an appointment as Professor of Psychology. A developmental psychologist, she has investigated contextual issues and the factors that have an impact on social behavior, especially in African-American communities. She is a fellow of the American Psychological Association (APA) and of the American Psychological Society, as well as former president of the APA Division of Psychology of Women and a former member of the Executive Council of the Division for the Psychological Study of Ethnic Minority Issues.

LESLEY J. ROGERS is Head of the Department of Psychology at the University of New England in Australia. She conducts research into the relationship between brain and behavior, and is particularly interested in environmental influences on brain development, the lateralization of brain structure and function, and mechanisms of memory formation. She recently coauthored a book on the evolution of brain asymmetry and its implications for language, tool use, and intellect. She has also held academic positions at Monash University and the Australian National University.

BETTY ROSOFF, an endocrinologist, is Professor Emerita of Biology at Stern College of Yeshiva University. She is a member of the International Committee against Racism and serves on the editorial board of the journal, *The Prostate.* She applies her expertise in endocrinology to the investigation of gender and biological determinism. She is a founding member of the Genes and Gender Collective.

GEORGINE SANDERS [Vroman] was born in Indonesia and studied medicine in Utrecht, the Netherlands, where she lived during World War II under the German occupation. She has lived in the United States since 1947 and is now a medical anthropologist working in cognitive rehabilitation of the elderly with memory problems and with brain injury survivors. She is a consultant at the Geriatric Clinic of Bellevue Hospital Center, New York, and an associate of Cognitive Rehabilitation Services, Sunnyside, New York. In recent years she has been publishing poetry under the name of Georgine Sanders in the Netherlands and the United States. She is a founding member of the Genes and Gender Collective.

SIMONA SHARONI is a Jewish-Israeli feminist, peace activist, and scholar. She received her Ph.D. in Conflict Analysis and Resolution from George Mason University. Her research interests include feminist perspectives on peace, security and conflict resolution, critical interpretations of the Israeli-Palestinian conflict, the interplay between gender and politics in the Middle East, and the relationship between militarism and sexism. Her book, *Gender and the Israeli-Palestinian Conflict: The Politics of Women's Resistance,* is forthcoming from Syracuse University Press.

ETHEL TOBACH is a comparative psychologist at the American Museum of Natural History and Adjunct Professor of Biology and Psychology at the Graduate Center of the City University of New York. Her research deals with evolution and the development of social-emotional behavior. She has written extensively on the role of science in societal processes leading to racism and sexism. She is a founding member of the Genes and Gender Collective.

CARMEN LUZ VALCARCEL is a doctoral candidate in the Counseling Psychology Department at Teachers College of Columbia University. She was born and raised in Puerto Rico and is interested in women's issues, cross-cultural issues, and race relations within the Puerto Rican culture. Her professional experience includes counseling in mental health settings, social work in educational institutions, and community activist work. She is a member of the board of the Violence Intervention Program (a community-based program for battered women) and a member of the Genes and Gender Collective.

REGINA E. WILLIAMS is a poet and writer. She is a founding member of the Metamorphosis Writers Collective and Ain't I a Woman Writing Collective. She is currently pursuing a master's degree in Applied Anthropology.

VAL WOODWARD has been a member of the Genetics and Cell Biology faculty at the University of Minnesota at St. Paul for twenty-seven years. During the first twenty years of his scientific career he studied gene-enzyme relations in *Neurospora crassa*, and during the past twenty years his primary research interest has been in human genetics, in particular critiques of the claims of simple cause-effect relationships between genes and individual and social behaviors. He has also taught at Rice University and Kansas State University, and, more briefly, at Stanford University and the University of California at Berkeley.

CHOICHIRO YATANI is Assistant Professor of Psychology at the State University of New York College of Technology at Alfred. He is a native-born Japanese now teaching introductory, social, and I/O psychology courses, and conducting research in the areas of personality and organizational behavior, total quality management, democracy in the workplace, and racial and sexual discrimination. American individualism and organizational and managerial behavior are his special interests. He has presented his work at national and international conferences and has published both in the United States and Japan.

The Feminist Press at The City University of New York offers alternatives in education and in literature. Founded in 1970, this nonprofit, tax-exempt educational and publishing organization works to eliminate stereotypes in books and schools and to provide literature with a broad vision of human potential. The publishing program includes reprints of important works by women, feminist biographies of women, multicultural anthologies, a cross-cultural memoir series, and nonsexist children's books. Curricular materials, bibliographies, directories, and a quarterly journal provide information and support for students and teachers of women's studies. Through publications and projects, The Feminist Press contributes to the rediscovery of the history and the emergence of a more humane society.

NEW AND FORTHCOMING BOOKS

The Answer/La Respuesta (Including a Selection of Poems), by Sor Juana Inés de la Cruz. Critical edition and translation by Electa Arenal and Amanda Powell. $12.95 paper, $35.00 cloth.

Australia for Women: Travel and Culture, edited by Susan Hawthorne and Renate Klein. $17.95 paper.

The Castle of Pictures and Other Stories: A Grandmother's Tales, Volume One, by George Sand. Edited and translated by Holly Erskine Hirko. Illustrated by Mary Warshaw. $9.95 paper, $19.95 cloth.

Folly, a novel by Maureen Brady. Afterword by Bonnie Zimmerman. $12.95 paper, $35.00 cloth.

Japanese Women: New Feminist Perspectives on the Past, Present, and Future, edited by Kumiko Fujimura-Fanselow and Atsuko Kameda. $15.95 paper, $35.00 cloth.

Shedding and Literally Dreaming, by Verena Stefan. Afterword by Tobe Levin. $14.95 paper, $35.00 cloth.

The Slate of Life: More Contemporary Stories by Women Writers of India, edited by Kali for Women. Introduction by Chandra Talpade Mohanty and Satya P. Mohanty. $12.95 paper, $35.00 cloth.

Songs My Mother Taught Me: Stories, Plays, and Memoir, by Wakako Yamauchi. Edited and with an introduction by Garrett Hongo. Afterword by Valerie Miner. $14.95 paper, $35.00 cloth.

Women of Color and the Multicultural Curriculum: Transforming the College Classroom, edited by Liza Fiol-Matta and Mariam K. Chamberlain. $18.95 paper, $35.00 cloth.

Prices subject to change. *Individuals:* Send check or money order (in U.S. dollars drawn on a U.S. bank) to The Feminist Press at The City University of New York, 311 East 94th Street, New York, NY 10128-5684. Please include $3.00 postage/handling for one book, $.75 for each additional book. For VISA/MasterCard orders call (212) 360-5790. *Bookstores, libraries, wholesalers:* Feminist Press titles are distributed to the trade by Consortium Book Sales & Distribution, (800) 283-3572.